handbook of

PEDIATRIC

EMERGENCY MEDICINE

handbook of

PEDIATRIC
EMERGENCY MEDICINE

Edited by:

P.O. Brennan
Department of Accident and Emergency Medicine,
Sheffield Children's Hospital, Sheffield, UK

K. Berry
Department of Accident and Emergency Medicine, Birmingham
Children's Hospital, Birmingham, UK

C. Powell
Department of Accident and Emergency Medicine,
Royal Melbourne Children's Hospital, Melbourne, Australia

M.V. Pusic
Division of Emergency Medicine,
British Columbia Children's Hospital, Vancouver, Canada

© BIOS Scientific Publishers Limited, 2003

First published 2003

All rights reserved. No part of this book may be reproduced or transmitted, in any form or by any means, without permission.

A CIP catalogue record for this book is available from the British Library.

ISBN 1 85996 242 4

BIOS Scientific Publishers Ltd
9 Newtec Place, Magdalen Road, Oxford OX4 1RE, UK
Tel. +44 (0)1865 726286. Fax +44 (0)1865 246823
World Wide Web home page: http://www.bios.co.uk/

Production Editor: Andrea Bosher.
Typeset by Phoenix Photosetting, Chatham, Kent, UK
Printed by Cromwell Press, Trowbridge, UK

Contents

Abbreviations

ADH	antidiuretic hormone
APLS	Advanced Pediatric Life Support
ASOT	antistreptolysin titre
AT	antitrypsin
BP	blood pressure
BSA	body surface area
CPAP	continuous positive airways pressure
CRP	C-reactive protein
CSE	convulsive status epilepticus
CSF	cerebrospinal fluid
CSU	catheter specimen of urine
CVP	central venous pressure
CXR	chest X-ray
DMSA	dimercapto-succino-acetic acid
ENT	ear nose and throat
ESR	erythrocyte sedimentation rate
FBC	full blood count
G6PD	glucose-6-phosphate dehydrogenase
GCS	Glasgow Coma Scale
GIT	gastrointestinal tract
HBIG	hepatitis B immunoglobulin
HbsAg	hepatitis B surface antigen
hCG	human choriogonadotropin
HDCV	human diploid cell vaccine
HIDA	^{99m}Tc-HIDA scan (imino-diacetic acid derivative)
HIV	human immunodeficiency virus
HRIG	human rabies immune globulin
ICP	intracranial pressure

ILCOR	International Liaison Committee on Resuscitation
INR	international normalized ratio
ITP	idiopathic thrombocytopenic purpura
LCP	Legg–Calve–Perthes disease
LFT	liver function test
LP	lumbar puncture
LRT	lower respiratory tract infection
MCP	metacarpal phalangeal joint
MCU	micturating cysto-urethrogram
MCV	mean corpuscular volume
MSBP	Munchausen syndrome by proxy
MSU	mid-stream urine
MVC	motor vehicle collisions
OD	osteochondritis dissecans
OI	osteogenesis imperfecta
PALS	Pediatric Advanced Life Support
PCEC	purified chick embryo cell culture
PDA	patent ductus arteriosus
PEEP	positive end expiratory pressure
PICU	Pediatric Intensive Care Unit
PK	pyruvate kinase
PTSD	post-traumatic stress disorder
RBC	red blood cell
RSV	respiratory syncytial virus
RVA	rabies vaccine adsorbed
SAH	subarachnoid hemorrhage
SCIWORA	spinal cord injury without radiological abnormality
SIDS	sudden infant death syndrome
SPA	suprapubic aspiration
SSSS	staphylococcal scalded skin syndrome
SVR	systemic vascular resistance
SVT	supraventricular tachycardia
TLC	total lung capacity
TPN	total parenteral nutrition
TSH	thyroid stimulating hormone
UKRC	United Kingdom Resuscitation Council
URTI	upper respiratory tract infection
UTI	urinary tract infection
VF	ventricular fibrillation
VSD	ventricular septal defect
VT	ventricular tachycardia
WBC	white blood count

Contributors

Editors

Dr Patricia O Brennan DCH, FRCP, FFAEM, FRCPCH
Consultant in Paediatric Accident and Emergency Medicine,
Children's Hospital, Sheffield, UK

Dr Kathleen Berry FRCP(C), FRCPCH, FFAEM
Consultant in Paediatric Emergency Medicine, Birmingham Children's
Hospital, Birmingham, UK

Dr Colin Powell DCH, MRCP(UK), FRACP, MD
Consultant Paediatrician, University Hospital of Wales, UK
Formerly, Consultant Paediatrician, Royal Children's Hospital,
Melbourne, Australia

Dr Martin V Pusic MD, MA, FRCP(C), FAAP
Assistant Professor of Pediatrics, Division of Emergency Medicine,
British Columbia Children's Hospital, Vancouver BC, Canada

Contributors

Dr Samina Ali MD, FRCPC, FAAP
Assistant Professor, Departments of Paediatrics and Emergency
Medicine, Paediatric Emergentologist, Stollery Children's Hospital,
University of Alberta Hospitals, Edmonton, Alberta, Canada

Dr Karen Black MD, FRCP(C)
Lecturer, Dalhousie University and Paediatric Emergency Physician, Isaak Walton Killam Hospital for Children, Halifax, Nova Scotia, Canada

Dr Sarah Denniston MB, BCh, MSc, MRCPCH
Senior House Officer, Birmingham Children's Hospital, Birmingham, UK

Dr Lisa Evered BSc, MD, FRCPC, FAAP
Assistant Professor, Departments of Paediatrics & Emergency Medicine, Paediatric Emergentologist, Stollery Children's Hospital, University of Alberta Hospitals, Edmonton, Alberta, Canada

Dr Alison M Freeburn MB, BCh, BAO, MRCPCH
Specialist Registrar in Paediatrics, Craigavon Area Hospital Group Trust, Craigavon, Northern Ireland

Dr Stephen Gordon MD
Assistant Attending Paediatrician, New York Presbyterian Hospital, Assistant Clinical Professor of Paediatrics, Columbia University College of Physicians and Surgeons, USA

Dr Katherine Lendrum DCH, MRCP(UK), FFAEM
Accident and Emergency Consultant, Chesterfield and North Derbyshire Royal Hospital, Chesterfield, UK

Mr William A McCallion BSc, MD, FRCSI, FRCSpaed
Consultant Paediatric Surgeon, Royal Belfast Hospital for Sick Children, Belfast, Northern Ireland

Mr David Moore MA, FRCS(Ed), FFAEM, DIMC (RCSEd), DFMS
Accident and Emergency Consultant, City Hospital & Birmingham Children's Hospital, Birmingham, UK

Dr Gayle Pearson FRCPCH, MRCP
Consultant Intensivist, Birmingham Children's Hospital, Birmingham, UK

Dr T Reade MBBS, BMedSc
Emergency Registrar, Western Hospital Sunshine, Victoria, Australia

Dr Michael Riordan BSc, MBChB (Hons.), MRCPCH
Specialist Registrar in Paediatric Accident and Emergency, Birmingham Children's Hospital, Birmingham, UK

Dr Michael Smith FRCPC, FRCPCH
Consultant Paediatrician, Department of Paediatrics, Craigavon Area
Hospital Group Trust, Craigavon, Northern Ireland

Dr Ben Stanhope MRCP (UK), MRCPCH
Clinical Fellow Paediatric Emergency Medicine, Hospital for Sick
Children, Toronto, Canada

Dr Sapna Verma MBChB, MRCP(Paeds), MRCPCH
Clinical Fellow, Paediatric Emergency Medicine, The Children's
Hospital at Westmead, Westmead, Sydney, Australia

Preface

The emergency presentation of children's illnesses and injuries is a worldwide problem. Casemix, workload and management vary from country to country. However, there is enough commonality to warrant the production of this international text. It is written by experienced practitioners from the United Kingdom, North America and Australia.

This concise book has been produced for junior doctors and other staff in Emergency Departments and will also be of use to trainee pediatricians and family practitioners. It covers the presentation, assessment, investigation and emergency management of life-threatening, serious and frequently presenting conditions. The format is mainly system-based, but it has some useful diagnostic symptom-based algorithms and covers pediatric medical, surgical and orthopedic conditions and trauma. There are also chapters on child abuse, pain management and medicolegal issues.

The book is based on evidence-based research where this is available and otherwise on a consensus view. Variations in management between healthcare systems are highlighted. The brief formulary is based on drug dosages set by the Royal College of Paediatrics and Child Health, in the UK, and by the Advanced Paediatric Life Support Group (2001). Local guidelines and formularies should be used where available. We are grateful to the Royal Children's Hospital, Melbourne, for their permission to use some of their clinical guidelines. These are web-based guidelines (http://www.rch.unimelb.edu.au/clinicalguide/). Many of the medical sections in this book are adapted from this source.

Acknowledgements

Our thanks go to many people, including our teachers, colleagues, patients and their parents. Particular thanks go to colleagues who gave helpful suggestions and criticisms, particularly Peter Bull, John Williamson and Mary Farnell. In addition, we must thank our spouses and children for their forbearance and constant support.

Chapter 1

Introduction

Patricia O. Brennan

Contents

1.1 Pediatric emergencies

When children fall ill or are injured, they often need urgent or emergency assessment and treatment. Healthcare systems vary. However, the common problem of ill and injured children has resulted in the development of specific services and protocols for their management in many countries. The specific illnesses and injuries vary from site to site, but there is sufficient commonality across the world for us to share knowledge and experience of good practice.

The role of an Emergency Pediatric Department may vary from place to place, but is generally to offer:
- an open access emergency facility
- diagnosis, or provisional diagnosis
- emergency/urgent investigation
- emergency management
- referral to next appropriate care, e.g.
  - intensive care
  - hospital inpatient care
  - community care
  - discharge with advice
- data collection for epidemiology and accident prevention
- training in emergency pediatrics
- audit and research

1.2 Workload

The whole range of conditions present to emergency departments, including medical conditions from the child with collapse, convulsions or severe respiratory difficulties, to the child with a mild pyrexia or an upper respiratory tract infection. Similarly presentation with trauma crosses the whole spectrum from major, multiple trauma, to the most minor trauma requiring no treatment.

The balance of medical, surgical, orthopedic and social conditions, and trauma that present is unique to each department. This book has been produced by the USA, the UK and Australia, and seeks to give a consensus view on investigation and management of commonly presenting conditions. However, policies and procedures and practice do vary, and individual departments will have their own policies.

1.2.1 Example: United Kingdom

An example is England and Wales, where 25–30% of all attenders to emergency departments are children under 16 years old, approximating to 2 million children per year. In one UK city there are over 37 000 attendances per annum to the pediatric Emergency Department out of the local population of approximately 100 000 under 16 years old. There are a few dedicated such departments within children's hospitals in the UK. However, most children are still seen within general departments, although there is an increasing trend to develop a sub-department for children, with appropriate facilities and staffing. The ratio of medical emergencies to injuries varies widely across the country, depending on other available healthcare provision in the vicinity.

1.3 The needs of the child and family

It cannot be stated too often that children are not just little adults. In addition, within the 'pediatric' workload, there are wide differences in childhood, from the neonatal period to adolescence in physical and psychological needs and in the presenting conditions, requiring appropriate medical and nursing skills and knowledge from the staff.

Children attending the hospital at a time when they are injured or unwell are often anxious and distressed by their condition and also by the hospital environment. Both the physical surroundings of the department and interactions with staff can help to reassure both the child and the parents. In addition, help and support at this time may help to reduce post-traumatic stress disorder (PTSD) (see Chapter 12).

Treatment of children is constantly being reviewed and ways developed to reduce trauma to the child from this source. We are programmed to 'treat' patients but staff must remember that 'no treatment' may be the best option for some children, e.g. in those with a viral tonsillitis or minor soft tissue injury. Parents are often reluctant to accept this, but will do so if given a simple, straightforward explanation. Distraction techniques, pain control and sedation are becoming increasingly important. New treatments for minor conditions are often less traumatic for the child, for example closing wounds with plaster strips or skin glue, and using removable splints rather than plaster casts for torus fractures of the radius.

Parents are usually correct in their assessment of their child's condition; however, occasionally a child presenting to an Emergency Department appears not to warrant emergency management by the medical and nursing staff. There may be many reasons for the attendance and staff need to understand the parents' perspective and manage the child and family with both medical and social needs in mind. These may include:

- parents' misplaced perception that their child is seriously ill/injured
- wish for second opinion
- convenience
- inability to get timely appropriate appointment elsewhere

Particularly after an injury to their child, parents experience a mixture of emotions, including worry, guilt and anger, and may vent these inappropriately on the staff of the Emergency Department. Training and experience will help staff to understand this and manage the situation appropriately.

It is rarely right to separate a child from the parent during the attendance. Each consultation is therefore geared to include both child and family in the assessment, investigation and management. The approach to child and family should be friendly and relaxed. Talk both to the child and family throughout the consultation. This will build confidence and help gain cooperation. Flattery, praise and distraction are other techniques that ease a consultation with a child, and experienced pediatricians develop their own favourite techniques particularly to interact and distract young children.

The physical examination should be adapted as necessary from the classical textbook-structured examination described for the adult. Infants and young children, for example, may be happiest and most compliant when examined on the mother's knee. Much can be observed by observing the child before any physical contact takes place. This may include alertness, responsiveness, respiratory rate, the work of breathing, and even power and coordination. The first physical contact with the child should be of a non-threatening nature – for example, holding the child's hand and chatting about any minor scratches visible and examination of ears and throat should be left until last.

1.4 Departmental design

A lot of work has gone into making emergency medical facilities acceptable to children and young people. They should be visually separate from adult facilities and have suitable décor and furnishings, with activities available for children and young people. Cots for infants and areas and activities appropriate for adolescents are particularly important and often forgotten. Toys and play reduce anxiety in young children and medical examination and treatment can be explained through play. Imaginative décor such as ceiling decorations in trolley and procedure areas can be used to distract even a child who is lying down.

Pediatric procedures and protocols must be available for the whole range of ages and conditions from simple weighing for all children so that medicines can be prescribed appropriately to guidelines for resuscitation.

The siting of the Emergency Department is important. It should be sited to give easy access to the population it serves while being supported by the services needed to give the patients the best service. Ideally, it should be within a pediatric facility, offering imaging services, intensive care, inpatient facilities, theatres, laboratories and the whole range of pediatric medical and nursing care.

1.5 Staffing

The value of appropriately trained and experienced staff is recognized in the emerging speciality of emergency pediatrics. Medical training programmes are available in the USA, the UK and Australia. These are constantly monitored and updated. Trainees benefit from having experience in both their own and in an overseas system. Both medical and nursing staff are usually trained in the almost universal systematic approach to resuscitation, the Advanced Pediatric Life Support Courses.

Programmes of training for emergency pediatric nurses are also being developed in some departments, so that they can work as independent practitioners for specific groups of patients. The value of other dedicated staff must be remembered. Play specialists, clerks and porters dedicated to working in pediatric Emergency Departments all influence the child and family's experience of the hospital attendance.

All staff need to be aware of some basic principles of pediatric emergency care:
- consider the whole child
- consider the child within the family
- consider each child's developmental needs
- don't make the attendance more traumatic than the presenting complaint

1.6 Triage

Children are triaged on presentation to the department, to determine whether there is an urgent need for treatment, such that the child should take priority over other children who are already waiting. Triage is usually undertaken by a senior nurse, supported by decision-making algorithms. The contact should be brief and focused and should determine urgency not diagnosis. However, analgesia can be given, investigations ordered and clinical observations done. These can be repeated during the wait to see the doctor, enabling the waiting time to be a useful part of the overall patient attendance.

Most departments have triage categories of urgency, which broadly convene into:
• emergency, immediate treatment
• urgent need
• routine need (i.e. can wait their turn)
• non-urgent

Each standard of urgency has an acceptable waiting time and this can be used to monitor one aspect of care in the department. Some have developed other categories, such as 'suitable for specialist nurse treatment' or 'primary care attender', and patients in these categories would be redirected appropriately.

Injury scores have been developed worldwide. These have been used for triage patients in the field, before they reach hospital. They predict the severity and outcome of the injury and can also be used to compare the effectiveness of care and patient populations and for epidemiological research.

1.7 Health promotion and accident prevention

In view of the numbers of children and families presenting to emergency facilities, there is, in theory, an excellent opportunity to give parents accident prevention and health promotion advice. However, this is not always appropriate at a time when parents are anxious about their child and often feeling guilty or angry about the accident. The department should have advice leaflets freely available, but staff should use judgement on whether to give specific advice about prevention of the condition at the time of the first presentation.

Worldwide, health promotion and accident prevention initiatives have proved effective. Epidemiology has proved that high-risk groups can be identified for certain accidents and there are similarities and differences across the world. Motor vehicle accidents remain a frequent cause of childhood death in developed countries. However, homicides from gunshot wounds are more common in the USA than in the UK. Pedestrian accidents in the USA are commonest in boys from low socioeconomic groups between the ages of 5 and 9 years old. Emergency Departments can support preventative work by developing databases on injuries. These databases should be compatible across many departments, and preferably across nations, to be most effective.

Chapter 2

Pediatric cardiopulmonary resuscitation and life-threatening emergencies

Kathleen Berry, Sapna Verma and
David Moore

Contents

2.1 Pediatric cardiopulmonary resuscitation

2.1.1 Introduction

Cardiopulmonary arrest is simply defined as the cessation of spontaneous respiratory effort and circulation manifest as apnoea, absence of central pulses and lack of responsiveness. Overall fewer than 10% of children suffering cardiopulmonary arrest survive to hospital discharge. As cardiopulmonary arrest is rarely seen in children, paramedics, the public and Emergency Department staff should familiarize themselves with national guidelines and published protocols. This has been made increasingly possible with the local availability of life support courses, namely Advanced Pediatric Life Support (APLS) and Pediatric Advanced Life Support (PALS).

The International Liaison Committee on Resuscitation (ILCOR) established in 1992 aimed to scrutinise existing scientific evidence, compare national differences and hence formulate recommendations that could subsequently be incorporated into international guidelines and used by individual resuscitation councils worldwide. ILCOR has the task of highlighting potential areas for future research and development and encouraging collaboration between the national resuscitation councils. The United Kingdom Resuscitation Council (UKRC) recommends all the algorithms detailed in this chapter.

2.1.2 Pathophysiology

In contrast to the adult, primary cardiac pathology is rarely responsible for cardiopulmonary arrest in a child. It is more often the end result of respiratory insufficiency or circulatory failure. A state of tissue hypoxia and acidosis rapidly develops if respiratory insufficiency is allowed to proceed unrecognized or untreated. Ischemia to the end organs, namely heart, brain and kidney, occurs and cardiopulmonary arrest is the end point of prolonged and severe myocardial damage. Circulatory failure secondary to fluid/blood loss or maldistribution of fluid within the circulatory compartment can also eventually lead to cardiac arrest, for example secondary to severe gastroenteritis, burns, overwhelming sepsis and traumatic hemorrhage. In children, a period of prolonged hypoxia occurs in the prearrest state unlike the sudden cardiac event experienced in adults. This accounts for the extremely poor neurological outcome in survivors.

2.2 Basic life support

The prehospital provision of basic life support is essential to maintain perfusion of the vital organs until the facilities for advanced life support become available. Hence it is vital that increased public awareness and further education, to increase the pool of basic life support providers in the community, is encouraged, and that advanced life support providers are proficient with basic life support techniques to enable its continuous provision during resuscitation. The exact techniques in children vary in accordance with the age of the child and currently three categories exist – infants (under 1 year), small children (1–8 years) and larger children (>8 years).

2.2.1 Assessment and treatment

The appropriate sequence of assessment and treatment is as follows:

Airway

Breathing

Circulation

Progression from airway to breathing should occur only when the airway has been appropriately assessed and secured, and similarly for breathing to circulation. Any deterioration in the child's condition should prompt a rapid reassessment of the airway and subsequently breathing and circulation.

Prior to assessment of the child, additional help should be summoned. It is paramount to take care when approaching the victim to prevent the rescuer from becoming a second victim. Only commence evaluation of airway, breathing and circulation after the victim has been freed from existing danger – the so-called SAFE approach (*Figure 2.1*). An assessment of responsiveness can be achieved by asking the simple question, 'Are you alright?', and gently shaking the arm. If there is a suspected cervical spine injury, a clinician should place a hand on the child's forehead to immobilize the head throughout resuscitation to prevent further damage. Children may respond either verbally signifying a patent airway or by opening the eyes.

2.2.2 Airway

In the unconscious child, the large tongue has a tendency to fall backwards and obstruct the pharynx. Blind sweeps are contraindicated in children as a partial obstruction can be converted into a complete obstruction. The tissues of the soft palate are very friable and their tendency to bleed can further obstruct the airway. Attempts to improve the obstructed airway can be performed by various airway opening manoeuvres, including head tilt and chin lift. The head should remain in the neutral position in the infant but in the 'sniffing the morning air' position in the child (*Figure 2.2a,b*). Employ the jaw thrust maneuver if spine

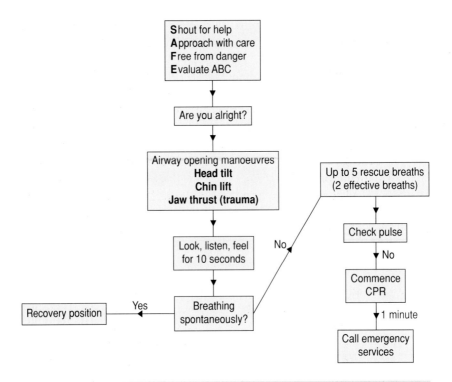

Figure 2.1 Algorithm for basic life support.

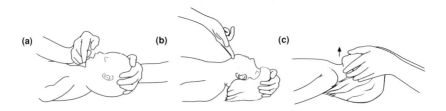

Figure 2.2 Airway opening manoeuvres. (a) Chin lift in infant; (b) chin lift in child; (c) jaw thrust.

trauma is suspected (*Figure 2.2c*). Only proceed to assessment of the breathing once the airway is patent.

2.2.3 Breathing

Assessment should take no longer than 10 seconds and involves **the look, listen and feel approach.** It is best performed by placing the head over the child's face with the ear near the child's nose and the cheek over the child's mouth looking along the line of the chest. This involves looking for chest movement, listening for air expulsion and feeling for expired breath on the cheek. If breathing does not resume within 10 seconds, exhaled air resuscitation should be performed by giving up to five exhaled breaths, at least two of which must be effective (*Figure 2.1*).

In the larger child, the rescuer should pinch the nose and place his or her mouth over the child's mouth and breathe out. In infants place the mouth over both nose and mouth. The lowest expiratory pressure to produce visible chest rise is all that is required and failure to achieve visible chest expansion may simply require a readjustment of position and repetition of the airway opening manoeuvres. Resist using excessive pressure as this results in gastric dilatation and increases the risk of aspiration. If spontaneous breathing is subsequently resumed the child should be placed in the recovery position. If despite everything adequate ventilation is not achieved, foreign body aspiration should be suspected and treated according to protocol.

2.2.4 Circulation

To test for adequate circulation, palpation of the brachial pulse in the antecubital fossa or the femoral pulse in the groin should be performed in infants, as the carotid pulse is difficult to locate in this age group. In children over a year of age the carotid can be palpated. The absence of a central pulse for 10 seconds or a pulse rate of less than 60 beats per minute in a poorly perfused child necessitates commencement of cardiac compressions. Ideally the child should be positioned on his or her back on top of a hard surface. Correct hand positioning for cardiac compressions varies according to the age of the child in three age bands:
• infant (<1 year)
• younger child (1–8 years)
• older child (>8 years) (see *Table 2.1*).

Common to all three age groups is a rate of compression of 100 per minute, the depth of compression of one-third of the depth of the chest wall. The ratio is one breath to five cardiac compressions in infants and young children, and two breaths to 15 compressions in the older child, regardless of number of rescuers (*Table 2.1*). Following completion of a minute or 20 cycles of cardiopulmonary resuscitation (CPR), the rescuer must seek assistance and call the emergency services if they have not already arrived. This is essential as basic life support merely supports perfusion of the vital organs and survival is virtually impossible unless the provision of advanced life support is ensured.

2.3 Advanced life support

Basic life support should continue uninterrupted until the arrival of appropriately trained personnel and equipment. Asystole is the primary rhythm encountered in pediatric practice, ventricular fibrillation

Table 2.1 Basic life support techniques

	Infants (<1 year)	Younger child (1–8 years)	Older child (>8 years)
Positioning	1 finger breadth below internipple line; thumbs overlying sternum	1 finger breadth above xiphisternum; heel of 1 hand	2 finger breadths above xiphisternum; heel of 2 hands
Compression rate	100 per minute	100 per minute	100 per minute
Breath:compression ratio	1:5	1:5	2:15

accounting for less than 10% of cases. Pulseless electrical activity also presents as cardiac arrest. The ambulance control center will notify the receiving Emergency Department in the event that resuscitation is in progress, to enable preparation of equipment and assembly of the designated arrest team. On arrival at the department, continue basic life support following reassessment of the airway, breathing and circulation, and simultaneously apply cardiac monitoring. Mucus, vomit or blood in the oropharynx can easily be suctioned and Magill's forceps can be used to remove visible foreign bodies.

2.3.1 Asystole and pulseless electrical activity

Asystole is the absence of a palpable pulse and of electrical activity (*Figure 2.3*), whereas pulseless electrical activity is failure to detect a pulse with the presence of electrical activity on the cardiac monitor. Pulseless electrical activity can deteriorate into asystole and together these account for the vast majority of cardiopulmonary arrests in childhood.

Treatment for both includes (*Figure 2.5*):
- 100% oxygen and ventilation, initially using bag and mask ventilation until definitive airway secured following intubation.
- Nasogastric tube insertion early on to decompress the stomach; if bag and mask ventilation continues, diaphragmatic splinting will occur and the risk of gastric aspiration is increased.
- Establish intravenous access (maximum of three attempts or 90 seconds), thereafter intraosseous access should be attempted if under 6 years of age.
- Epinephrine (adrenaline) administration at an initial dose of 0.1 ml kg^{-1} of 1/10 000 (10 micrograms kg^{-1}). If this is ineffective, it should be repeated after 3 minutes of ongoing CPR. An increased dose of epinephrine (adrenaline) has not been shown to increase success and it can lead to myocardial damage.
- Epinephrine (adrenaline) can be inserted down the endotracheal route while vascular or intraosseous access is being established.

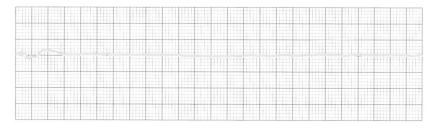

Figure 2.3 ECG showing asystole.

2.3.2 Ventricular fibrillation and pulseless ventricular tachycardia

Ventricular fibrillation (VF) (*Figure 2.4*) and pulseless ventricular tachycardia (pulseless VT) are rarely encountered in the childhood population, accounting for 10% of cardiac arrest rhythms. Pre-existing cardiac pathology, hypothermia following drowning and ingestion of tricyclic antidepressants all predispose to their development. The management of VF and pulseless VT follow the same algorithm (*Figure 2.5*).

If the arrest is witnessed, a precordial thump can be given in attempt to restart the heart. Prior to defibrillation gel pads should be applied to the apex and right sternal edge of the chest. If the child is under 10 kg, use pediatric paddles. If these are unavailable defibrillation can still be achieved by placing one paddle on the front and the other on the back of the chest.

Defibrillation with DC shock should proceed as in *Figure 2.6*.

If the arrhythmia persists, give 0.1 ml kg^{-1} 1/10 000 epinephrine (adrenaline) (10 µg kg^{-1}) and follow with 1 minute of CPR before giving further three shocks of 4 J kg^{-1}. If the VF and pulseless VT is still resistant, amiodarone at a dose of 5 mg kg^{-1} in a bolus is the treatment of choice followed by 4 J kg^{-1} DC shock 60 seconds after administration. CPR should continue with, stopping only to deliver shocks.

2.4 Drugs

In a cardiorespiratory arrest, drugs are usually given intravenously. However, prior to obtaining vascular or intraosseous access, many drugs can be administered via the tracheal route, namely epinephrine (adrenaline), lignocaine, naloxone and atropine. At least two to three times the intravenous dose, and, in the case of epinephrine (adrenaline), 10 times, the dose should be mixed with 2–3 ml of 0.9% saline. The dose is usually administered via a tracheal suction catheter, which is advanced past the

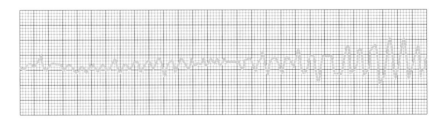

Figure 2.4 ECG showing ventricular fibrillation running into ventricular tachycardia.

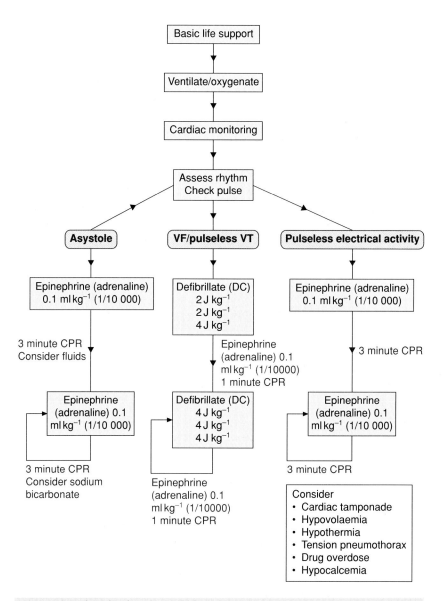

Figure 2.5 Algorithm for advanced life support of cardiac arrest.

trachea in order to maximise delivery of the drug. This route is a last-resort drug delivery and absorption from this route is very unpredictable.

2.4.1 Atropine

Persistent myocardial hypoxia results in bradycardia, which, left untreated, will lead to a cardiopulmonary arrest. Atropine in a dose of $20\,\mu g\,kg^{-1}$ is useful to antagonise the vagally induced bradycardia during

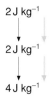

2 J kg^{-1}

2 J kg^{-1}

4 J kg^{-1}

Figure 2.6 Defibrillation with DC shock.

tracheal intubation. The pupils should be examined prior to the administration of atropine as it causes bilateral pupillary dilatation and hence interferes with neurological assessment in head injuries.

2.4.2 Epinephrine (adrenaline)

Despite experience with cardiopulmonary resuscitation over the last 30 years, epinephrine (adrenaline) still remains the sole drug effective in restoring circulation in patients following cardiac arrest. Its alpha-receptor activity is thought to be responsible for increasing the aortic diastolic pressure and subsequently coronary artery perfusion. Peripheral arterial vasoconstriction increases the afterload and myocardial perfusion but also has a tendency to increase myocardial oxygen demand. Enhancement of the contractile state of the heart and stimulation of spontaneous cardiac contractions is responsible for the successful return of circulatory activity. It has been postulated that a drug with pure alpha-receptor agonist properties may in fact be more effective, but studies comparing epinephrine (adrenaline) with norepinephrine (noradrenaline) have shown no clear benefit.

2.4.3 Sodium bicarbonate

Metabolic acidosis rapidly develops during cardiopulmonary resuscitation as a result of anaerobic metabolism owing to the absence of oxygen. Myocardial contractility is inevitably depressed by this state of acidosis. The use of alkalising agents, namely sodium bicarbonate, is not routinely recommended in the initial stages of resuscitation as it can produce a transient increase in intracellular acidosis. The generation of carbon dioxide, whose elimination is already impaired will result in a left shift in the oxygen dissociation curve and further limit the supply of oxygen. Sodium bicarbonate can reliably be used in the treatment of hyperkalemia and, as worsening acidosis renders epinephrine (adrenaline) ineffective, its use may be advocated if return of spontaneous circulation has not occurred after the second dose of epinephrine (adrenaline).

2.4.4 Fluid administration

In the pre-arrest state, the tissues are often poorly perfused and administration of $20\,ml\,kg^{-1}$ of crystalloids (0.9% saline) or colloid (4.5% human albumin solution) as a fluid bolus will result in rapid expansion of the circulatory volume. The controversy regarding crystalloid versus colloid administration in resuscitation will continue until published evidence is available.

2.4.5 Glucose

Once vascular access has been obtained, blood should be taken to check the blood glucose as hypoglycemia ($< 3\,mmol\,l^{-1}$) can develop following cardiac arrest. Prompt correction with $5\,ml\,kg^{-1}$ bolus of 10% dextrose is essential as the hypoglycemic state may worsen neurological outcome.

2.5 Post-resuscitation stabilization

Following the return of spontaneous circulation, damage still continues by way of reperfusion injury, hence stabilization is essential. The child will need complete ventilatory support until cardiac stability is achieved in a designated intensive care unit. Often inotropic support with dopamine, dobutamine and epinephrine (adrenaline) will be required in the immediate post-arrest state to maintain adequate tissue perfusion.

The patient needs monitoring and investigations as in *Boxes 2.1* and *2.2.*

The facilities for these may not be readily available until transfer to the intensive care unit but the following investigations should be carried out immediately post-resuscitation.

Box 2.1 Monitoring

- Pulse and rhythm
- Invasive and non-invasive blood pressure monitoring
- Respiratory rate
- Pulse oximetry
- Transcutaneous CO_2 monitoring
- Arterial blood gases
- Skin and core temperature
- Central venous pressure
- Urine output

Box 2.2 Post-resuscitation investigations

- Full blood count
- Urea, creatinine and electrolytes
- Liver function tests
- Blood glucose
- Arterial blood gases
- Clotting
- 12-lead ECG
- Chest X-ray

2.6 Prognosis

Despite 30 years of experience, the outcome of pediatric cardiopulmonary arrest remains very poor. Improved outcomes are associated with the following:
- witnessed arrests
- bystander CPR
- arrival of emergency medical services in less than 10 minutes
- isolated respiratory arrests
- resuscitation lasting less than 20 minutes and requiring less than two doses of epinephrine (adrenaline)

Studies also reveal that 30% of children suffering a VF arrest survive to hospital discharge in stark contrast to only 5% for asystolic arrests.

Techniques in basic and advanced pediatric life support have already been clearly outlined in the previous sections. Owing to the relative rarity of cardiac arrest in childhood previous research has included only small retrospective studies and more research from prospective multi-centre studies is needed. It should also be focused in preventing progression of the pre-arrest to the arrest state. This may best be achieved by increasing lay public awareness and the availability of life support courses.

2.7 The choking child

2.7.1 Introduction

Every year, hundreds of children die, particularly in the preschool age group, after inhaling a foreign body, the commonest cause of accidental death in the under 1-year-old group.[1] Consumer product safety standards have helped decrease this number by dictating the minimum size of toys and their components suitable for this at-risk under 4-year-old age group, [2] or by modifying previously dangerous items such as ballpoint pen tops. In addition, responsible manufacturers have withdrawn some of the dangerous elements of their product range. Tragically, however, children still choke on a host of things around the home, including food such as hot dog, crisps, nuts and buttons with resultant avoidable deaths. Small children will put almost any object in their mouths and the potential for a choking accident always exists.

2.7.2 Diagnosis

The diagnosis of foreign body inhalation is not always obvious, especially if unwitnessed. It should be suspected in any infant or child who develops sudden onset respiratory distress, particularly if associated with coughing, gagging, stridor or wheeze. A collapsed apnoeic child with foreign body aspiration may also present with a chest that cannot be inflated despite adequate airway opening manoeuvres and rescue breaths. The differential diagnosis includes a number of important infections, such as croup and epiglottitis with upper airway edema and obstruction. They should be suspected in children who, in addition to upper airway obstruction, present with features such as fever, lethargy, hoarseness or drooling. Incorrect diagnosis leading to inappropriate management can be disastrous and may result in worsening obstruction and possible death. These children should be taken to an appropriate hospital facility as a matter of urgency.

Small inhaled objects may well pass down into the distal bronchial tree and, if a careful history and examination are not performed, they could be mistaken for asthma. Unilateral wheeze and air trapping on chest X-ray are helpful clues. Bronchoscopic retrieval of even a small asymptomatic foreign body is necessary to prevent infection developing.

2.7.3 Management (*Figure 2.7*)

A child suspected of foreign body inhalation should be managed as a priority in a calm and reassuring manner. When foreign body aspiration is either witnessed or strongly suspected and the child is still able to cough, he or she should be encouraged to do so for as long as a forceful cough is maintained.

In the absence of an effective cough or respiratory effort with the development of stridor, cyanosis and unconsciousness and in the presence of obstructed breathing, other techniques are used to try and dislodge an inhaled foreign body. The technique depends on the age of the victim.

They are all designed to create an artificial cough by rapidly increasing intrathoracic pressure, thereby expelling air to expel the foreign body.

Blind finger sweeps in a child's mouth are not recommended and should not be performed. They are likely to cause the child to panic all the more or even push a foreign body at the back of the throat further down into the airway making it more difficult to remove. In addition the soft palate is easily damaged and blood tracking down into the airway increases obstruction.

In the unconscious apnoeic child, airway opening manoeuvres should be performed. In addition to the standard techniques, the tongue–jaw lift is useful and is achieved by grasping the tongue and lower jaw between finger and thumb and pulling forwards. This pulls the tongue off the back of the throat and may relieve the obstruction and make visualisation of a foreign body easier. If the foreign body is visible it should be removed preferably with Magill's forceps.

Infants
A combination of back blows and chest thrusts only is recommended in this age group. Infants have a relatively large liver and abdominal thrusts could potentially result in abdominal injury.

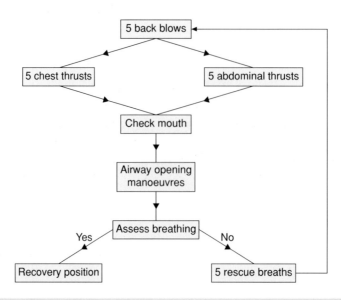

Figure 2.7 Algorithm for choking child (chest thrusts alternate with abdominal thrusts only in children older than 1 year).

The rescuer should place the baby prone and head down over the out-stretched arm with the forearm resting on the thigh, supporting the baby's head. Five back blows, with the heel of the free hand, are then delivered between the baby's shoulder blades. Should this be unsuccessful the baby is turned over, again head down and cradled on the outstretched arm. Five chest thrusts are then delivered using the same landmarks and techniques as for cardiac massage, only more slowly. Larger infants can be dealt with the same way but with the child resting over the lap.

Children

In the older child, back blows are carried out as in the larger infant with the child lying over the lap. If the victim is conscious, abdominal thrusts (the Heimlich manoeuvre) [3] can then be used with the child sitting, standing, lying or kneeling. If unconscious, the victim should be managed lying in the supine position. When the child is in other than the lying position, the rescuer should stand behind and place the arms around the child's torso with a clenched fist against the abdominal wall between the xiphisternum and umbilicus. The other hand is then placed over the fist and both hands are thrust rapidly upwards into the abdomen. This is performed five times or less if the foreign body is expelled.

To carry out abdominal thrusts with the child lying supine, the rescuer kneels to one side or astride the child and places the heel of one hand on the abdominal wall between the umbilicus and xiphisternum. The free hand is then placed onto the first hand and five vigorous midline upward thrusts are carried out or until the foreign body is expelled.

2.8 Anaphylaxis

Anaphylaxis is a potentially life-threatening systemic allergic reaction mediated by IgE antibody, resulting in the release of histamine, leukotrienes and vasoactive mediators. The commonest etiologies are specific environmental allergens, e.g. food, insect bites, drugs, blood products and radiocontrast media. Most reactions occur within 30 minutes of exposure and require prompt assessment and aggressive treatment.

2.8.1 Signs and symptoms

A prodrome of flushing, facial swelling, urticaria, wheeze and stridor may precede airway obstruction or shock. The life-threatening features are shown in *Table 2.2*.

The child may also have pruritis, nausea, vomiting, abdominal cramps and diarrhea.

Table 2.2 Life-threatening features of anaphylaxis and their cause

Feature	Cause
Stridor	Laryngeal and pharyngeal edema (tongue, lips and uvula)
Cough and wheeze	Bronchospasm
Hypotension	Systemic vasodilatation and hypovolemia (capillary leak)

2.8.2 Immediate management

Epinephrine (adrenaline) and the ABC approach are the mainstays of treatment.

Epinephrine
Give epinephrine (adrenaline) s.c. i.m. (0.01 ml kg^{-1} of 1:1000) or slowly i.v. (0.1 ml kg^{-1} of 1:10 000)

Improvement should be seen within 2 minutes. The dose of epinephrine (adrenaline) should be repeated if the effect is incomplete.

Airway/breathing
The child should be given:
- oxygen by facemask
- nebulized epinephrine (adrenaline) 5 ml of 1/1000 may be used in conjunction with intravenous epinephrine, or alone for mild upper airway obstruction
- intubation if airway obstruction is severe

Call for urgent anesthetic and ENT assistance as the child may need urgent intubation and, very rarely, a surgical airway.

Circulation
Intravenous access should be secured with a wide bore cannula. Circulation should then be supported.
- Give 20 ml kg^{-1} of normal saline, for hypotension.
- If hypotension continues, give further fluid bolus of 20 ml kg^{-1} and not colloid doses and repeat epinephrine (adrenaline) dose every 5 minutes or consider i.v. epinephrine (adrenaline) infusion 0.1 µg kg^{-1} min^{-1} with the child on continuous oxygen saturation, ECG and BP monitoring. Senior emergency and intensive care staff should be called.

2.8.3 Further management

All patients with anaphylaxis should be admitted for observation as they may deteriorate after the initial episode. They may need further treatment, including:
• steroids: hydrocortisone 4 mg kg^{-1}.

2.9 Drowning

2.9.1 Definition

Drowning is defined as death by asphyxiation following submersion in a fluid, which is usually water. During the initial resuscitation it does not seem to make any difference whether this is fresh or salt water. Near-drowning occurs when the victim recovers, however briefly, following submersion.

2.9.2 Epidemiology

Bodies of water act as a strong draw for children and are a favored play area. Every year hundreds of children drown and this is a significant cause of death particularly in the under 4-year-olds who are often oblivious to the potential dangers. Carers should be ever mindful of this and should never leave children unsupervised especially if they suffer with epilepsy. Whether it be the garden pond or the unattended bathtub, they are all potential death traps. Children should be encouraged to learn to swim from an early age.

2.9.3 Pathophysiology

In drowning accidents, the primary event is a respiratory arrest eventually leading to a secondary cardiac arrest. A child submerged in water will initially hold their breath and their heart rate slows as part of the diving reflex. If this process continues, hypoxia develops and the child then becomes tachycardic. Eventually the child will take a breath and inhale water, which on contact with the glottis results in laryngospasm and secondary apnoea. In about 10% of cases no water actually enters the lungs in what is known as 'dry drowning'. In the remaining cases, secondary apnoea is followed by the disappearance of laryngeal spasm and the development of involuntary respiration. Water and debris are then drawn down into the lungs. The child becomes progressively more hypoxic and acidotic, with a terminal bradycardia or arrhythmia acting as the prelude to eventual cardiac arrest.

2.9.4 Management

Treatment of the victim of near-drowning can be attempted even before rescue from the water. Having said this, basic life support is difficult unless the rescuer has a firm foothold. Rescuers must always make a safe approach, otherwise further unnecessary deaths may occur.

Once on dry land the child's airway should be opened and cleared but attempts at emptying the lungs of water are time wasting and futile. Fluid filled lungs have reduced compliance and so require higher inflation pressures. Resuscitation follows standard guidelines and most survivors will usually start to breathe after about 5 minutes.

The stomach is often full of water and vomiting often follows successful resuscitation attempts. Stomach decompression and intubation guards against this and both should be achieved once resuscitation has got underway. Once the child has been intubated, continuous positive airways pressure (CPAP) and positive end expiratory pressure (PEEP) are useful in ventilating stiff lungs.

Near-drowning can be complicated by a number of other factors, which must be borne in mind during resuscitation attempts. Many drowning incidents result from children falling or diving into water. In these circumstances the child could also have been injured and the rescuer should assume this until it can be ruled out. Particularly when there has been a diving accident in shallow water, there is significant risk of a cervical spine injury and the neck must be adequately immobilized until this possibility can be excluded.

The large surface area:volume ratio of children means that even during warm weather hypothermia is a common feature of near-drowning. A core temperature should be determined at an early stage during resuscitation using a low reading thermometer. Hypothermia is a mixed blessing. Although its presence hampers resuscitation attempts, rapid cooling slows the metabolic rate and protects the vital organs. Children have survived long periods of submersion in cold water and resuscitation attempts should be equally prolonged. Survival has been recorded in children after an hour following submersion in cold water. Cardiac arrhythmias are frequently seen at low body temperatures, which also make them all the more difficult to treat. Ventricular fibrillation is often refractory at core temperatures below 30°C. Resuscitation should not be abandoned until the child has been rewarmed to at least 33°C. A child should not be declared dead until it is 'warm and dead'.

Rewarming

The techniques used to rewarm a child depend on the degree of hypothermia. Methods are divided into external and core rewarming but must not hamper CPR.

External rewarming alone is usually adequate where core temperature is more than 32°C. Below 32°C, core warming is necessary. The means used depend on the skills of the rescuers and the facilities available (*Boxes 2.3, 2.4*).

Box 2.3 Means of external rewarming, temperature > 32°C

- Remove wet clothing
- Dry child
- Wrap in warmed blankets
- Use radiant heat lamp

Box 2.4 Means of core rewarming, temperature < 32°C

- Infusion of warm intravenous fluids (at 43°C)
- Ventilation with warm gases (at 43°C)
- Instillation of warm fluids into body cavities (at 43°C)*
- Cardiac bypass

*Instillation of warm fluids into body cavities is used by some, but thought to confer no advantage to others.

2.9.5 Indicators of outcome

Abandoning resuscitating is always a difficult decision and should ideally be made by a senior doctor. As already mentioned, despite an initially poor outlook, children have still survived. A number of factors may help when coming to a decision. The majority of successful resuscitations occur in children who have had submersion times of less than 10 minutes (see *Boxes 2.5* and *2.6*).

Box 2.5 Indicators of good outcome

- Submersion for < 10 minutes
- Submersion in cold water
- Initial core temperature below 33°C preserves vital organ (especially brain) function
- Initial spontaneous breath in first few minutes

Box 2.6 Indicators of poor outcome

- No spontaneous respiratory attempt within 40 minutes
- Arterial pO_2 less than 8.0 kPa (60 mmHg) despite resuscitation
- Blood pH below 7.0 despite resuscitation
- Persisting coma

2.9.6 Investigations

Once the child has been successfully resuscitated a chest X-ray should be performed, both to confirm the position of any tubes and to act as a baseline in the detection of any subsequent pulmonary complications. Blood gases during and after resuscitation in addition to electrolytes, glucose and blood cultures are also useful in further management.

2.9.7 Complications

Following successful resuscitation the patient should be observed for a minimum of 6 hours for a number of potential, mainly respiratory complications. Abnormal respiratory signs should be assumed to indicate the aspiration of water. In these cases pulmonary edema may develop and require intensive care and ventilation. The wheezy child should be treated with a nebulized bronchodilator.

Early onset of fever is not uncommon but one developing after 24 hours often indicates Gram-negative infection and should be treated once blood cultures have been taken.

Children who have made a rapid recovery after immersion can appear clinically stable. It may be possible to discharge them but only after a minimum of 6 hours of observation and if they are quite well with no respiratory symptoms or fever. The clinical chest examination and radiograph must be completely clear and blood gases normal whilst they are breathing air.

2.9.8 Conclusion

Drowning is an important and avoidable cause of death in childhood. Recovery is possible even after prolonged immersion particularly when it has occurred in cold water. Hypothermia is a common complicating feature, which should be actively treated. Particularly when there has been a fall or a diving accident into water, cervical spine injuries should be assumed to be present.

References

1. The American Academy of Pediatrics and Mannio, V.P. (1999) Program Coordinator/Public Educator.
2. American Heart Association. (1997) *Pediatric Advanced Life Support.*
3. Advanced Life Support Group.(2000) *Advanced Pediatric Life Support – The Practical Approach*, 3rd Edn, BMJ Publishing Group, London.

Suggested Further Reading

American Heart Association. (1992) Guidelines for cardiopulmonary resuscitation and emergency cardiac care. *J. Am. Med. Ass.*

Heimlich, H.J. A life-saving manoeuvre to prevent food-choking. *J. Am. Med. Ass.* **234:** 398–401

Macnab, A., Macrae, D., Henning, R. (1999) *Care of the Critically Ill Child.* Churchill Livingstone, Edinburgh.

Patterson M.D. (1999) Resuscitation update for the pediatrician. *Ped. Clinics N. Am.* 1999, **46:** 1285–99.

Young K.D., Seidel T.S. (1999) Pediatric cardiopulmonary resuscitation. A collective review. *Ann. Emerg. Med.* **33:** 195–205.

Chapter 3

Shock

Ben Stanhope

Contents

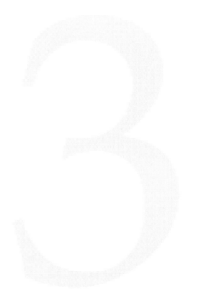

3.1 Introduction

Shock is most simply conceptualised as failure of the circulation to provide adequate delivery of oxygen and essential nutrients to the tissues to ensure normal cell respiration. The process leading to this state may be single or multifactorial. In the management of sick and injured children, the emphasis lies in swift recognition of shock followed by rapid assessment of the nature of the circulatory failure. The latter is essential because avoidance of significant morbidity and mortality relies on the clinician's ability to determine the origin(s) of the shock accurately and initiate appropriate and specific management.

At a cellular level inadequate oxygen delivery leads to lactic acid formation and the development of metabolic acidosis. Up to a point the body compensates for this by redistributing blood flow away from non-essential tissues (e.g. mesenteric circulation, skin) to the **vital organs** (e.g. brain and heart). This state of **compensated shock** is completed by increased extraction of oxygen from the blood by these essential organs to maintain oxygen delivery. **Uncompensated shock** develops when despite these mechanisms the pathological insult makes it impossible for the body's vital organs to overcome the inadequacy of oxygen delivery. Untreated, uncompensated shock will inevitably lead to a spiralling deterioration. An inflammatory cascade ensues at the endothelium causing cellular tissue damage. If prolonged, this damage becomes irreversible and indeed restoration of adequate circulation at this stage may lead to reperfusion injury, itself exacerbating the damage. Multi-organ failure will follow, which in many cases will be unrecoverable. However, compensated and early, uncompensated shock are treatable and so this chapter focuses on the clinician's recognition, assessment and initial management of shock in the Pediatric Emergency Department.

3.2 The heart in shock

Shock can be thought of in terms of three key elements that affect the heart's ability to provide an adequate circulation, namely preload, contractility and afterload.

3.2.1 Preload

Preload refers to the degree of tension placed upon the cardiac muscle as it begins to contract. It is usually considered to be the end-diastolic pressure at the completion of ventricular filling. A sufficient degree of stretch to the myocardium is required to produce a level of contraction as governed by the Frank–Starling mechanism. This stretch is produced by venous return, itself inherently linked to actual circulating volume. A fall in circulating volume will reduce venous return, myocardial stretch, force of myocardial contraction and cardiac output.

3.2.2 Contractility

The force generated during ventricular contraction defines ventricular contractility. Contractility is maximised in a neutral homeostatic environment when myocardial oxygen delivery is adequate, acidosis absent, electrolytes in balance, etc. Improvement in contractility increases cardiac output through improved stroke volume.

3.2.3 Afterload

Afterload may be thought of as the resistance against the heart as it exerts its force during contraction. It is actually the pressure created in the artery leading from the ventricle during ventricular systole. Whilst it is true that too high an afterload would result in a reduction in the output by the ventricle, too low an afterload itself poses significant problems since adequate organ perfusion relies on a finely balanced relationship between preload, contractility and afterload.

3.3 Classification of shock

The diagnosis of shock is purely clinical. It is possible to classify shock into physiological categories but in reality there is usually overlap between these in individual patients. Classification may be useful in diagnosis since clinical signs may differ between types, as may treatment. Shock is most commonly classified by the anatomical site of the circulation failure (*Figure 3.1*).

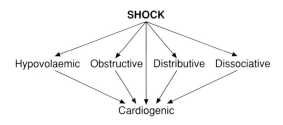

Figure 3.1 A classification of shock.

Hypovolemic shock results from a fall in actual circulating volume within the intravascular space. In children there are:

- *Common causes*
  - dehydration, e.g. diarrhea and vomiting
  - hemorrhage
  - sepsis (due to fluid redistribution secondary to increased capillary permeability)
- *Less common*
  - burns
  - peritonitis

Compensatory mechanisms will be employed in response to a fall in circulating volume. Cardiac output is maintained or augmented by tachycardia and peripheral vasoconstriction, the latter maintaining afterload. Renal perfusion is reduced as blood is diverted to the brain and heart, resulting in activation of the renin–angiotensin system and a subsequent increase in circulating volume by sodium and water reabsorption.

Cardiogenic shock refers to situations where myocardial contractility is compromised resulting in reduced cardiac output and tissue perfusion. It is less common than hypovolemia as the primary etiology in the shocked child but, since reduced perfusion will always eventually affect myocardial function, it is an inevitable consequence wherever shock is prolonged (see *Figure 3.1*). Causes are as follows:
- heart failure
- cardiac surgery
- intrinsic myocardial disease, e.g. acute viral myocarditis, cardiomyopathy
- drug toxicity
- electrolyte and acid-base disturbances
- dysrhythmias.

Reduction in cardiac output brings about compensatory manoeuvres as with hypovolemia.

Obstructive shock describes a scenario where despite adequate contractility the heart is unable to pump out an adequate volume of blood to be oxygenated and/or distributed to the tissues. Causes include:
- obstructive congenital cardiac lesion, e.g. aortic coarctation or critical aortic valve stenosis
- tension pneumothorax
- cardiac tamponade.

Distributive shock is usually a complication of severe infection. It is the principal pathophysiological process that defines septic shock. In the presence of overwhelming sepsis an unchecked, generalised inflammatory response develops. Inflammatory mediators such as TNFα, inter-leukin-1 and lipopolysaccharide endotoxin are produced causing local cell damage particularly to vascular endothelium. The vasoactive effects of these mediators on the endothelium produce variation in vascular tone. Whilst areas of vasoconstriction and vasodilatation may coexist side-by-side, the overall effect is that of peripheral vasodilatation and a fall in systemic vascular resistance (SVR). This means that blood is not distributed efficiently to the tissues despite a state of high cardiac output, which may exist in septic shock. Adults in septic shock secondary to Gram negative bacteremia classically present with this picture where good peripheral perfusion mediated by profound vasodilatation gives rise to the description of 'warm shock'. In children, however, the more common presentation is that of cold peripheries, skin mottling and pro-longed capillary refill time. Causes of distributive shock include:

- *Septic*
  - meningococcemia
  - Gram negative bacteremia
  - streptococcal infection (group B streptococcus in neonates, pneumo-coccus in older children)
- *Non-septic*
  - anaphylaxis
  - neurogenic, e.g. following transection of the spinal cord
  - drugs, e.g. vasodilators or anesthetics

Dissociative shock occurs when there is inadequate oxygen capacity. It occurs in:

- profound anemia
- methemoglobinemia
- carbon monoxide poisoning

3.4 **Recognition of shock**

Most physical signs are consistent regardless of the origin of shock; there are some exceptions. *Table 3.1* presents the principal clinical findings in the shocked child.

Physical examination may give clues as to the etiology of shock, which may aid management, e.g.

- meningococcemia   purpuric and petechial rash
- cardiac failure   gallop rhythm/hepatomegaly
- dehydration   dry mucous membranes, oliguria, reduced skin turgor
- anaphylaxis   angioedema, pallor, urticaria, wheeze, stridor

Table 3.1 Clinical signs of shock

System	Sign	Comments
Respiratory	Tachypnea Increased work of breathing Apnea Cyanosis	Grunting; inter/subcostal retraction; use of accessory muscles Particularly in neonates/babies NB: Central cyanosis is a preterminal sign in children
Cardiovascular	Heart rate Pulse volume Blood pressure Skin appearance*	Tachycardia is a sensitive marker of hypovolemia. Bradycardia may be preterminal Reduced or absent NB: Hypotension is a late and preterminal sign in children Cool and mottled peripheries progressing distal to proximal as shock worsens Prolonged capillary refill time (> 2 s)
Neurological	Irritability Reduced conscious level Coma	Neurological deterioration will mirror deteriorating shock from irritability to a fall in conscious level and eventually coma
Renal	Oliguria/anuria	Acceptable urine output is generally defined as: Infants: at least 2 ml kg^{-1} hour^{-1} Young children: at least 1 ml kg^{-1} hour^{-1} Older children/adolescents: at least 0.5 ml kg^{-1} hour^{-1}

* In 'warm' septic shock, vasodilatation and high cardiac output may produce warm seemingly well-perfused peripheries, despite shock.

3.5 Management of shock

Figure 3.2 shows how the presence of shock is managed.

3.5.1 Airway and breathing

The resuscitation mantra of Airway, Breathing, Circulation or 'ABC' remains the management priority in the shocked child as in any other. Before assessment of the nature or severity of shock can be made, the clinician must ensure that the airway is patent and that the patient is breathing adequately without assistance. If this is not so then appropriate steps should be taken to stabilise the airway and ensure adequate breathing. Intubation and judicious positive pressure ventilation can benefit the shocked child when significant myocardial dysfunction exists and will reduce oxygen consumption caused by increased work of breathing. High flow oxygen should be administered via a facemask with

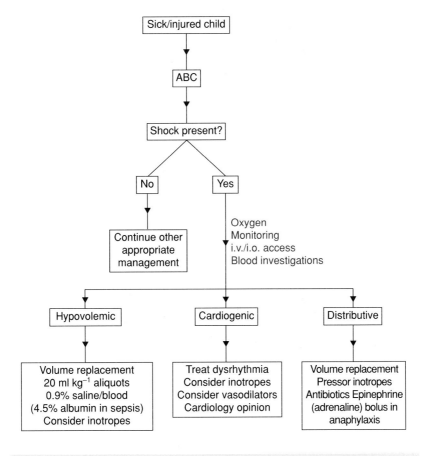

Figure 3.2 Algorithm for the management of shock.

a reservoir bag to maximise oxygen concentration. The shocked child must not be allowed to become hypoxic by the omission of a simple treatment such as oxygen therapy.

As the airway and breathing are being managed, the following monitoring should take place:
• Pulse oximetry
• 3 lead electrocardiogram monitoring
• Blood pressure

3.5.2 Circulation

The clinician should pay particular attention to:
• Pulse rate, rhythm and volume
• Peripheral skin color, temperature, capillary refill time, rashes
• Respiratory rate and work of breathing
• Signs of cardiac failure
• Neurological state
• Signs of injury that might have caused hemorrhage (limb fracture, abdominal trauma, head trauma)
• Urine output

Whilst relatively uncommon in children, the presence of cardiac dysrhythmia associated with shock will require immediate management. The definitive management of dysrhythmia is covered in other chapters.

Vascular access should be achieved as quickly as possible. At least one, but preferably two, large-bore venous cannule should be sited. If poor perfusion makes this impossible then intraosseous, central venous (femoral or internal jugular vein) or peripheral venous cutdown are acceptable alternatives. At the time of vascular access appropriate blood samples should be taken:
• Full blood count and film
• Blood cross-match – in hemorrhage; most children with septic shock will require transfusion
• Coagulation screen – particularly in septic shock
• Plasma urea, creatinine and electrolytes
• Serum calcium
• Plasma glucose and lactate
• Blood gas estimation – arterial or central venous gases are most useful
• Blood culture and microbial sensitivities

A bedside blood glucose test should also be performed and hypoglycemia corrected promptly. Once assessment and monitoring have been completed (in the acutely sick child this should take no more than 1–2 minutes), the clinician then moves on to definitive management of the shock state. With reference to the three factors involved in the shocked heart there are three objectives of treatment:

1. Correction of hypovolemia (preload)
2. Optimising the cardiac pump (contractility)
3. Ensuring peripheral distribution of blood (afterload)

Following restoration of circulation, a secondary survey for organ specific signs should be carried out.

3.5.3 Correction of hypovolemia

The objective of volume replacement in shock is to optimise preload. The hypovolemic child should be managed initially with a rapid intravenous infusion of warmed fluid of 20 ml kg^{-1}. The approximate weight of a child can be calculated by using the formula:

$$\text{Weight of child (kg)} = 2 \, (\text{age in years} + 4)$$

The selection of fluid is a matter of departmental policy and no little controversy in the literature. The author recommends 0.9% saline as the fluid of choice in volume resuscitation except in suspected meningococcemia and septic shock when 4.5% human albumin solution is preferred. This is because albumin offers a more logical approach and a theoretically longer duration of action in the presence of the profound capillary leak that occurs, particularly in meningococcal sepsis. Close attention should be made to the effect of the fluid bolus on heart rate, pulse volume and, to a lesser extent, blood pressure. A lack of or very transient fall in heart rate should be followed by a second similar fluid bolus. Further boluses of 10–20 ml kg^{-1} may be required depending on clinical response. Prompt consideration of definitive airway support and intensive care unit admission will be required for these patients as the risk of pulmonary edema is very high. If available, reference to serial blood gas and plasma lactate measurements may aid assessment of progress and invasive monitoring of central venous pressure (CVP) is a marker of preload in the unobstructed heart. A CVP higher than that usually acceptable (i.e. > 10 mmHg) will be required to optimise cardiac performance in myocardial dysfunction which is universal in septic shock. Important management notes are listed in *Box 3.1*.

> **Box 3.1** Important management notes
>
> - When hemorrhage is suspected, no more than 40 ml kg^{-1} of crystalloid should be given before blood is used as the replacement fluid
> - In meningococcemia and septic shock, 4.5% albumin is preferred to crystalloid
> - In infants with gastroenteritis, 4.5% albumin should be used after 40 ml kg^{-1} crystalloid, and other diagnoses considered, e.g. volvulus, peritonitis
> - Children with meningococcal sepsis often require up to and over 100 ml kg^{-1} fluid in resuscitation

3.5.4 Optimising the cardiac pump

Inotropic support may be required when shock persists despite significant fluid replacement. This may not apply when hemorrhage is the cause of hypovolemia. In this case surgical management of the bleed will be required whilst the child continues to receive blood as volume replacement. Patients in septic shock commonly demonstrate poor myocardial contractility and concurrent low SVR in the presence of metabolic acidosis and endothelial injury. These children benefit from agents producing strong inotropy and peripheral vasoconstriction. *Table 3.2* lists commonly used inotropes, their principal actions and therapeutic dose ranges.

Choice of inotropic agent is not without controversy and is an issue for departmental consideration. Dopamine is widely used as the first line inotrope in the shocked child, followed by epinephrine (adrenaline) if response to dopamine is inadequate. In cases of septic shock, where low SVR is likely, there is logic in choosing first an agent that produces vasoconstriction. Epinephrine (adrenaline) (often in conjunction with norepinephrine (noradrenaline) offers positive inotropy and peripheral vasoconstriction, and its early use in the septic shocked child can be very valuable. The dose of inotrope should be titrated according to clinical response. Once this level of cardiac support has been instituted, the patient is likely to have been intubated and ventilated and requires invasive blood pressure monitoring and definitive intensive care management.

3.5.5 Ensuring peripheral distribution of blood

Afterload can be too great or too low to allow normal delivery of blood to the tissues. In the vasodilated child, such as in sepsis, norepinephrine

Table 3.2 Actions and dose ranges of common inotropic drugs

Agent	Actions and comments	Dose range
Epinephrine (Adrenaline)	α, β_1 and β_2 agonist Positive inotrope and chronotrope Increases afterload by increasing SVR	0.05–1.0 μg kg^{-1} min^{-1} by i.v. infusion
Dobutamine	β_1 and β_2 agonist Improves contractility and increases heart rate Relatively few effects on SVR Reduced effect seen in infants	1–20 μg kg^{-1} min^{-1}
Dopamine	β_1, β_2 and dopaminergic agonist increases heart rate and vasoconstricts (high dose) Vasodilatation at low doses Release of endogenous norepinephrine (noradrenaline)	5–20 μg kg^{-1} min^{-1} 1–15 μg kg^{-1} min^{-1}
Enoximone	Phosphodiesterase inhibitor Improves contractility Reduces afterload by vasodilatation Weak inotrope – an 'inodilator'	0.5–1.0 μg kg^{-1} min^{-1}
Isoproterenol (Isoprenaline)	β agonist Increases heart rate and contractility Vasodilatation Useful in infants	0.02–1.0 μg kg^{-1} min^{-1}
Norepinephrine (Noradrenaline)	α and β_1 agonist Potent vasoconstrictor Improves blood pressure	0.02–1.0 μg kg^{-1} min^{-1}

Note: Clinicians should consult local drug policy advice prior to using these agents.

(noradrenaline) and epinephrine (adrenaline) provide vasoconstriction to improve SVR and reduce maldistribution. In the child with cardiogenic shock, such as in those following cardiac surgery, the afterload is relatively high as the injured heart struggles to pump efficiently. Vasodilators such as sodium nitroprusside can 'off-load' ventricular work improving cardiac output. More recently phosphodiesterase inhibitors, such as enoximone and milrinone, are increasingly used, as they provide low-level inotropy in conjunction with vasodilatation to enhance cardiac output.

3.5.6 Specific therapies

Individual problems require action in addition to the general principles of management employed in most cases of shock. The following are for consideration:
- Antimicrobial drugs as clinically indicated, e.g. in meningococcemia or the immunocompromised
- Coagulopathy – correct with fresh frozen plasma or cryoprecipitate
- Metabolic acidosis – can improve with volume replacement or might require alkalising agents
- Electrolyte disturbances – correct as necessary

3.6 Summary

The child presenting in shock carries a high risk of morbidity and mortality. Prompt medical treatment offers the best chance of recovery even in uncompensated shock. Emphasis is placed on expedient management to arrest the pathophysiological cascade and avoid hypotension, a sinister marker for mortality in the critically ill child. *Figure 3.2* gives an aide-memoir for the clinician presented with the shocked child.

Suggested reading

Advanced Life Support Group. (2001) *Advanced Pediatric Life Support – The Practical Approach*, 3rd edn. BMJ Publishing Group, London.

Cochrane Injuries Group Albumin Reviewers. (1998) Human albumin administration in critically ill patients: systematic review of randomised controlled trials. Why albumin may not work. *BMJ* **317**: 235–240.

Petros *et al.* (1998) Human albumin administration in critically ill patients (letter). *BMJ* **317**: 882.

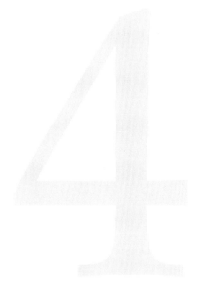

Chapter 4

Cardiac emergencies

Colin Powell

Contents

4.1 **Supraventricular tachycardia**

Supraventricular tachycardia will usually present with signs of congestive cardiac failure or shock, but will also depend on the age of the child. Sinus tachycardia can be up to about 200 beats per minute. Supraventricular tachycardia (SVT) is usually above 220 beats per minute.

4.1.1 Assessment

Symptoms
Infants usually present with pallor, dyspnea and poor feeding. Older children have palpitations and chest discomfort.

Signs
In SVT (*Figure 4.1*) there is a regular tachycardia with a heart rate usually 180–300 per minute. Hypotension might be present but is often compensated early on in presentation. Heart failure with hepatomegaly with gallop rhythm occurs, especially in infants.

Consult cardiology urgently if tachycardia is broad complex or irregular.

4.1.2 Management

The child must be monitored with continuous ECG trace and frequent measurements of blood pressure. The options for treatment are listed below.
- If necessary apply oxygen 10 l min⁻¹ by facemask
- If child is shocked (i.e. hypotensive, poor peripheral perfusion, impaired mental state) proceed to direct current cardioversion (see below)
- If child is not shocked treat with intravenous adenosine

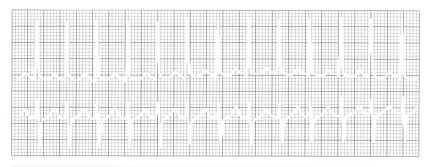

Figure 4.1 A 12-lead ECG showing regular narrow complex tachycardia.

Shocked child

If the child is shocked, then direct current cardioversion is needed. You must:

- Call ICU. Ensure experienced staff and full resuscitative measures are present
- Ensure child is on oxygen, and has intravenous access
- Administer diazepam intravenously if there is any chance of awareness
- DC revert using a synchronised shock of 0.5 J kg^{-1}. If this is unsuccessful, increase dose to 1 J kg^{-1} and then to 2 J kg^{-1} if still unsuccessful
- An unsynchronised shock is necessary for ventricular fibrillation or polymorphic ventricular tachycardia

Stable child

If the child is stable, vasovagal maneuvers and adenosine should be tried:

- **Vagal maneuvers** – use the Valsalva maneuver if child old enough, the gag or icepack/iced water for infants (apply to face for a maximum of 30 seconds). Do not use eyeball pressure.
- **Intravenous adenosine**
  - Insert cannula into a large proximal peripheral vein (the cubital fossa is ideal) with a 3-way tap attached
  - Draw up starting dose of adenosine 50 µg kg^{-1}. If necessary dilute to 1 ml with normal saline
  - Draw up 10 ml saline flush
  - Turn on the ECG trace recorder
  - Administer adenosine as a rapid i.v. push followed by the saline flush
  - Repeat procedure at 2-minute intervals, until tachycardia terminated, increasing the dose of adenosine by 50 µg kg^{-1} to a total dose of 300 µg kg^{-1} for infants of less than 1 month, and to a total dose of 500 µg kg^{-1} to children between 1 month and 12 years.
  - Perform 12-lead ECG postreversion

The recorded strip at the time of conversion to sinus rhythm should be inspected and saved, for concealed pre-excitation may only be revealed during the first few beats after conversion to sinus rhythm. After a patient has been reverted, a 12-lead ECG should be performed to look for pre-excitation and other abnormalities. Rapid re-initiation of tachycardia is not uncommon, mostly because of premature atrial contractions stimulated by the adenosine. If this occurs consider trying adenosine again. Side effects including flushing and chest tightness or discomfort are not uncommon but they are usually brief and transient. Rarely atrial fibrillation or prolonged pauses may occur. Adenosine is contraindicated in adenosine–deaminase deficiency (rare immune deficiency) and patients taking dipyridamole (Persantin). Care is required in asthma, as it may cause bronchospasm. If these measures fail to revert the SVT, consult a cardiology specialist.

Disposition

A follow-up plan should be made in consultation with cardiology. Some children may be started on beta blockers. There may be an underlying conduction abnormality such as Wolff–Parkinson–White syndrome.

4.2 Syncope

A syncopal attack is brief, usually with sudden loss of consciousness and muscle tone caused by cerebral ischemia or inadequate oxygen or glucose to the brain.

4.2.1 Features

- It usually lasts only a few seconds
- The child limp and unresponsive
- Tonic–clonic movements can occur with prolonged unconsciousness
- The patient is back to normal on awakening

4.2.2 Cause

There are several causes, including (*Figure 4.2*):
- Vasovagal (fainting)
- Orthostatic or postural hypotension
- Cardiac
  - structural (e.g. critical aortic stenosis, tetralogy of Fallot, atrial myxoma etc.)
  - arrhythmia (e.g. prolonged QT, AV block, sick sinus syndrome)
- Respiratory (e.g. cough, hyperventilating, breath holding)
- Metabolic (e.g. anemia, hypoglycemia, hysteria etc.)

4.2.3 Management

A history of the surrounding events is important. Orthostatic hypotension usually occurs on standing suddenly. Vasovagal collapse is usually associated with environmental or emotional stresses. Structural cardiac lesion is more likely if the syncope is exertional. The patient should be examined for cardiac anomaly (e.g. murmur, heaves etc). Investigations should include an ECG to look for dysrythmias, short/abnormal PR interval (e.g. Wolff–Parkinson–White syndrome) or prolonged QT syndrome.

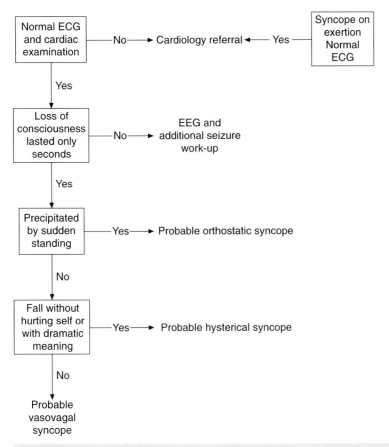

Figure 4.2 Diagnosis of syncope.

If unconsciousness lasts more than a few seconds and the patient is not fully awake immediately after the event, then consider seizures as a cause (*Table 4.1*). The patient may need an EEG to clarify this issue. Hysterical syncope generally occurs in front of an audience, patients do not hurt themselves and there is associated moaning or non-rhythmical jerking.

4.2.4 Follow up

All patients who have unexplained syncope should be reviewed in outpatients.

4.3 Kawasaki disease

Kawasaki disease is a systemic vasculitis that predominantly affects children under 5 years old. Although the specific etiological agent remains unknown, it is believed that Kawasaki disease is a response to some form

Table 4.1 Differentiating syncope from seizures

Sign	Syncope	Seizures	Hypoglycemia
Period of unconsciousness	Usually seconds	Frequently 5 min or longer	Usually over a few minutes
Incontinence	Absent	May be present	Absent
Confusion on waking	Absent	Marked for 20–30 min	Usually, slow to improve
Tonic–clonic movements	Occasionally and brief, particularly if unconsciousness is prolonged	Frequently present	Frequently absent
EEG	Normal	Frequently abnormal if done soon after event	Normal

of infection (although it is not transmitted from person to person). Diagnosis is often delayed because the features are similar to those of many viral exanthems.

The diagnostic criteria for Kawasaki disease are fever for 5 days or more, plus four out of five of the following:
• polymorphous rash
• bilateral (non-purulent) conjunctival infection
• mucous membrane changes, e.g. reddened or dry cracked lips, strawberry tongue, diffuse redness of oral or pharyngeal mucosa
• peripheral changes, e.g. erythema of the palms or soles, edema of the hands or feet, and in convalescence desquamation
• cervical lymphadenopathy (> 15 mm diameter, usually unilateral, single, non-purulent and painful)

and exclusion of diseases with a similar presentation: staphylococcal infection (e.g. scalded skin syndrome, toxic shock syndrome), streptococcal infection (e.g. scarlet fever, toxic shock-like syndrome not just isolation from the throat), measles, other viral exanthems, Stevens–Johnson syndrome, drug reaction and juvenile rheumatoid arthritis. The diagnostic features of Kawasaki disease can occur sequentially and may not all be present at the same time. Moreover, it is recognised that some patients with Kawasaki disease do not develop sufficient features to fulfil the formal diagnostic criteria. Clinical vigilance and recognition of this possibility are necessary to recognise these 'incomplete' or 'atypical' cases. This is important because the atypical cases are probably at similar risk of coronary complications and require treatment. Other relatively common features include arthritis, diarrhea and vomiting, coryza and cough, uveitis, and gallbladder hydrops. Some patients get myocarditis.

4.3.1 Investigations

All patients should have the following investigations:
- ASOT/anti-DNAase B
- echocardiography (at least twice: at initial presentation and, if negative, again at 6–8 weeks)
- platelet count (marked thrombocytosis is common in second week of illness).

Other tests are not diagnostic or particularly useful. The following may be seen:
- neutrophilia
- raised ESR + CRP
- mild normochromic, normocytic anemia
- hypoalbuminemia
- elevated liver enzymes.

Thrombocytosis and desquamation appear in the second week of the illness or later. Their absence earlier does not preclude the diagnosis.

4.3.2 Management

Patients require admission to hospital if Kawasaki disease is diagnosed or strongly suspected. **Intravenous immunoglobulin** ($2 \, g \, kg^{-1}$ over 10 hours) should be given, preferably within the first 10 days of the illness, but should also be given to patients diagnosed after 10 days of illness if there is evidence of ongoing inflammation, for instance with fever or raised ESR/CRP.

Aspirin ($3–5 \, mg \, kg^{-1}$ once a day) should be given for at least 6–8 weeks. Some give a higher dose ($10 \, mg \, kg^{-1}$ 8 hourly for the first few days) but this probably adds nothing over immunoglobulin.

4.3.3 Follow up

Pediatric follow up should be arranged on discharge. At least one further echocardiogram should be performed at 6–8 weeks. If this is normal, no further examinations are needed.

4.4 Cyanotic episodes

Cyanotic episodes occur in children with cyanotic congenital heart disease, in particular tetralogy of Fallot and pulmonary atresia. There may be a previous history of squatting. The episodes usually occur early in the morning, or in the context of stress or dehydration with periods of increased oxygen demand or increased oxygen use. The pathophysiology is not fully understood, but relates to decreased pulmonary blood flow. Most episodes are self-limiting but cause hypoxic–ischemic brain injury or indeed may be fatal.

4.4.1 Assessment

The assessment includes consideration of the severity of the cyanosis or pallor with either distress and hyperpnea (not tachypnea), or lethargy and a depressed conscious state. There may be evidence of structural heart disease occasionally with lessening or absence of a previously documented heart murmur.

4.4.2 Management

This can be divided into initial measures for short periods of cyanosis and measures for more prolonged problems.

Initial measures
- Put the child in knee to chest position
- Give high flow oxygen via mask or headbox
- Avoid exacerbating distress
- Give morphine $0.2 \, mg \, kg^{-1}$ s.c.
- Do continuous ECG and oxygen saturation monitoring and frequent blood pressure measurements
- Correct any underlying cause/secondary problems, which may exacerbate episode, e.g. cardiac arrhythmia, hypothermia, hypoglycemia.

If the attack is prolonged
- Consult a pediatrician or a cardiologist
- Give intravenous fluids – $10 \, ml \, kg^{-1}$ bolus followed by maintenance fluids
- Give sodium bicarbonate 2–$3 \, mmol \, kg^{-1}$ i.v. (ensure adequate ventilation)
- Consider admission

4.5 Cardiac failure and congenital heart disease

4.5.1 Presentation

Congenital heart disease may present as heart failure with or without shock or cyanosis. However, there are many causes of cardiac failure, including non-congenital reasons such as myocarditis. These may present with signs of heart failure, such as breathlessness, hepatomegaly, pallor and sweating, or may be severe enough to present as cardiogenic shock. Remember that heart failure in an infant can mimic bronchiolitis and the child may have contracted bronchiolitis. This in turn may be the precipitating cause of the heart failure. The likely causes are in *Box 4.1*.

In infancy heart failure is usually secondary to congenital structural heart disease. As pulmonary pressures reduce after birth over the first few hours to days of life, increased pulmonary flow from lesions such as VSD or PDA will become apparent. These infants are likely to have a cardiac murmur audible. Rarer duct-dependent lesions, such as pulmonary atresia or transposition of the great vessels, will also present after a few days to weeks as the duct closes. These infants may have a large liver but may not have a cardiac murmur audible. Coarctation and severe aortic stenosis will also present as the duct closes.

Box 4.1 Causes of cardiac failure

- Primary pump failure
  - Myocarditis
  - Cardiomyopathy
- Left-sided outflow obstruction
  - Aortic stenosis
  - Coarctation of the aorta
  - Hypoplastic left heart syndrome
  - Hypertrophic cardiomyopathy
- Left ventricular overload or excessive pulmonary blood flow
  - Ventricular septal defect (VSD)
  - Atrioventricular septal defect
  - Patent ductus arteriosus (PDA)
- Rhythm disturbance
  - Supraventricular tachycardia
  - Complete heart block

4.5.2 Investigation

- CXR may be helpful to demonstrate cardiomegaly with pulmonary plethora or a characteristic cardiac shape and size

- 12-lead ECG
- Cardiac echocardiography and cardiac consultation
- Infection screen as above
- 4-limb blood pressure

4.5.3 Management

Shock

If there are signs of shock then treat as in the cardiogenic shock section.

Heart failure

If the ventilation is adequate, then oxygen by facemask will be sufficient. However, if breathing is inadequate, intubation and artificial ventilation with PEEP will be required. If oxygenation improves with this maneuver, then the likely problem is that of pulmonary congestion secondary to increased flow from a VSD or PDA etc. A heart murmur may be heard and chest X-ray might be helpful in confirming the diagnosis (see below). Treatment needs to be discussed with the cardiologists. It will include oxygenation and reducing the preload with diuretics (with, for example, frusemide 1 mg kg^{-1} i.v., repeated if no response after 2 hours). Consideration will be given to improving cardiac contractility (using, for example, digoxin or inotropes, such as dopamine or dobutamine) or decreasing the afterload with vasodilatation (using, for example, captopril).

Cyanosis

Increasing breathlessness and cyanosis in the first few days of life is the presentation of the rarer duct-dependent disease, such as tricuspid or pulmonary atresia. In these conditions, oxygen may cause the duct to close further but, if it is considered necessary for ventilation, it should be carefully titrated. Intravenous prostaglandin E1 (0.01–0.1 µg kg^{-1} per min) should keep the duct open until cardiac opinion is available. Once a response occurs, the infusion rate should be titrated down. Prostaglandins may cause apnea and so the child should be ventilated during its administration.

All these children require careful monitoring by ECG, pulse oximetry and non-invasive blood pressure measurement. Remember to check blood pressure in lower limbs as well as upper limbs. It is essential to consider sepsis as a differential diagnosis of cardiac failure in infancy and most infants will require a full infection screen and possible antibiotic cover. These children need admission and assessment by the cardiology team.

4.6 Pericarditis and myocarditis

Pericarditis and myocarditis can be bacterial, caused by *Hemophilus influenzae* or *Staphylococcus aureus*, or viral, caused by, for example, Coxsackie B. Children can present ill-looking, and should be considered in the differential diagnosis of sepsis in infancy.

Suggested reading

Penny, D.J. and Sherkerdemian, L.S. (2001) Management of the neonate with symptomatic congenital heart disease. *Arch. Dis. Child. Fetal. Neonatal Ed.* **84:** F141–145.

Chapter 5

Respiratory emergencies

Colin Powell

Contents

5.1 Asthma

Acute asthma is one of the commonest reasons for presentation to an emergency department and admission to a hospital. Consider acute asthma when a child presents with signs of increased work of breathing, widespread wheezing and shortness of breath. There are other causes to consider such as *Mycoplasma pneumonia*, aspiration, inhaled foreign body, and cardiac failure. In the setting of a child with a previous history of asthma or when asthma seems the most likely diagnosis, then perform a primary assessment of severity and institute the initial resuscitation and treatment.

5.1.1 Primary assessment and initial resuscitation and management

Table 5.1 shows the clinical signs and management of asthma at varying degrees of severity.

The arterial oxygen saturation (SaO_2) may be reduced in the absence of significant airway obstruction by factors such as atelectasis and mucous plugging of airways. SaO_2 is purely a measure of oxygenation, which may be preserved in the presence of deteriorating ventilation (with CO_2 retention).

Consider transferring the child to a pediatric intensive care unit if the child:
• is in impending respiratory failure
• requires continuous nebulizers for > 1 hour
• requires salbutamol more frequently than every 30 minutes after 2 hours
• is becoming exhausted.

Consider ventilation if:
• PCO_2 is > 8 kPa
• there is persistent hypoxemia with PO_2 < 8 kPa in inspired oxygen of 60%
• there is increasing exhaustion despite emergency treatment.

Note that exhaustion, a silent chest, cyanosis, bradycardia and hypotension are preterminal signs.

5.1.2 History

Inquire specifically about the duration and nature of symptoms, treatments used (relievers, preventers), trigger factors (including upper

Table 5.1 Assessment and management of asthma

Severity	Primary signs	Secondary signs	Management
Mild	Normal mental state Subtle or no accessory muscle use/recession	O₂ saturation >95% in air Able to talk normally	Salbutamol by MDI/spacer* – once and review after 20 min. Ensure device/technique appropriate Good response – discharge on β2-agonist as needed. Poor response – treat as moderate Oral prednisolone (1 mg kg⁻¹ daily for 1–3 days) if on prophylaxis or episode has persisted over several days Provide written advice/action plan on what to do if symptoms worsen. Consider overall control and family's knowledge. Arrange follow up as appropriate See discharge below
Moderate	Normal mental state Some accessory muscle use/recession	O₂ saturation = 92–95% in air Tachycardia Some limitation of ability to talk	Give O₂ if O₂ saturation is <92%. Need for O₂ should be reassessed Salbutamol by MDI/spacer* – 3 doses, every 20 min; review 10–20 min after 3rd dose decide on admission or discharge Oral prednisolone (1 mg kg⁻¹ daily for 3–5 days) The children of moderate severity who can go home must be discussed with the registrar and should not leave Emergency until at least 1 hour after their last dose of salbutamol Arrange home treatment and follow-up as above

continued

Table 5.1 Assessment and management of asthma – *continued*

Severity	Primary signs	Secondary signs	Management
Severe	Agitated/distressed Moderate/marked accessory muscle use/recession	O_2 saturation <92% in air Tachycardia Marked limitation of ability to talk Note: wheeze may lessen with tiring	Oxygen Salbutamol by MDI/spacer* – 3 doses every 20 min; review on-going requirements 10–20 min after 3rd dose – if improving, reduce frequency; if no change, continue every 20 min; if deteriorating at any stage, treat as critical Ipratropium by MDI/spacer** Oral prednisolone (1 mg kg⁻¹ daily); if vomiting give i.v. methylprednisolone Involve senior staff Arrange admission after initial assessment and management
Critical	Confused/drowsy Maximal accessory muscle use/recession Exhaustion	O_2 saturation <90% in air Marked tachycardia Unable to talk	Involve senior staff in the management early on High flow oxygen Continuous nebulized salbutamol (0.5% undiluted) Nebulized ipratropium 250 µg 3 times in 1st hour only (every 20 min, added to salbutamol) Methylprednisolone 1 mg kg⁻¹ i.v. 6 hourly If deteriorating give i.v. salbutamol 5 µg kg⁻¹ per minute over 10 min then 1–5 µg kg⁻¹ per minute

If poor response to i.v. salbutamol give aminophylline 10 mg kg^{-1} i.v. (maximum dose 250 mg) over 60 min. Following loading dose, give continuous infusion (1–9 years: 1.1 mg kg^{-1} per hour, 10+ years: 0.7 mg kg^{-1} per hour)

See notes for indications for transfer to PICU

Note: If currently taking oral theophylline, do not give i.v. aminophylline in the Emergency Department – take serum level.

* Salbutamol 6 puffs if <6 years, 12 puffs if >6 years. Note nebulized salbutamol can also be used at a dose of 2.5–5 mg as described above.

** Ipratropium (Atrovent Forte 40 µg per puff) 2 puffs if <6 years, 4 puffs if >6 years.

respiratory tract infection, allergy, passive smoking), pattern and course of previous acute episodes (e.g. admission or ICU admissions), parental understanding of the treatment of acute episodes, and the presence of interval symptoms (see the section on discharge below).

Consider other causes of wheeze (e.g. bronchiolitis, mycoplasma, aspiration, foreign body).

5.1.3 Examination

The most important parameters in the assessment of the severity of acute childhood asthma are general appearance and mental state, and work of breathing (accessory muscle use, recession), as indicated in *Table 5.1*.

Initial SaO$_2$ in air, heart rate and ability to talk are helpful but less reliable additional features. Wheeze intensity, pulsus paradoxus and peak expiratory flow rate are not reliable features. Lung function is hard to measure during an acute attack particularly if the child is tired, is young (<7 years) or if the child has not seen a peak flow meter or spirometer before; focus on the above signs in the assessment.

Asymmetry on auscultation is often found due to mucous plugging, but might be due to a foreign body.

5.1.4 Investigation

Chest X-ray is not generally required (discuss with registrar/consultant if you are considering it). Arterial blood gas and spirometry are rarely required in the assessment of acute asthma in children.

5.1.5 Discharge

Time spent planning a discharge either from the emergency department or the ward will reduce the likelihood of readmission and may also reduce morbidity. When you are organizing discharge, consider the factors in *Box 5.1*.

Review need for preventative treatment
Consider preventative treatment, initially with inhaled steroids, if:
• Wheezing attacks are less than 6 weeks apart
• Attacks are becoming more frequent and severe
• Interval symptoms are increasing

Check inhaler technique
Emergency attendance or admission should provide the patient and family with the opportunity to use a spacer device and MDI. Make sure

> **Box 5.1** Discharge pack
>
> - Review need for preventative treatment
> - Check inhaler technique
> - Family education
> - Prescription
> - Follow up
> - Written action plan
> - Communication with general practitioner or primary care pediatrician

the child can use the device adequately and the child and family know the importance of using it for all preventative therapy and treatment for significant exacerbations.

Family education

On discharge from the Emergency Department or ward it is important that families understand the immediate management of their child's asthma and care of spacers etc. It is not appropriate to educate them on all aspects of asthma during an acute episode. This is best reserved for a visit to an outpatient clinic or doctor's rooms at a time more distant from the acute episode. A reasonable amount of time must be allocated and it is more likely that the information will be understood and retained. Go over the action plan and give the brief parent information handout.

Prescription

A prescription for all medications should be provided at the time of discharge. In most cases this should include a prescription for a short course of prednisolone for a future attack. The use of this steroid supply should be discussed when the action plan is provided.

Follow up

All patients should have a clear follow up plan. For some it will be appropriate that they visit their general practitioner (GP) for an early review, particularly if their condition deteriorates or fails to improve significantly within 48 hours.

At discharge all patients should have an outpatient appointment or appropriate follow up arranged with a pediatrician within 4–6 weeks. This visit will be used for medical review and, most importantly, appropriate education about asthma management.

Written action plan

All patients should have an individual written action plan and the discharging doctor should spend time going over the plan with the family.

Communicate with GP

For every emergency attendance or discharge, there should be communication with the patient's GP or pediatrician. If possible this should be by fax, telephone or even email. The GP should receive a copy of the action plan.

5.2 Bronchiolitis

This is an acute viral lower respiratory infection. Varying definitions throughout the world cause confusion when doctors are assessing useful treatments. The etiological agent is usually respiratory syncytial virus but can also be adenovirus or parainfluenza 3. The infection usually affects children under 1 year old. It occurs in about 10% of all infants and 2–3% are admitted to hospital. Younger infants are usually more seriously affected. The illness usually peaks on day 2–3 with resolution of wheeze and respiratory difficulty over 7–10 days. The cough may persist for weeks and postbronchiolitic respiratory symptoms may cause much concern. Management involves a primary assessment of severity and initiation of resuscitation and treatment. Assessment and management are illustrated in *Table 5.2.*

5.2.1 History

The child presents with cough and wheezing. A lethargic, exhausted child may feed poorly, be hypoxemic, and is at risk of respiratory failure. Risk factors include age, infants with bronchopulmonary dysplasia or congenital heart disease.

The time course is important. Is the child improving, stable, or likely to deteriorate over the next few days? Peak severity is usually at around day 2–3 of the illness. If the child is early on in the illness, consider admission to hospital.

5.2.2 Examination

Clinical signs include cough, tachypnea and hyperinflation. There may be audible wheeze. Auscultation reveals widespread crepitations and wheeze and signs of accessory muscle use. Cyanosis always indicates severe disease. Acyanotic infants may also be hypoxemic. If O_2 saturation is less than 90%, the infant should receive supplementary O_2 during the examination.

Table 5.2 Primary assessment and initial management of bronchiolitis

Severity	Signs	Treatment
Mild	Alert, pink in air Feeding well No underlying cardiorespiratory disease O$_2$ saturation >92%	Can be managed at home. Advise parents of the expected course of the illness, and when to return if there are problems – give smaller, more frequent feeds. Review by GP within 24 hours
Moderate	Any one of: poor feeding, lethargy, marked respiratory distress, underlying cardiorespiratory disease, O$_2$ saturation <92% or age <6 weeks	Admit Administer O$_2$ to maintain adequate saturation Consider i.v. fluids at 75% maintenance (inappropriate ADH). 2 hourly observations
Severe	As above but with increasing O$_2$ requirement or signs of tiring or CO$_2$ retention (sweaty, irritable or apneas)	Cardiorespiratory monitor Consider arterial blood gas Inform PICU – may require CPAP or ventilation

5.2.3 Investigations

A routine NPA (nasopharyngeal aspirate) or chest X-ray is not required for children with a typical clinical picture of bronchiolitis. If a chest X-ray is taken it may demonstrate hyperinflation, peribronchial thickening, and often patchy areas of consolidation and collapse.

Consider whether this may be early asthma. Nebulized salbutamol may help in the older infant. Currently there is little evidence supporting the use of bronchodilators or antibiotics in bronchiolitis. Steroids were not thought to be of benefit, although some recent work from Toronto suggests that they may help.

5.3 Acute upper airways obstruction

Discuss all cases of upper airway obstruction with the Emergency Registrar or Emergency Consultant.

5.3.1 Examination and assessment

A harsh barking cough with stridor in a child with minimally raised temperature suggests croup (see below). **Cough with low pitched expiratory**

stridor and drooling suggests epiglottitis. Sudden onset of coughing, choking, drooling and aphonia suggests a laryngeal foreign body (this is extremely rare). Swelling of the face and tongue with wheeze and urticarial rash suggests anaphylaxis. The differential diagnosis is seen in *Table 5.3.*

5.3.2 Examination

The mouth and throat should not be examined if signs of partial upper airway obstruction are present, as complete obstruction can ensue during the examination. Partial acute upper airways obstruction is characterised by stridor and increased work of breathing. Signs of deterioration are those of hypoxia (worried, restless), fatigue, decreased conscious state, and increased and then decreased work of breathing. Heart rate may be rapid or indeed slow. A child's general appearance is more useful.

5.3.3 Treatment

Allow the child to settle quietly on the parent's lap and observe closely with minimal interference. Treat specific cause (see croup/anaphylaxis guidelines). Call the Pediatric Intensive Care Unit (ICU) if the child's condition is worsening or there is severe obstruction, or call for senior doctors (ENT/anesthetics) if an ICU is not available in your hospital.

Table 5.3 Differential diagnosis of upper airway obstruction

Symptoms	Likely diagnosis
High fever, toxic Anxious Drooling	Epiglottitis
High fever Hyperextension of neck Dysphagia, pooling of secretions in throat	Retropharyngeal/peritonsillar abscess
Sudden onset with aphonia	Laryngeal foreign body
Markedly tender trachea 'Toxic' appearance	Bacterial tracheitis
Pre-existing stridor(infant)	Congenital abnormality, e.g. floppy larynx Subglottic hemangioma/stenosis

Note: There is a high degree of overlap in clinical presentation between epiglottitis, bacterial tracheitis and upper airway abscess.

Oxygen may be given while you are awaiting transfer transport. It can be falsely reassuring because a child with quite severe obstruction may look pink with oxygen. **Note that:**

- Intravenous access should be deferred – upset can cause increasing obstruction.
- Lateral X-rays do not assist in management. In severe airways obstruction, X-rays cause undue delay in definitive treatment and may be dangerous (positioning may precipitate respiratory arrest).
- Do not examine the throat with a tongue depressor.
- If intubation is considered necessary, this should be done by the most experienced medical personnel present, using a smaller than normal endotracheal tube (*Table 5.4*). This should ideally be done in the operating room with tracheostomy equipment and a surgeon in attendance.
- Once the airway is protected, then full blood count (FBC)/blood cultures, i.v. cannulation and antibiotics can be started.

Table 5.4 Size of endotracheal tube in upper airways obstruction

Age	ET tube size
Neonate	2.5–3 mm
< 6 months	3.0 mm
6 months–2 years	3.5 mm
2–5 years	4.0 mm
> 5 years	Half to one size smaller than usual

Note: The usual size (mm) = 4 + age/4; this may clearly be too large.

5.4 Croup (laryngotracheobronchitis)

This tends to occur in a previously well child aged 3 months to 6 years but can occur in older children. The term croup refers to a clinical syndrome characterised by barking cough, inspiratory stridor and hoarseness of voice. It results from viral infection, most often with parainfluenza virus with inflammation of the upper airway, including larynx, trachea and bronchi; hence the term laryngotracheobronchitis.

The symptoms are typically worse at night and peak on about the second or third night. Differentiating spasmodic croup from viral croup is difficult and often not useful. Consider other causes of acute stridor, such as epiglottitis (much rarer since Hib vaccine), bacterial tracheitis (rare), or laryngeal foreign body (very rare). Refer to upper airways obstruction section.

The primary assessment of croup is shown in *Table 5.5*.

5.4.1 History

The loudness of the stridor is not a good guide to the severity of obstruction. Children with pre-existing narrowing of the upper airways (e.g. subglottic stenosis, congenital or secondary to prolonged neonatal

Table 5.5 Primary assessment and initial management of croup

Severity	Signs	Management
Mild	No stridor at rest Not distressed No sternal retraction No signs of hypoxia	Can be managed at home. No specific treatment is usually required, although steroids can be considered if the patient is seen early in the course of the illness. Explanation to parent needed
Moderate	Stridor at rest Distressed Sternal retraction at rest Normal breath sounds No signs of hypoxia	Administer steroids** Observe and settle child with minimal interventions Consider use of nebulized epinephrine (adrenaline) (1% eye drop solution 0.05 mg kg^{-1} or 1:1000 preparation 0.5 ml kg^{-1} (max 2 ml)* If settles well after prednisolone consider discharge (see notes on discharge)
Severe	Marked stridor at rest or may be soft Very distressed Marked increase work of breathing Reduced breath sounds Evidence of hypoxia (restless, lethargy, pallor, cyanosis)	Continually assess the child and response to therapy Involve senior staff early on Administer nebulized epinephrine (as above*) Administer steroids** Rarely will require intubation Admission to PICU

*See Epinephrine (adrenaline) section on p. 67.
**See Steroid section on p. 67.

ventilation) or children with Down syndrome are prone to more severe croup and admission should be considered even with mild symptoms.

5.4.2 General management

Avoid distressing procedures, e.g. examining throat, because anxiety exacerbates croup. Nurse the child on the parent's lap. Blood tests, pulse oxymetry, or O_2 mask are rarely indicated. A routine nasopharyngeal aspirate (NPA) is not required for children with a typical clinical picture of croup.

Steroids
There is little evidence supporting the use of steroids in mild croup, although the current studies are underpowered. However there is good evidence for the efficacy of corticosteroids for the treatment of moderate to severe croup. There are a number of ways of administering the steroids: use nebulized budesonide, oral prednisolone or dexamethasone or i.m. dexamethasone. Varying doses have been suggested in the literature and all are effective in the treatment of the acute symptoms. Cost and availability may influence the treatment choice. Suggested doses are prednisolone ($1\,mg\,kg^{-1}$), nebulized budesonide $2\,mg$, dexamethasone ($0.15\,mg\,kg^{-1}$).

Epinephrine (adrenaline)
There has been a change in the use of nebulized epinephrine (adrenaline) in the last few years and nebulized epinephrine (adrenaline) no longer needs to be reserved only for children with severe croup. Current evidence would support the use of nebulized epinephrine (adrenaline) in children with moderate and severe croup. In a number of selected children following observation in the Emergency Department for 3 hours after the administering of nebulized epinephrine (adrenaline) and the start of steroid treatment, it may be safe to discharge the child home. Nebulized epinephrine (adrenaline) may cause circumoral pallor.

5.4.3 Admission or discharge

The decision to admit a child is made after initial treatment and observation. As is usual with other children, the time of the day, parent's anxiety and access to transport, and ability of early review should be taken into account if admission or discharge is being considered. Some centres will suggest that if the child still has stridor at rest after treatment, he or she should be admitted. It has been suggested that if there is no sign of increased work of breathing and no sternal recession but minimal stridor at rest, then they could be discharged with adequate explanation and follow up.

5.5 Foreign bodies in the airway

5.5.1 Upper airway foreign body

The child will have had a sudden onset of coughing, choking and possibly vomiting. If the obstruction is total, then this will lead to unconsciousness and cardiorespiratory arrest. You will need to consider the diagnosis in a child in a cardiorespiratory arrest if you are unable to ventilate.

If obstruction is total

Open the airway and, under direct vision, check in the mouth for a foreign body and remove with Magill's forceps. Place the child prone down, apply five firm blows to the infrascapular area using an open hand. Turn the child face up. Give five chest thrusts and check the mouth. Do an airway chin-lift or jaw thrust and assess the breathing. If this is not successful, repeat the sequence in infants under the age of 1 year. In older children, repeat the cycle, but alternate the five chest thrusts with abdominal thrusts. A surgical airway might be necessary if the foreign body cannot be removed. Note, abdominal thrusts and the Heimlich maneuver should only be used in older children (see section 2.7 on Choking).

If obstruction is partial

Do not try the above maneuvers. Keep the child in the most comfortable position and arrange urgent removal of foreign body in theatre by ENT.

5.5.2 Lower airway foreign body

History

Children between the ages of 6 months and 4 years are at greatest risk of foreign body aspiration. There may have been an episode of choking, coughing or wheezing while eating or playing, but many episodes are unwitnessed. Symptoms may include persistent wheeze, cough, fever or dyspnea not otherwise explained. Recurrent or persistent pneumonia may be the presenting feature. The child may be asymptomatic after the initial event.

Examination

There may be asymmetrical chest movement, tracheal deviation, chest signs such as inspiratory wheeze or decreased breath sounds. The respiratory examination may be completely normal.

Radiology

Request inspiratory and expiratory chest X-ray. Look for:

- an opaque foreign body
- segmental or lobar collapse
- localized emphysema in expiration (ball valve obstruction)

The chest X-ray may be normal.

Management
Any child who is suspected of inhaling a foreign body should be discussed with the Emergency Registrar or a consultant, even if asymptomatic and the chest X-ray normal.

5.5.3 Prevention

No child under 15 months old should be offered foods such as popcorn, hard candies, raw carrot or apples. Children under the age of 4 years should not be offered peanuts.

Encourage the child to sit quietly while eating and offer food one piece at a time. Avoid toys with small parts for children under the age of 3 years.

5.6 Pneumonia

Pneumonia is common, but the cause may vary with age. The commonest bacterial causes are:
- *Staphylococcus aureus* in children < 1 year
- *Streptococcus pneumoniae* in children < 4 years
- *Hemophilus influenzae* in children < 10 years
- Group A streptococcus in children > 10 years

Viral infection with RSV (respiratory syncytial virus) and parainfluenza occurs in children, especially in those under 2 years of age, and with influenza virus in older children. Mycoplasma infection is more common in older children.

In a previously well child older than 1 month, consider pneumonia in infants and children with the following signs and symptoms (*Box 5.2*).

Chest X-ray (AP) should be performed to confirm or exclude pneumonia. Patients with wheeze and air trapping most commonly have bronchiolitis or asthma. Neonates who are unwell, or have a temperature over 38°C, should have a chest X-ray as part of a septic work-up, especially if the respiratory rate is elevated or there are other signs of respiratory embarrassment.

> **Box 5.2** Clinical signs and symptoms of pneumonia
>
> • Fever and cough (or difficulty breathing)
> • Tachypnea, nasal flaring
> • Lower chest indrawing or recession
> • Clinical signs of consolidation or effusion
> • Persistent fever
> • Fever and abdominal pain

5.6.1 Management of pneumonia

Pneumonia can be managed with inpatient or outpatient care depending on the severity of the condition. This is illustrated in *Figure 5.1* and *Figure 5.2*.

5.7 Pleural effusion

A pleural effusion may occur, especially in infections with *Staphylococcus aureus*, *Hemophilus influenzae* and occasionally with *Streptococcus pneumoniae*. It is managed together with the underlying pneumonia (*Figure 5.3*).

5.8 Empyema

Empyema or pus in the pleural cavity can occur in pneumonia with *S. aureus* or *H. influenzae* from direct extension, lymphatic spread or from the septicemic process. Management of empyema is controversial. The four approaches to empyema are:
• conservative, with long courses of intravenous antibiotics
• aggressive, with early thoracotomy and surgical removal of the collection
• intrapleural urokinase or streptokinase via chest drain
• thorascopic drainage.

There are no clear data on the best approach. Management will vary from centre to centre.

5.9 Pneumothorax

A pneumothorax is defined as the presence of air in the intrapleural space. Spontaneous pneumothorax is unusual. It is often associated

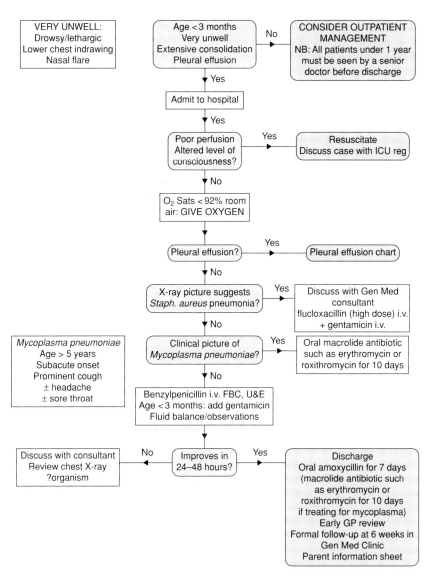

Figure 5.1 The management of pneumonia in previously well child >1 month old. Abbreviations: FBC, full blood count; ICU, intensive care unit; U&E, urea and electrolytes.

with trauma but can be spontaneous, particularly if a person has a marfanoid habitus. It can occur secondary to a bullous or a cyst. Children with cystic fibrosis are more at risk of developing pneumothoraces. Consider pneumothorax in a child presenting with pleuritic chest pain or shortness of breath. There may be a previous history of pneumothorax. On examination, there may be reduced air entry and a deviated trachea (away from the collection) and hyper-resonance, but no added breath sounds.

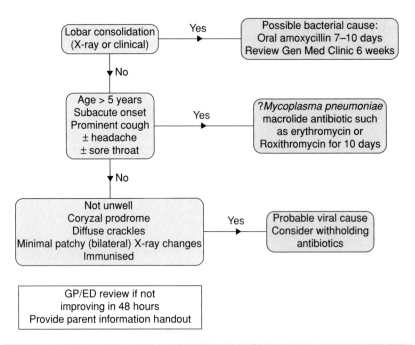

Figure 5.2 Outpatient management of pneumonia in previously well child >1 month old. Abbreviation: ED, Emergency Department.

5.9.1 Management

In small pneumothoraces, a conservative approach is appropriate. Where there is less than 30% reduction of total lung capacity (TLC), initial high flow oxygen will help absorb the intrapleural air and in most cases the pneumothorax will resolve over a 1–2 week time scale. Where there is between 30–50% reduction in TLC there are three steps depending on response:

- Oxygen therapy in cases where there are no major symptoms and observation and repeat X-ray over 12 hours.
- Oxygen therapy and a needle thoracocentesis using a small catheter attached to a 3-way tap. This is inserted in the second intercostal space above the rib and in the mid-clavicular line. Air is aspirated, the tap is closed off and chest X-ray repeated over the following 6 hours. If the air has not reaccumulated, the catheter can be removed and the patient reviewed 24 hours later with repeat X-ray.
- Insertion of an intercostal drain with a valve or underwater seal. This should be placed in the anterior axillary line in the fourth intercostal space.

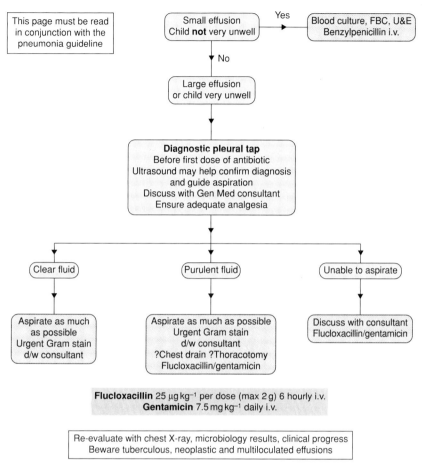

Figure 5.3 Inpatient management of pleural effusion. Abbreviations: FBC, full blood count; U&E, urea and electrolytes.

Suggested reading

General reading

Phelan, P.D., Olinsky, A., Robertson, C.F. (1994) *Respiratory Illness in Children*. 4th edn. Oxford: Blackwell Science.

Specific reading

Croup

Geelhoed, G.C. (1997) State of the art: Croup. *Ped. Pulmonol.* **23:** 370–374.

Geelhoed, G.C. (1996) Sixteen years of croup in a Western Australian teaching hospital: Effects of routine steroid treatment. *Ann. Emerg. Med.* **28:** 621–626.

Powell, C.V.E., Stockell, R.A. (2000) Changing hospital management of croup; what does this mean for general practice? *Austr. Family Phys.* **29:** 915–919.

Pneumothorax

Baumann, M.H., Strange, C., Heffner, J.E. *et al.* (2001) Management of spontaneous pneumothorax: an American College of Chest Physicians Delphi consensus statement. *Chest* **119**:590–602.

Miller, A.C., Harvey, J.E. (1993) Guidelines for the management of spontaneous pneumothorax: Standards of Care Committee, British Thoracic Society. *B.M.J.* **307**:114–116.

Asthma

National Asthma Council of Australia Guidelines (2002) www.nationalasthma.org.au

Powell, C.V.E., Maskell, G., Marks, M.K., South, M., Robertson, C.F. (2001) Research evidence into clinical practice: successful implementation of spacer treatment guideline for acute asthma. *Arch. Dis. Child.* **84**:142–146.

Chapter 6

Neurological emergencies

Colin Powell

Contents

6.1 Coma

Coma is a symptom, not a diagnosis. The aim of management is to minimise any ongoing neurological damage. History, examination, investigation and treatment will be simultaneous.

6.1.1 Immediate resuscitation and management

The primary assessment should be as for any seriously ill child. A structured approach to the primary survey is particularly important; if a problem is found during the initial ABCDE assessment, then immediate treatment and resuscitation should start, remembering to treat the treatable as you progress through the primary survey. Supporting an inadequate airway, ineffective breathing or compromised circulation should reduce the likelihood that the reduced conscious level is secondary to hypoxia and fluid loss and of any further deterioration of conscious level due to these two mechanisms. Thus, you must clear and protect the airway and assist the breathing as necessary (see Chapter 2, Resuscitation section). If a traumatic cause for the symptoms is likely, immobilise the cervical spine and arrange urgent neurosurgery involvement. Check the pulse and insert an intravenous line and perform a blood sugar test; if blood glucose is less than $2.5 \, mmol \, l^{-1}$ in a person who is not diabetic, send specific blood tests (see Section 8.2 Hypoglycemia) and administer 10% dextrose i.v., $5 \, ml \, kg^{-1}$ bolus. Consider naloxone, $0.1 \, mg \, kg^{-1}$ (max 2 mg) if pupils are small.

Assess and monitor pulse, respiratory rate, BP, temperature, oximetry and conscious state. Consider signs of raised intracranial pressure and look for subtle signs of continuing convulsions.

6.1.2 History and examination

Consider the onset and duration of symptoms. Is there a past history? Relevant conditions include seizures, diabetes, adrenal insufficiency, infection and cardiac problems. Other signs and symptoms may suggest the cause of the coma (*Box 6.1*).

6.1.3 Investigations and further management

Consider these investigations in the light of the possible diagnoses, if not already done:
• full blood examination
• urea and electrolytes
• glucose
• liver function

Box 6.1 Clues to the cause of coma	
In the presence of:	**Consider:**
Scalp bruising or hematoma	Head injury
Inconsistent history, retinal hemorrhage	Non-accidental injury
Fever, seizures	Meningitis, encephalitis
Focal neurological signs, focal seizures, papilledema, asymmetric pupils	Focal intracerebral pathology, e.g. tumor
Shunted hydrocephalus	Blocked shunt
Renal disease	Hypertensive encephalopathy
Nil obvious cause	Poisoning

- arterial blood gas
- urine drug ± metabolic screen
- urine antigens
- blood and urine culture
- ammonia
- cortisol
- coagulation screen
- ECG

6.1.4 Investigation and management of coma

Figure 6.1 shows the investigation and management of coma. It is important that raised intracranial pressure is always excluded before lumbar puncture in all cases.

6.1.5 Ongoing care

Continue to assess and support the airway, breathing and circulation. Care will depend on the diagnosis, level of consciousness and degree of ventilatory and circulatory support required. Consider an early transfer to a pediatric intensive care unit.

6.2 Convulsions

6.2.1 Afebrile convulsions and status epilepticus

Most convulsions are brief and do not require any specific treatment. Convulsions may be generalized and tonic–clonic in nature but can also be focal. Generalized convulsive status epilepticus (CSE) is currently defined as a convulsion lasting 30 minutes or more or when successive

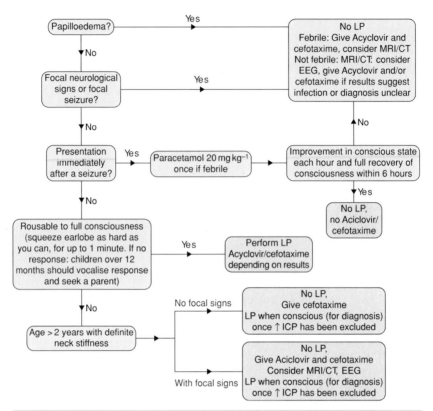

Figure 6.1 Lumbar puncture, imaging and antibiotics in coma. Abbreviations: CT, computed tomography; EEG, electroencephalogram; ICP, intracranial pressure; LP, lumbar puncture; MRI, magnetic resonance imaging.

convulsions occur so frequently that the patient does not recover consciousness between convulsions. Tonic–clonic status occurs in up to 5% of patients with primary epilepsy and about 5% of children with febrile seizures may present with CSE.

Management of the convulsion

The primary assessment should be as for any seriously ill child. A structured approach to the primary survey is particularly important; if a problem is found during the initial ABCDE assessment then immediate treatment and resuscitation should occur, remembering to treat the treatable as you progress through the primary survey. In a fitting child never forget to check the glucose and treat hypoglycemia appropriately.

If a convulsion occurs, position the child in a semiprone position to minimise the chance of aspiration. If necessary and possible, clear the airway with gentle suction and give oxygen via the facemask.

If the convulsion continues for more than 10 minutes then follow the flow chart in *Figure 6.2*.

Give high-flow oxygen via facemask, monitor oxygen saturation and test the glucose level. A short acting benzodiazepine should then be administered. The nature and dose of the drug will depend on whether intravenous access had been obtained and on departmental guidelines. Some antiepileptics such as paraldehyde are used in some countries but not others.

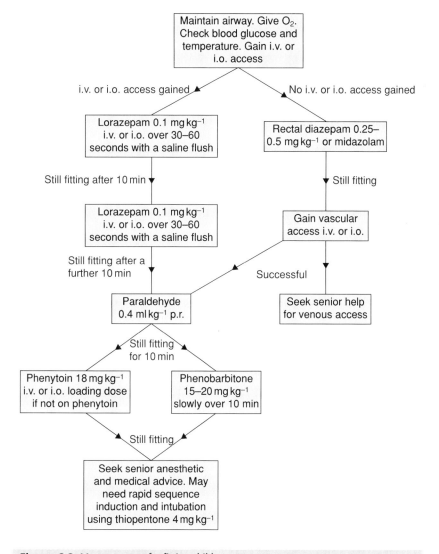

Figure 6.2. Management of a fitting child.

If venous access or intraosseous access has been obtained

The following drugs can be given in sequence if fitting continues:

- Lorazepam 0.1 mg kg^{-1} i.v. or intra-osseous (i.o) can be given and repeated after 10 minutes if necessary. This is currently the drug of choice in the latest Advanced Pediatric Life Support Guidelines in the UK, USA and Australia. Diazepam 0.25 mg kg^{-1} or midazolam 0.15 mg kg^{-1} are alternatives to lorazepam. They can be repeated after 5 minutes if seizures continue. The child needs to be monitored carefully for respiratory depression.
- Paraldehyde 0.4 ml kg^{-1} per rectum (p.r.) is given 10 minutes after the benzodiazepines if necessary, but is not available in Australia.
- Phenytoin 18 mg kg^{-1} i.v. or i.o. as a loading dose in normal saline over 30 minutes can then be given with ECG monitoring. If the child is already on phenytoin, then i.v. phenobarbitone 15–20 mg kg^{-1} can be used over 10 minutes. In neonates, phenobarbitone is often used as the drug of choice.
- If fitting still continues, seek senior anesthetic and medical advice and assistance. The child may require rapid sequence induction and intubation with thiopentone 4 mg kg^{-1} i.v. or i.o. Muscle relaxants should not be used long term.

If venous access has not been obtained

- Diazepam 0.25–0.5 mg kg^{-1} rectally or midazolam 0.15 mg kg^{-1} i.m. can be given.
- After 10 minutes, give paraldehyde 0.4 ml kg^{-1} p.r. (0.4 ml of paraldehyde plus 0.4 ml of olive oil = 0.8 ml kg^{-1} of prepared solution), but this is not a choice in Australia.
- Seek medical assistance as above for vascular access and RSI.

Notes

Non-convulsive status may occur. It manifests as decreased conscious state with or without motor accompaniments. It may occur particularly in the Lennox–Gastaut syndrome, or in other children with developmental delay.

Pyridoxine-dependent seizures should be considered in any infant under 18 months with recurrent or refractory afebrile seizures. A clinical trial of pyridoxine 100 mg i.v. is warranted. If it is going to be effective it will work within 10–60 minutes. If it is not effective in 10 minutes begin other standard anticonvulsants as above.

After the convulsion

First seizures, even if unprovoked, rarely require continuous anticonvulsant medication. Discuss with the Registrar or a Consultant. Parents should be warned that all children or adolescents who have had seizures should be supervised when bathing, swimming, or riding a bicycle on the road, and that children should avoid tree-climbing. Parents should be advised of first-aid measures should the seizure recur.

In some centres, children with their first afebrile seizure are referred to the general pediatric outpatient clinic for follow up. If the child has not fully recovered, or there are concerns about the underlying etiology, he or she should be admitted to hospital.

6.2.2 Febrile convulsions

A simple febrile convulsion is a brief (< 15 min) generalized convulsion in a febrile ($> 38°C$) child aged between 6 months and 6 years, with no previous afebrile seizures, no progressive neurological condition and no central nervous system infection. Febrile convulsions are common, and occur in 3% of healthy children between the ages of 6 months and 6 years. They are usually associated with a simple viral infection. The onset of the convulsion may be sudden with little evidence of preceding illness. The convulsion may be terrifying for the parents to observe – they frequently believe that their child is dying and may attempt CPR or other resuscitative measures. Febrile convulsions are benign, with minimal morbidity and essentially no mortality.

Most febrile convulsions are brief and do not require any specific treatment. The initial management of the convulsion is described in the afebrile seizure section.

After the convulsion
A septic work-up including lumbar puncture is mandatory in children under 6 months of age; by definition a febrile convulsion should not be diagnosed in a child under 6 months. Lumbar puncture should be very strongly considered in those aged 6–12 months.

Possible clinical scenarios and management include those shown in *Box 6.2*.

Most children with simple febrile convulsions who have recovered sufficiently do not need to be admitted to hospital. If a patient is discharged home following a febrile convulsion, it is important to give the family advice regarding fever control and what to do in the event of a future convulsion. Verbal advice should be reinforced with written advice. Follow up during the next 24 hours is advisable to assess the progress of the child's illness and to allow parents the opportunity for further discussion.

Box 6.2 Possible clinical scenarios and management following febrile convulsions

- Full recovery from a simple febrile convulsion with the child appearing well
  - Focus of infection identified
    - Investigations as appropriate for focus (e.g. none if URTI)
    - Explanation and reassurance to parents
    - Home and follow up by family doctor
  - No focus of infection identified
    - Follow fever guidelines
    - Possible FBC and blood culture
    - Dipstick urine – if positive for nitrites or leucocytes, obtain clean catch, suprapubic aspiration (SPA) or catheter sample for microscopy and culture
    - Explanation and reassurance to parents. Home and follow up by family doctor
- Complex features, e.g. prolonged (> 15 minutes), focal, multiple seizures or incomplete recovery or child looks unwell on recovery
  - Consider other diagnoses (e.g. meningitis, encephalitis) and take: FBC/differential; blood culture; clean catch, SPA or catheter urine for microscopy and culture; LP if fully conscious and no focal neurological signs during or after convulsion.

Repeated convulsions during the same illness occur in about 10–15% of children. The child should be reassessed in hospital. There are usually no serious implications; however, a period of observation might be required to clarify the progress of the illness.

Fever control

Clothing should be minimal – a nappy alone or light outer layer depending on ambient temperature. Tepid sponging, baths and fans are ineffective in lowering core temperature, and are not recommended. Paracetamol has not been shown to reduce the risk of further febrile convulsions. It may be used for pain or discomfort or as an antipyretic associated with febrile illnesses such as otitis media. The parents should understand the reasons for its use and be discouraged from trying to get their child's fever down.

Long-term issues

Recurrence rate depends on the age of the child – the younger the child at the time of the initial convulsion, the greater the risk of a further febrile convulsion.

Epilepsy. Risk of future afebrile convulsions is increased by a family history of epilepsy, any neurodevelopmental problem or complex, very prolonged or focal febrile convulsions (*Box 6.3*).

Box 6.3 Risk of afebrile convulsions following a febrile convulsion

- No risk factors: 1% risk of future epilepsy, similar to the general population
- 1 risk factor: 2% increased risk
- More than 1 risk factor: 10% increased risk

Anticonvulsant treatment. Children who have recurrent prolonged convulsions (which are rare) may benefit from having a rectal diazepam kit available at home, which their parents can administer if a convulsion does not cease spontaneously within 5 minutes.

Long-term anticonvulsants are not indicated except in rare situations with frequent recurrences. It may be appropriate to offer a review appointment with a general pediatrician.

6.3 Headaches

Headache is a common symptom in children, affecting 80–90% by the age of 15. The common causes are systemic illness with fever, local ENT problems, migraine and tension headache. Meningitis, raised intracranial pressure (ICP), e.g. from tumors, and subarachnoid hemorrhage (SAH) are much rarer causes but these need to be considered. Any headaches that wake a child from sleeping or that are associated with focal signs such as a hemiplegia require investigation as an inpatient.

6.3.1 Assessment

History
It is useful to classify headache as acute or recurrent. The following list gives the causes and key features to help make a diagnosis, based on careful history and examination:

Acute
- Systemic: fever and general illness (e.g. 'flu, pneumonia, septicemia)
- Local sinusitis, dental caries, otitis media
- Trauma: head injury

- Meningitis: reduced conscious level, toxicity, photophobia, neck stiffness
- SAH: sudden onset, severe occipital pain; possible reduced conscious level, neck stiffness

Recurrent
- Migraine: aura, nausea, vomiting, pallor, family history
- Tension: throbbing pain (involving neck muscles) at end of day
- Behavioral: family/social/school problems (may be difficult to identify)
- Raised ICP: morning headaches ± vomiting, worse with coughing/sneezing/bending
- Progressively worsening raised ICP: personality or behavioral changes, focal neurological symptoms
- Benign intracranial hypertension, systemic hypertension, uremia, recurrent hypoglycemia, recurrent seizures, lead or CO poisoning.

It may be useful to make out a possible family headache patterns diagram to help identify the nature of the headache.

Examination
As part of the examination it is important to document the following:
- ABC: blood pressure, heart rate
- General: toxic, unwell, temperature, rash
- Neurology: conscious level, fundi, visual fields, cerebellar signs, neurocutaneous stigmata, neck stiffness, cranial bruits
- Local causes: cervical lymphadenopathy, teeth, sinus, ears
- Growth and puberty: head growth, height, weight, growth velocity, pubertal status.

Investigations
In the acute situation, the two most important questions to answer are:
- **Does the child need an urgent computerised tomography (CT) scan of the head?** and
- **Should a lumbar puncture (LP) be performed?**

In making the decision, you should consider the following factors:
- If the child has altered state of consciousness, focal neurological signs, raised blood pressure or papilledema, consider management of raised ICP and CT scan of head. Discuss this with senior medical staff.
- Consider LP (in the absence of the contraindications) if you are concerned about meningitis or SAH. You may need to do a CT scan first (discuss with consultant).

- If there are no symptoms and signs suggesting raised ICP/SAH/ meningitis and the story is suggestive of migraine, then treat symptomatically (see below).
- If other causes are suspected, do the appropriate investigations (e.g. septic screen, urea, carboxyhemoglobin or lead level [wrist X-rays], blood sugar profile).

Management
If there is a specific diagnosis such as meningitis, SAH, tumor, systemic infection or local infection, then treat as appropriate. Most recurrent headaches can be managed by a pediatrician and do not need to be referred to a neurologist.

6.3.2 Migraine

Abort attack
Avoid opiates. Initially try simple oral analgesics such as paracetamol (20 mg kg^{-1} stat then 15 mg kg^{-1} per dose every 4 hours, to a maximum of 4 g per day) or codeine (1 mg kg^{-1} per dose every 4 hours) or NSAID (ibuprofen 2.5–10 mg kg^{-1} per dose 6–8 hourly). For adolescents give 1 g of aspirin, 1 g of paracetamol, 10 mg of metoclopramide. Some, but not all, pediatricians use intravenous anti-emetics in severe vomiting. For example, if vomiting is a prominent feature in children over 10 years give slow i.v. prochlorperazine (0.1–0.2 mg kg^{-1}).

Prophylaxis
Refer to a local doctor or general pediatric outpatient clinic for long-term management. Consider beta blockers, pizotifen or calcium channel blockers. Non-pharmacological interventions (e.g. avoidance of triggers, relaxation) often play an important role in prevention. Consider getting the child or parents to make a headache diary.

Headache patterns
It may be a good idea with the use of the chart below to explore the pattern of the child's headaches (*Figure 6.3*).
- *Acute recurrent* includes migraine (common, classical, complicated).
- *Chronic non-progressive* includes tension (stress related); muscle contraction; anxiety; depression; somatisation headaches.
- *Chronic progressive* includes headaches from tumor; benign intracranial hypertension; brain abscess; hydrocephalus.
- *Acute on chronic non-progressive* includes tension headache with co-existent migraine.

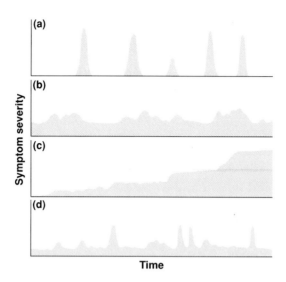

Figure 6.3 Headache patterns. (a) Acute recurrent; (b) chronic non-progressive; (c) chronic progressive; (d) acute on chronic non-progressive.

6.4 Meningitis

The presentation of a child with meningitis varies with age. Infants with meningitis frequently present with non-specific signs and symptoms such as fever, irritability, lethargy, poor feeding and vomiting. The fontanelle may or may not be full. Older children may complain of headache or photophobia. Neck stiffness may be present (although this is not a reliable sign in young children). A purpuric rash is suggestive of meningococcal septicemia. It is important to examine for spinal and cranial abnormalities such as dermal sinuses, which may have predisposed the child to meningitis.

Note: This guideline is not for use in children with spinal abnormalities or ventriculoperitoneal shunts where the neurosurgical team should be consulted.

6.4.1 Assessment

Assess airway, breathing and circulation (see Chapter 2, Resuscitation section). Monitor pulse, blood pressure, respiratory rate, oxygen saturation and consciousness. Insert intravenous line and take blood for glucose, FBC and blood cultures and U&Es, meningococcal PCR, and CRP (C-reactive protein). Do nose and throat swabs, as occasionally the organism is isolated from these. If the clinical diagnosis is meningitis and there are contraindications for a lumbar puncture give intravenous antibiotics without delay.

Lumbar puncture (LP)

An LP is used to confirm the diagnosis of bacterial meningitis and to identify the organism and its antibiotic sensitivities. In some cases it should be postponed because of the risk of coning. There are contraindications to performing an LP, including:
- Coma – Glasgow Coma Scale (GCS) < 13 or rapid deterioration in conscious state or absent or non-purposeful responses to painful stimuli (squeeze earlobe hard for up to 1 minute. Children should localise response and seek a parent).
- Focal neurological signs
- Papilledema
- Cardiovascular compromise
- Evidence of coagulopathy.

If any of these signs are present the patient is in danger of coning, and management in Intensive Care is usually required. Notify a PICU immediately (for retrieval or transfer), perform blood cultures, commence antibiotics.

Remember cerebrospinal fluid (CSF) findings in early bacterial meningitis may mimic a viral pattern or even be normal (see *Table 6.1*). In a traumatic tap, allow 1 white blood cell for every 500 red blood cells, and $0.01\,g\,l^{-1}$ of protein for every 1000 red cells. Request culture and analysis for bacterial antigens (this is non-urgent as it does not change immediate management and there is no need for it to be performed out of hours).

Table 6.1 Normal CSF values for children over 2 months of age

Meningitis type	White cells (mm^{-3})	Protein (g l^{-1})	Glucose (mmol l^{-1})
Normal (age > 3 months)	< 5	< 0.4	> 2.5 or 50% blood level
Partially-treated meningitis	1–10 000 mainly neutrophils	> 0.4	< 2.5
Bacterial meningitis	usually thousands (mainly neutrophils)	usually > 1.0	< 2.5
Viral meningitis	usually < 1000 neutrophils early, then lymphocytes	> 0.4	Normal or < 2.5

6.4.2 Management

Admission to a PICU

Admission to PICU should be discussed with the consultant in the following circumstances (*Box 6.4*):

Box 6.4 Meningitis: Factors requiring consultant opinion

- Age less than 2 years
- Coma
- Cardiovascular compromise
- Intractable seizures
- Hyponatremia

Antibiotics

In a child aged over 2 months the usual organisms causing bacterial meningitis are *Streptococcus pneumoniae*, *Neisseria meningitidis* and *Hemophilus influenzae* type b (HiB – uncommon after the age of 6 and the incidence is reduced following HiB vaccination).

Empirical treatment consists of cefotaxime (50 mg kg^{-1} per dose up to a maximum of 3 g, 6 hourly) given prior to determination of the organism responsible and its sensitivities. Chloramphenicol may be used in children with a type 1 hypersensitivity to cephalosporins. You may need to consider the addition of vancomycin if pneumococcus is suspected in an area of high incidence of penicillin-resistant pneumococcus.

Continue empirical treatment until cultures are known to be negative or an organism and its sensitivity pattern are known. A positive culture result with sensitivities should lead to narrower spectrum treatment (*Box 6.5*).

In a child aged under 2 months, the organisms to consider in this age group include group B streptococcus, *Escherichia coli* and other Gram negative organisms, *Listeria monocytogenes*, *Streptococcus pneumoniae*, *Neisseria meningitidis* and *Hemophilus influenzae* type b.

Initial therapy is with i.v. benzylpenicillin (50 mg kg^{-1} per dose, 6 hourly), and i.v. cefotaxime (50 mg kg^{-1} per dose, 6 hourly), and i.v. gentamicin (dose according to age). Ongoing therapy is modified according to culture and sensitivity results. Consult local guidelines.

Box 6.5 Treatment in meningitis with positive cultures with sensitivities

Neisseria meningitidis – give i.v. benzylpenicillin 50 mg kg^{-1} per dose up to a maximum of 3 g, 4 hourly for 7 days (in penicillin-sensitive cases)
Streptococcus pneumoniae – give i.v. benzylpenicillin 50 mg kg^{-1} per dose up to a maximum of 3 g, 4 hourly for minimum of 10 days (in penicillin-sensitive cases)
Hemophilus influenzae – give i.v. cefotaxime 50 mg kg^{-1} per dose up to a maximum of 3 g, 6 hourly for 7–10 days, or i.v. amoxycillin 50 mg kg^{-1} per dose 4 hourly for 7–10 days (depending on sensitivities)
Other – if an organism is not isolated, but significant CSF pleocytosis is present, a minimum of 7 days treatment with i.v. cefotaxime is recommended.

Fluid management

Careful fluid management is important in the treatment of meningitis as many children have increased antidiuretic hormone (ADH) secretion. The degree to which fluid should be restricted varies considerably from patient to patient depending primarily on their clinical state.

Shock should be corrected with 20 ml kg^{-1} of normal saline. A patient who is not in shock and whose serum sodium is within the normal range should be given 50% of maintenance fluid requirements as initial management. If the serum sodium is less than 135 mmol l^{-1} give 25–50% of maintenance requirements. The serum sodium should be repeated every 6–12 hours for the first 48 hours and the total fluid intake altered accordingly. If the serum sodium is less than 135 mmol l^{-1}, reduce the fluid intake.

General measures

- Neurological observations including blood pressure should be performed every 15 minutes for the first 2 hours and then at intervals determined by the child's conscious state.
- Weight and head circumference should be monitored on a daily basis.
- Control seizures.
- Early consultation with intensive care unit is necessary for any child who is experiencing a deterioration in conscious state, hemodynamic instability or seizures.
- Electrolytes should be checked every 6–12 hours until the serum sodium is normal.

- Ensure adequate analgesia (e.g. paracetamol) for children in the recovery phase who may have significant headache.
- The role of steroids is still controversial and we have opted generally not to use them, although they may be indicated in Hemophilus meningitis.

6.4.3 Isolation

Children with meningococcal disease require isolation until they have had 24 hours treatment. Other children with meningitis can be nursed on the open ward.

6.4.4 Fever persisting for more than 7 days

This may be due to nosocomial infection, subdural effusion or other foci of suppuration. Uncommon causes include inadequately treated meningitis, a parameningeal focus or drugs.

6.4.5 Contact chemoprophylaxis

Practice differs in different countries. Below is one regime used in Australia (*Box 6.6*). It is important that prophylaxis be given early to both the index case and contacts as follows:
- Index Case and all household contacts if household includes other children under 4 years of age who are not fully immunized.
- Index Case and all household contacts in households with any infants under 12 months of age, regardless of immunization status.
- Index Case and all household contacts in households with a child 1–5 years of age who is inadequately immunized.
- Index Case and all room contacts including staff in a child-care group if Index Case attends over 18 hours per week and any contacts under 2 years of age who are inadequately immunized. (NB. Inadequately immunized children should also be immunized.)
- Index Case (if treated only with penicillin) and all intimate, household or day-care contacts who have been exposed to the Index Case within 10 days of onset.
- Any person who gave mouth-to-mouth resuscitation to the Index Case.

6.4.6 Notification

All cases of *Neisseria meningitidis* and *Hemophilus influenzae* type b disease should be notified to the Public Health Department.

> **Box 6.6** Australian contact chemoprophylaxis regimen
>
> ***Hemophilis influenzae* type b** – give rifampicin 20 mg kg⁻¹ orally as a single daily dose to a maximum 600 mg) for 4 days.
>
> For *infants < 1 month* give rifampicin 10 mg kg⁻¹ orally daily for 4 days.
>
> In *pregnancy* or *contraindication to rifampicin* give ceftriaxone 125 mg kg⁻¹ i.m. (< 12 years) or 250 mg kg⁻¹ i.m. (> 12 years) as a single dose.
>
> ***Neisseria meningitidis*** – give either:
> rifampicin 10 mg kg⁻¹ orally 12 hourly up to a maximum 600 mg for 2 days.
>
> For *infants < 1 month* give rifampicin 5 mg kg⁻¹ orally 12 hourly for 2 days.
>
> In *pregnancy* or *contraindication to rifampicin* give ceftriaxone 125 mg kg⁻¹ i.m. (< 12 years) or 250 mg kg⁻¹ i.m. (> 12 years) as a single dose.
>
> or ciprofloxacin 500 mg orally as a single dose.
>
> ***Streptococcus pneumoniae*** – there are no increased risks to contacts, so no antibiotic required.
>
> Rifampicin may cause orange-red discoloration of tears, urine and contact lenses, skin rashes and itching, and gastrointestinal disturbance. It negates the effect of the oral contraceptive pill and should not be used in pregnancy or severe liver disease.

6.4.7 Follow up

All children with bacterial meningitis should have a formal audiology assessment 6–8 weeks after discharge (earlier if there are concerns regarding hearing). Neurodevelopmental progress should be monitored in outpatients.

6.4.8 Viral meningitis

For CSF findings see *Table 6.1*. Admission is required if the diagnosis is in doubt and/or antibiotics or intravenous hydration are required. Ensure adequate analgesia.

Chapter 7

Gastroenterological emergencies and abdominal pain

Michael Smith, William A. McCallion and Colin Powell

Contents

7.1 Abdominal pain

7.1.1 Causes of abdominal pain in childhood

Abdominal pain is one of the more common reasons for parents to bring their child to the Emergency Department. While many diagnoses traverse all age groups, some are more age specific (*Table 7.1*).

7.1.2 Assessment of abdominal pain

The assessment of the child with acute abdominal pain depends on a good history and careful examination. The nature of the pain itself must be carefully elicited, including its characteristics, relieving and precipitating factors. Truly severe colicky pain suggests an obstruction of the gastrointestinal, genitourinary or hepatobiliary tract. Pain can be referred from elsewhere such as the testes and the lungs. Associated features must also be elicited such as gynecological symptoms in adolescent girls. A full and careful but sensitive examination must follow. If acute activity precipitates pain, it suggests peritonitis. Acute serious problems need rapid combined surgical and medical assessment and management. The algorithm (*Figure 7.1*) may be used as a guide to the systematic consideration of various categories of causes of acute abdominal pain. Typical features of some important causes of acute abdominal pain in children are described in the following table (*Table 7.2*).

Notes:
- **Acute appendicitis** must be considered in any child with severe abdominal pain, aggravated by movement such as walking, or a bumpy car ride. The child is often flushed, with a tachycardia and a mildly elevated temperature. In the very young child, in whom the risk of perforation is higher, the presenting symptoms are less specific. The diagnosis is clinical – no laboratory or radiological tests are required, although there is usually an elevated white cell count.
- The peak age for **intussusception** is 6–12 months. The child may present in shock. Plain anterior chest X-ray may show signs of bowel obstruction, with decreased gas in the right colon. The diagnosis is confirmed by air insufflation or barium enema, with reduction usually possible by the same means (unless there are signs of peritonitis, which increase the risk of perforation).
- **Mid-gut volvulus** is commonest in the newborn period, but can occur in later childhood. Predisposing factors include malrotation and abnormal mesentery.
- Vomiting is rarely due to **constipation**.
- Some children suffer **recurrent non-specific abdominal pain**, with no organic cause identifiable. Constipation is often an important

Table 7.1 Causes of abdominal pain by age

Age group	Classification	Cause
Neonate	Functional	Colic (excessive infant crying)
		Constipation
	Inflammatory/infective	Gastroenteritis
		Urinary tract infection
		Omphalitis
	Mechanical	Mid-gut volvulus
	Other	Milk intolerance
Infant	Functional	Colic
		Constipation
	Inflammatory/infective	Gastroenteritis
		Urinary tract infection
	Mechanical	Mid-gut volvulus
		Intussusception
	Other	Milk intolerance
		Trauma/abuse
Preschool age	Functional	Constipation
	Inflammatory/infective	Gastroenteritis
		Urinary tract infection
		Pneumonia
		Appendicitis
	Mechanical	Mid-gut volvulus
		Intussusception
		Urinary calculi
		Trauma/abuse
	Other	Henoch–Schönlein purpura
		Diabetic ketoacidosis
		Neoplasm
School age and adolescent	Functional	Recurrent abdominal pain
		Constipation
	Inflammatory/infective	Appendicitis
		Mesenteric adenitis
		Gastroenteritis
		Urinary tract infection
		Inflammatory bowel disease
		Pancreatitis
		Pelvic inflammatory disease
	Mechanical	Mid-gut volvulus
		Urinary calculi
		Trauma/abuse
	Other	Henoch–Schönlein purpura
		Diabetic ketoacidosis
		Neoplasm
		Ovarian/testicular pathology

Table 7.2 Assessment of abdominal pain

Diagnosis	Typical features	
	History	Examination
Acute appendicitis	Abdominal pain becomes increasingly severe, and often localises to RIF	Tenderness, guarding, and rebound usually greatest in right iliac fossa, though may be more diffuse
Intussusception	Intermittent colicky abdominal pain, vomiting and the passage of blood and/or mucus per rectum. There is frequently a preceding respiratory or diarrheal illness	Pallor, lethargy. A sausage-shaped mass is palpable in about 2/3 of cases, crossing the mid-line in the epigastrium or behind the umbilicus
Mid-gut volvulus	Bowel obstruction – abdominal pain; usually bile-stained vomiting	The abdomen may be flat and non-tender. Abdominal X-ray shows no gas because the obstruction is proximal duodenum
Constipation	Can present with quite severe abdominal pain in children; often recurrent	Firm stool palpable in lower abdomen (sometimes entire colon)
UTI	*Infants*: fever, vomiting, lethargy *Older children*: dysuria, hematuria	Fever; suprapubic tenderness; loin tenderness if associated pyelonephritis; full ward testing may be +ve (leucocyte esterase, nitrites)
Pneumonia	Fever; possibly cough; vomiting	Fever; tachypnea, recession; focal signs at one base
Gastroenteritis	Vomiting, diarrhea, fever	Tenderness, increased bowel sounds; signs of dehydration

contributing factor. Psychogenic factors (e.g. family, school issues) need to be considered. These children should be referred for general pediatric assessment.

- Some less common diagnoses need to be considered in patients with certain underlying chronic illnesses. Hirschsprung disease can be complicated by **enterocolitis**, with sudden painful abdominal distension and bloody diarrhea. These patients can become rapidly unwell with dehydration, electrolyte disturbances, and systemic toxicity, and are at risk of colonic perforation. Primary bacterial peritonitis can occur in children with nephrotic syndrome, splenectomy and those with VP shunts.

7.1.3 Management

An algorithm for abdominal pain management is given in *Figure 7.1*.

Intravenous access should be established. The electrolytes should be measured in a child who appears dehydrated and blood and stool

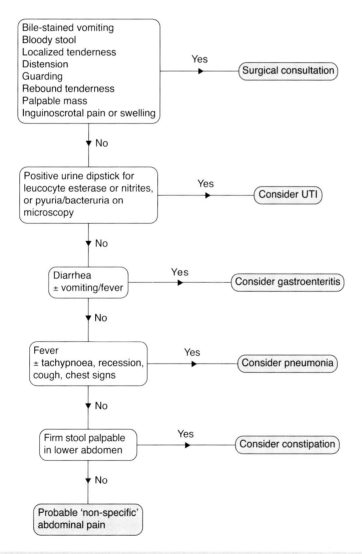

Figure 7.1 Algorithm for management of abdominal pain. Abbreviation: UTI, urinary tract infection.

cultures obtained if the child is potentially septic. The patient should be given and fasted until a surgical opinion has been sought. In addition, a nasogastric tube will be needed if there is bowel obstruction.

7.2 Constipation

Constipation is defined as hard stools that are difficult to pass. Defecation may be painful and may be less frequent than normal. There is a wide range of normal stool frequency: normal breastfed infants may have a stool following each feed or only one every 7–10 days; bottle-fed infants and older children will usually have a bowel action at least every 2–3 days. Constipation occurs more commonly in older children when they have been switched from breast milk or formula to cow's milk. Constipation may be associated with abdominal pain, reduced appetite and irritability. Vomiting is rarely a sign of constipation alone.

Children may develop constipation as a result of:
• a natural tendency related to reduced gut motility
• a poor diet
• a toddler behavior pattern
• inadequate fluid intake (sometimes after acute illness)
• reduced activity
• painful anal conditions, e.g. fissures
• sometimes following sexual abuse.

Organic causes are rare after early infancy.

7.2.1 Assessment

All infants under 3 months should be discussed with the registrar or consultant. They may require referral for exclusion of Hirschsprung disease. Suggestive symptoms and signs include delayed passage of meconium, vomiting, failure to thrive, abdominal distension and a positive family history.

Do not perform a rectal examination – it is rarely helpful and usually traumatic to the child. An inspection of the anus is important to exclude painful conditions. Acute anal fissures are generally posterior and may occur after passage of a large stool or may complicate inflammation of the perianal skin, e.g. in pinworm (or threadworm) infestation. Perianal cellulitis is caused by group A streptococcal infection and is characterised by induration and marked erythema of the perianal skin with mucopurulent exudate. An abdominal X-ray is not helpful in the initial assessment and should not be ordered. Remember that urine infections are more common in constipated children and should be sought if symptoms are suggestive (see urinary tract infection guidelines).

For the assessment of a child with constipation, see *Figure 7.2.*

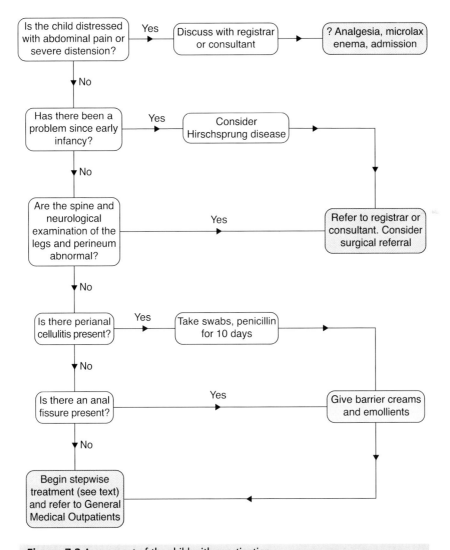

Figure 7.2 Assessment of the child with constipation.

7.2.2 Management

Carers need to be reassured about the safety of laxatives in children. Rectal medications should be avoided in the first instance and not pre-scribed without discussion with a consultant. Management can be divided into three main steps (*Box 7.1*).

Box 7.1 Management of constipation in children

Step 1
Initially give a high fibre diet with adequate fluid intake, adequate exercise and regular toileting.

Step 2
The child will need laxatives, including a stool softener and an aperient.

A suggested regime is: Parachoc **or** Lactulose; plus sennakot
- *Liquid paraffin* (< 5 years: 10 ml daily; 6–12 years: 15 ml daily). Parachoc should be avoided if there is an increased risk of aspiration, e.g. in cerebral palsy with bulbar involvement. Children may be given up to 25 ml of Parachoc per dose.
- *Lactulose* (< 5 years: 5 ml b.i.d.; > 5 years: 10 ml b.i.d.). Children may be given up to 25 ml of Lactulose per dose.
- *Senna* granules: (2–6 years: 1/2 teaspoon nocte; 6–12 years: 1 teaspoon nocte). The maximum daily dose of Sennakot granules should be 3 teaspoons per day.

Abdominal pain may occur as a side effect. Increased doses may be required in some children with chronic constipation. The dose should be titrated to achieve at least one soft stool per day.

If overflow incontinence is present, warn families that it may worsen initially with treatment.

Step 3
Rarely patients may require admission to achieve bowel emptying. Treatment will involve a bowel preparation agent either Picoprep (Picolax in the UK) sachets (sodium picosulphate 10 mg, magnesium oxide 3.5 mg, citric acid 12.0 g, aspartame 36 mg): < 2 years – 1/4 sachet; 2–4 years – 1/2 sachet; 4–9 years – 3/4 sachet, repeating in 6 hours if no response; or colonic lavage solution (e.g. Golytely: orally or via a nasogastric tube).

Chronic constipation can result in fecal overload, overflow incontinence and considerable secondary emotional and behavioral difficulties. Chronic fecal retention causes rectal dilatation, reduced sensation of fullness and sphincter disturbance, such that soft stool percolates down from the proximal colon and is passed without control. Encopresis or soiling is usually the result of constipation. Treatment needs to continue for a sufficient length of time for colonic size and sensation to return to normal. Many children will require months of treatment.

7.2.3 Disposition

All patients should be referred for follow up in a general pediatric clinic within 7 to 10 days.

7.3 Diarrhea and vomiting

Most diarrhea and vomiting in children is due to infective gastroenteritis (*Table 7.3*) but not all. It may be the presentation of a urinary tract infection (UTI), meningitis, appendicitis, intussusception or systemic illness. In the unwell child, especially if anuric, consider hemolytic uremic syndrome (hemolytic anemia, acute renal failure and thrombocytopenia).

Table 7.3 Common causes of infective gastroenteritis

Types	Organisms	Characteristics
Food poisoning	*Staphylococcus aureus* *Salmonella* spp. *Clostridium* spp.	Acute diarrhea and vomiting, often with abdominal pain, usually better within 24 hours
Viral gastroenteritis	Rotavirus Norwalk virus Enterovirus Adenovirus	Watery diarrhea
Bacterial gastroenteritis	*Clostridium jejuni* (under 5 years) *Escherichia coli* (undercooked meat) *Shigella* (high fever with seizures under age 5) *Salmonella* (undercooked poultry)	Bloody diarrhea with mucus, often with sheets of polymorphonuclear cells, usually minimal vomiting
Antibiotic-induced diarrhea	*Clostridium difficile* toxin	Persistent diarrhea with crampy pain
Parasitic gastroenteritis	*Giardia lamblia* *Entamoeba histolytica*	Mild diarrhea with flatulence and bloating, sometimes with blood and mucus

7.3.1 Assessment

There are essentially two aspects to the assessment of a child with gastroenteritis:
- *Diagnosis*: Does the child have a cause other than infective gastroenteritis?
- *Degree of dehydration*: Does the child need admission to hospital? Is there any reason why oral rehydration is not appropriate?

An initial weight measurement should form part of the initial assessment of any child who presents with diarrhea and vomiting.

Any child who is toxic, vomiting blood or bile or has severe abdominal pain or abdominal signs needs immediate consultant referral. Be especially careful of those children with chronic illnesses and poor growth, and of the very young.

You must assess degree of dehydration on clinical signs and change in body weight (if recent weight available).
- With mild dehydration (< 4%) there are no clinical signs.
- Moderate dehydration (4–6%) tends to be accompanied by dry mucous membranes and sunken eyes.
- With increasing severity to 7–9%, the signs of dehydration are more pronounced with cool peripheries, decreased skin turgor, impaired peripheral circulation and acidotic breathing.
- A shocked child needs immediate intravenous resuscitation.

Fecal samples should be collected for microbiological culture if the child has significant associated abdominal pain or blood in the motions, as a bacterial cause of gastroenteritis is more likely.

7.3.2 Management

The child with diarrhea should continue to be fed unless severely dehydrated. Most children can be rehydrated with oral or nasogastric feeds unless shocked. **Do not** give medications to reduce the vomiting or diarrhea. They do not work and may be harmful.

Oral rehydration

There is no evidence that milk, or other foods, should be diluted or excluded during the diarrheal illness, unless there is documented lactose intolerance, although a short period without food will not harm children. Breastfeeding should continue.

For **mildly dehydrated children**, increased frequency of normal drinks, giving small amounts often, will be adequate. Do not give fizzy drinks or fruit juice as their osmolarity is too high. For **moderately dehydrated** children, who are still drinking, small frequent amounts of fluids should be given according to the volumes given on the charts below. The fluids should be oral rehydrating fluids. Commercially available preparations usually have 35–50 mmol sodium l^{-1}. Examples include Diorylate or Rehydrat. Clear instructions and a written information sheet should be given to the parents together with an indication of when to seek review. Indications for admission are:

- refusal to take fluid
- severe pain
- bilious vomiting
- abdominal distension
- blood in the motions
- altered level of consciousness
- increasing dehydration
- parents coping poorly

Nasogastric rehydration

Nasogastric rehydration is a safe and effective way of rehydrating most children with moderate to severe dehydration, even if the child is vomiting. There are a number of possible regimens. Current practice is to replace deficit over 6 hours and then give daily maintenance over the next 18 hours using oral rehydration solution. To calculate hourly rates see *Table 7.4*. However, recent recommendations from the American Academy of Pediatrics say that rapid nasogastric rehydration over a 4-hour period is safe and effective. Using 100 ml kg^{-1} over 4 hours for a moderately dehydrated child or for more severe even 150 ml kg^{-1} over 4 hours is an appropriate replacement rate. In most cases it is not necessary to check electrolytes.

Intravenous rehydration

Any child with severe dehydration requires immediate boluses of 20 ml kg^{-1} normal saline until circulation restored (i.v. or i.o.). Urgent U&Es, glucose, FBC, blood gas and urinalysis. Consider whether a septic work-up and parenteral antibiotics are needed or a surgical consultation.

Always remember the ABC approach to a sick child. If serum Na^+ is between 130 mmol l^{-1} and 150 mmol l^{-1}, aim to replace deficit and maintenance over 24 hours after the circulation has been restored by fluid boluses. Reassess clinically and reweigh on the ward at 6 and 12 hours.

Contact a gastroenterology consultant if the child is hemodynamically unstable, has a past history of gut surgery or other significant disease.

If serum Na^+ is less than $130\,mmol\,l^{-1}$ or more than $150\,mmol\,l^{-1}$, aim to replace deficit carefully over 48–72 hours, and consult with senior staff.

Table 7.4 Recommended hourly rate for oral or nasogastric rehydration in gastroenteritis

Weight on admission (kg)	Degree of dehydration			
	Moderate (4–6%)		Severe (>7%)	
	$ml\,h^{-1}$ 0–6 h	$ml\,h^{-1}$ 7–24 h	$ml\,h^{-1}$ 0–6 h	$ml\,h^{-1}$ 7–24 h
3.0	25	20	45	20
4.0	35	30	60	30
5.0	45	35	75	35
6.0	55	40	90	40
7.0	60	45	100	45
8.0	70	50	115	50
9.0	80	55	130	55
10	90	60	150	60
12	105	65	175	65
15	135	70	220	70
20	175	85	290	85
30	260	90	440	90

7.4 Jaundice in early infancy

There are many causes of jaundice in early infancy (see *Box 7.2*). It is clinically defined as the yellow colouration of the skin and sclera. The best approach is to define it, if it is unconjugated or a conjugated jaundice, as this will dictate the approach to investigation and treatment.

Physiological jaundice
Jaundice is very commonly noted in the first 2 weeks of life. It is part of a normal physiological process and affects 50–70% of babies. Mild jaun-

---

Box 7.2 Causes of neonatal jaundice

Unconjugated
Breast milk jaundice: 3–5% of breastfed babies
Prematurity: exaggerated physiological pattern; may last 4 weeks
Bruising or cephalohematoma: breakdown of heme
Hemolysis (Rhesus, ABO, G6PD or pyruvate kinase (PK) deficiency, spherocytosis): early onset for ABO, Rhesus
Sepsis: rarely presents with jaundice alone (occasional for UTI); usually unwell
Metabolic (e.g. hypothyroidism): prolonged jaundice, can be mixed conjugated/unconjugated
Polycythemia: delayed cord clamping, twin-to-twin transfusion
Gilbert or Crigler–Najjar: rare, usually presents as prolonged jaundice
GI obstruction (e.g. pyloric stenosis)

Conjugated – pale stools/dark urine, raised conjugated bilirubin ($> 25\%$ total or $> 25\ \mu mol\ l^{-1}$)
Biliary atresia
Choledochal cyst
Neonatal hepatitis (congenital infection, alpha-1 antitrypsin deficiency; often idiopathic)
Metabolic (galactosemia, fructose intolerance – ask about sucrose/fructose in food/medication)
Complication of total parenteral nutrition (TPN)

---

dice with onset after 24 hours of life and which is fading by 14 days needs no investigation or treatment.

Breast milk jaundice

This is the most common cause of prolonged jaundice beyond 14 days but other causes should be eliminated before this diagnosis is made. A breastfed baby with prolonged unconjugated jaundice, normal stool and urine colour, normal FBC, blood film and Coombs test who is well and thriving probably has breast-milk jaundice. Do not stop breastfeeding. The child should have a review in a general pediatric clinic if not improving or if there are any changes – especially in stool colour.

Conjugated hyperbilirubinemia

This must be excluded as the causes of this pattern need urgent evaluation and treatment. Surgery for biliary atresia is most successful when the condition is diagnosed and treated early. **Don't forget to ask about the color of urine and stools. View a dirty nappy yourself if possible.**

Phototherapy or rarely exchange transfusion

This may be necessary in a baby with severe unconjugated jaundice associated with prematurity, hemolytic disease, or rare disorders such as Crigler–Najjar. Outside of these conditions, unconjugated jaundice is unlikely to lead to CNS or hearing problems, and no treatment is usually necessary.

7.4.1 Investigation of the jaundiced baby

This is shown in *Figure 7.3*.

7.5 Adolescent gynecology – Lower abdominal pain

Always remember the following gynecological issues in cases of abdominal pain in a young adult female.

7.5.1 Assessment

Assessment (*Figure 7.4*) should include:
- Menstrual history (last menstrual period, duration, flow, pain)
- Sexual activity (if the patient is active sexually, discuss safe sex and contraception)
- Associated symptoms (bowel, bladder, fever, nausea, vomiting).

Consider performing an human choriogonadotropin (hCG) test in all patients, and always consider urinary or gastrointestinal etiology.

7.6 Adolescent gynecology – Menorrhagia

This is defined as greater than 80 ml blood loss during menstruation. It equates to needing to change a super pad/tampon more frequently than every 2 hours.

7.6.1 Assessment

- Menstrual history (last menstrual period, frequency, duration, flow, pain)
- FBC if recurrent/severe
- Clotting disorders are rare. Consider coagulation profile (PT, PTT, fibrinogen, von Willebrand screen) if recurrent or severe, or associated with epistaxis/easy bruising or positive family history

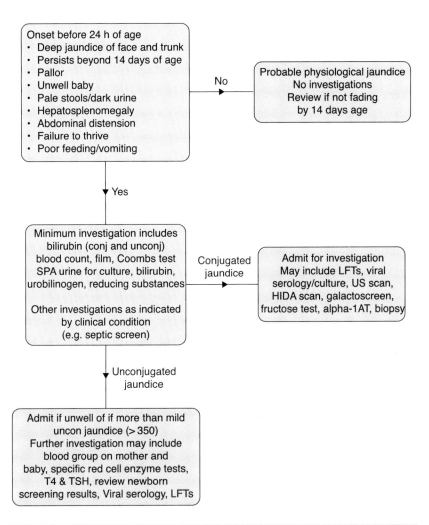

Figure 7.3 Investigation of neonatal jaundice. Abbreviations: AT, antitrypsin; LFT, liver function test; SPA, suprapubic aspirate; T4, TSH, thyroxine, thyroid stimulating hormone; US, ultrasound.

- hCG levels if sexually active + delayed menses (possible threatened abortion or ectopic pregnancy).

7.6.2 Management

The on-call gynecologist should be consulted for all cases of menorrhagia in the young. Some non-hormonal drugs help in the short term, namely:

- Give iron supplements if the patient is anemic or has recurrent or severe bleeding

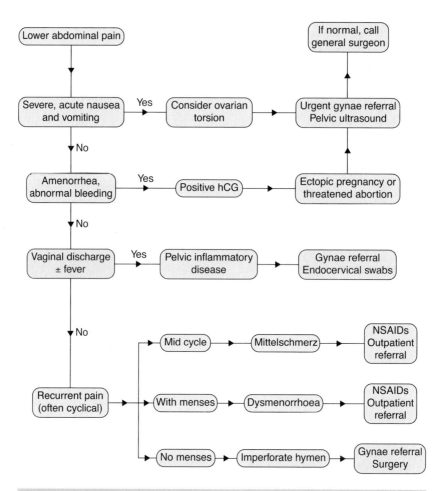

Figure 7.4 Assessment of lower abdominal pain in adolescent girls. Abbreviation: NSAID, non-steroidal anti-inflammatory drug.

- First line treatment to decrease flow:
  - NSAIDS (Naprogesic, Ponstan, Brufen) – also good if there is dysmenorrhea (antiprostaglandin). These can decrease flow up to 30% if taken regularly every 4–6 hours during the first 48 hours of menstruation
  - Cyklokapron (tranexamic acid, 500 every 8 hours), an antifibrinolytic, can decrease flow by 50%
- Hormonal forms of treatment will help in the longer term:
  - Progesterone (norethisterone – Primolut; medroxyprogesterone acetate – Provera) is good with anovulation (infrequent periods) from the lack of progesterone; acute treatment: 5–10 mg for 21 days (note the patient will bleed when medication is stopped!); prophylactic treatment: 7–10 days/month

- Combined oral contraceptive pill: can decrease flow by 50% and is good with anovulation/irregular menses
- Depo-Provera (75% amenorrhea after 1 year's use)
- For acute severe bleeding: Premarin i.v. (25 mg i.v. every 4 hours) will require admission

Suggested reading

Liebelt, E.L. (1998) Clinical and laboratory evaluation and management of children with vomiting, diarrhea and dehydration. *Curr. Opin. Ped.* **10:** 461–469.

Mackenzie, A., Barnes, G. (1991) Randomised controlled trial comparing oral and intravenous rehydration in children with diarrhea. *B.M.J.* **303:** 393–396.

Mason, J.D. (1996) The evaluation of acute abdominal pain in children. *Emerg. Clin. N. Amer.* **14:** 629–644.

Murphy, M.S. (1998) Guidelines for managing acute gastroenteritis based on a systemic review of published research. *Arch. Dis. Child.* **79:** 279–284.

Chapter 8

Endocrine emergencies

Colin Powell

Contents

Endocrine diseases occasionally present acutely to the Emergency Department. They must be included in the differential diagnosis of many acute presentations since, if they are present, urgent management can be life-saving.

8.1 Adrenal crisis

An adrenal crisis is a physiological event caused by an acute relative insufficiency of adrenal hormones. It may be precipitated by physiological stress, such as infection or surgery in a susceptible patient. It should be considered in patients with:
• congenital adrenal hyperplasia
• hypopituitarism with replacement therapy
• previous or current prolonged steroid therapy
• a history of central nervous system pathology or neurosurgical procedures.

8.1.1 Assessment

Signs of both glucocorticoid deficiency and mineralocorticoid deficiency should be looked for if adrenal insufficiency is suspected. In the history and examination, you should look for the following:
• **glucocorticoid deficiency** presenting with weakness, anorexia, nausea and/or vomiting, hypoglycemia, hypotension (particularly postural) and shock
• **mineralocorticoid deficiency** presenting with dehydration, hyperkalemia, hyponatremia, acidosis and prerenal renal failure.

8.1.2 Investigations

Prompt treatment is essential and should be based on the following investigations:
• immediate blood glucose using a Dextrostix
• serum glucose, urea, sodium and potassium
• arterial or capillary acid base

Where the underlying diagnosis of adrenal insufficiency is suspected, you should collect at least 2 ml of clotted blood for later analysis (cortisol and 17-hydroxyprogesterone). The results are unlikely to be available to help in the emergency management of the patient.

8.1.3 Management

Susceptible patients who present with vomiting
Susceptible patients who present with vomiting but who are not other-

wise unwell should be considered to have incipient adrenal crisis. To prevent this from possibly developing further:
- Administer i.v. or i.m. hydrocortisone 2 mg kg^{-1}.
- Give oral fluids and observe for 4–6 hours before considering discharge.
- Discuss with appropriate consultant.

For all other children

For all other children where adrenal insufficiency is suspected, the various abnormalities should be considered, namely, fluid requirements, hydrocortisone requirements, hypoglycemia, hyperkalemia and precipitating causes such as sepsis.

1. Give intravenous fluids

The level of dehydration should be assessed and intravenous fluids given accordingly. For management of various levels of dehydration, see *Box 8.1.*

Box 8.1 Management of dehydration in adrenal insufficiency

For shock and severe dehydration
- Normal saline 20 ml kg^{-1} i.v. bolus. Repeat until circulation is restored.
- Administer remaining deficit plus maintenance fluid volume as normal saline in 5% dextrose evenly over 24 hours.
- Check electrolytes and glucose frequently.
- After the first few hours, if serum sodium is >130 mmol l^{-1}, change to half normal saline.
- 10% dextrose may be needed to maintain normoglycemia.

For moderate dehydration in adrenal insufficiency
- Normal saline 10 ml/kg i.v. bolus. Repeat until circulation is restored.
- Administer remaining deficit plus maintenance fluid volume as normal saline in 5% dextrose evenly over 24 hours.

For mild dehydration in adrenal insufficiency
- No bolus.
- 1.5 times maintenance fluid volume administered evenly over 24 hours.

---

2. Give hydrocortisone

Hydrocortisone must be given intravenously. If intravenous access is difficult, hydrocortisone should be given intramuscularly while you are establishing the intravenous line, in the following doses:

- *Neonate*: hydrocortisone 25 mg stat and then 50 mg m^{-2} per 24 hours by continuous infusion
- *1 month – 1 year*: hydrocortisone 25 mg stat, then 50 mg m^{-2} per 24 hours by continuous infusion
- *Toddlers (1–3 years)*: hydrocortisone 25–50 mg stat then 50 mg m^{-2} per 24 hours by continuous infusion
- *Children (4–12 years)*: hydrocortisone 50–75 mg stat, then 50 mg m^{-2} per 24 hours by continuous infusion
- *Adolescents and adults*: hydrocortisone 100–150 mg stat, then 50 mg m^{-2} per 24 hours by continuous infusion

When the patient is stable, you should reduce the intravenous hydrocortisone dose, and then switch to triple dose oral hydrocortisone therapy, gradually reducing to maintenance levels (10–15 mg m^{-2} per day).

In patients with mineralocorticoid deficiency, start fludrocortisone at maintenance doses (usually 0.1 mg daily) as soon as the patient is able to tolerate oral fluids.

3. Treat hypoglycemia
Hypoglycemia is common in infants and small children. Treat with an intravenous bolus of 5 ml kg^{-1} 10% dextrose in a neonate or infant and 2 ml kg^{-1} of 25% dextrose in an older child or adolescent. Maintenance fluids should contain 5–10% dextrose.

4. Treat hyperkalemia
Hyperkalemia usually normalises with fluid and electrolyte replacement.
- If potassium is above 6 mmol l^{-1}, perform an ECG and apply a cardiac monitor as arrhythmias and cardiac arrest can occur.
- If potassium is above 7 mmol l^{-1} and hyperkalemic ECG changes are present (e.g. peaked T waves, wide QRS complex), give 10% calcium gluconate 0.5 ml kg^{-1} i.v. over 3–5 minutes. Commence an infusion of insulin 0.1 units kg^{-1} per hour i.v. together with an infusion of 50% dextrose 2 ml kg^{-1} per hour.
- If the potassium is above 7 mmol l^{-1} with a normal ECG, give sodium bicarbonate 1–2 mmol kg^{-1} i.v. over 20 minutes, with an infusion of 10% dextrose at 5 ml kg^{-1} per hour.

5. Identify and treat potential precipitating causes such as sepsis.

6. Admit to appropriate inpatient facility.

8.1.4 Prevention

The prevention of a crisis is usually possible in susceptible individuals. Situations likely to precipitate a crisis should be anticipated and the patient given:
- triple normal oral maintenance steroid dose for 2–3 days during stress (e.g. fever, fracture, laceration requiring suture)
- intramuscular hydrocortisone when absorption of oral medication is doubtful (e.g. in vomiting or severe diarrhea)
- increased parenteral hydrocortisone (1–2 mg kg^{-1}) before anesthesia, with or without an increased dose postoperatively.

8.2 Hypoglycemia

There should be a low threshold for performing a Dextrostix test in the acutely unwell child in the Emergency Department. Beyond the neonatal period, hypoglycemia is defined as a blood glucose less than 2.5 mmol l^{-1}. In children who have had a seizure, hypoglycemia can be the cause of the seizure, or the result of a prolonged seizure.

8.2.1 Effects of hypoglycemia

The effects of the hypoglycemia itself, from whatever cause, are mainly effects on the central nervous system and those of adrenergic overdrive as *Table 8.1*.

Other clinical signs will depend on the cause of the hypoglycemia and a thorough clinical examination is required, including height and weight. *Table 8.2* lists some of the causes with characteristic signs.

Other inborn errors of metabolism may also present with hypoglycemia.

Table 8.1 Effects of hypoglycemia	
Central nervous system effects	**Effects from adrenergic overdrive**
Irritability	Tremor
Coma	Jitteriness
Depressed level of consciousness	Pallor
Convulsions	Sweating

Table 8.2 Other causes and signs of hypoglycemia

Cause	Clinical signs
Hypopituitarism	Mid-line defects, micropenis, optic nerve hypoplasia
Galactosemia	Cataracts
Glycogen storage disease	Hepatomegaly
Adrenal insufficiency	Hyperpigmentation
Beckwith syndrome	Hemihypertrophy, exomphalos, macroglossia, transverse creases

8.2.2 Investigation

Blood and urine must be taken off for metabolic investigation as soon as the child presents, before treatment is commenced. Investigations are listed in *Box 8.2.*

Note that:
- Hyperinsulinism is the commonest cause of hypoglycemia in children under 2 years old. This diagnosis is excluded by ketonuria.
- 'Accelerated starvation' (idiopathic ketotic hypoglycemia) is the commonest cause of hypoglycemia after the age of 2 years, but may present earlier. The diagnosis can be established when fasting-induced hypoglycemia is accompanied by elevated urinary ketones,

Box 8.2 Urine and blood investigations in hypoglycemia

Blood
- Glucose and lactate: fluoride oxalate tube (1 ml)
- Insulin, cortisol, growth hormone: plain tube (2–4 ml)
- Ammonia: heparinised tube (1 ml)
- Ketones and free fatty acids: fluoride oxalate (BLF) tube (1 ml)
- Amino acids, electrolytes: heparinised (1–2 ml), if enough blood available
- Acid-base: capillary sample
- Blood drops onto a Guthrie test card (for acylcarnitine profile)

Urine
- Ketones, glucose, reducing substances,
- Amino acids and organic acids

in the absence of other pathology. It is treated by frequent high protein and carbohydrate meals.

8.2.3 Management

Symptomatic hypoglycemia should be treated with an i.v. bolus of 5 ml kg^{-1} of 10% dextrose (0.25–0.5 mg kg^{-1}). The expected maintenance infusion rate is 3–5 ml kg^{-1} h^{-1} of 10% dextrose (6–8 mg kg^{-1} min^{-1}). A required infusion rate of 10–20 mg kg^{-1} min^{-1} is consistent with hyperinsulinism.

8.3 Diabetes mellitus

8.3.1 Ketoacidosis

Thirty per cent of children with diabetes present with vomiting and secondary dehydration from the development of acidosis and ketosis. Diabetic ketoacidocis is a medical emergency. The clinical presentation may vary from polydipsia and polyuria or abdominal pain and vomiting to dehydration and weight loss with rapid acidotic breathing. It is important to check the blood glucose in any child who presents with any of these signs or symptoms.

8.3.2 Assessment

Assessment includes the clinical assessment, particularly of the level of dehydration and the laboratory investigations. The level of dehydration is often overestimated.

8.3.3 Degree of dehydration

- Mild–nil (<4%): no clinical signs
- Moderate (4–7%): easily detectable dehydration, e.g. reduced skin turgor, poor capillary return
- Severe (>7%): poor perfusion, rapid pulse, reduced blood pressure, i.e. shock.

8.3.4 Investigations

- Blood glucose, urea, electrolytes.
- Arterial or capillary acid/base
- Urine: ketones, culture
- Check for precipitating cause, e.g. infection (urine, FBC, blood cultures; consider CXR)
- Islet cell antibodies and insulin antibodies in newly diagnosed patients.

8.3.5 Management

Fluid requirements

If hypoperfusion is present, give normal saline at $20\,ml\,kg^{-1}$ stat. This should be repeated until the patient is hemodynamically stable with warm, pink extremities and rapid capillary refill time. If more than $30\,ml\,kg^{-1}$ is needed, call for senior advice. Rehydration should continue with normal saline.

$$\text{Requirement} = \text{deficit} + \text{maintenance}$$
$$\text{Deficit} = \%\text{ dehydration} \times \text{body weight (kg)}$$

The child should be kept nil by mouth (except ice to suck) until alert and stable. A nasogastric tube should be inserted if he or she is comatose or has recurrent vomiting. It should be left on free drainage. Rehydration can be completed orally after the first 24–36 hours if the patient is metabolically stable.

Maintenance fluids

If the blood sugar falls very quickly, i.e. within the first few hours, you should change to normal saline with 5% dextrose. When the blood sugar reaches $12–15\,mmol\,l^{-1}$, use 0.45% NaCl with 5% dextrose. You should aim to keep the blood sugar at $10–12\,mmol\,l^{-1}$.

If the blood glucose falls below $10–12\,mmol\,l^{-1}$ and the patient is still sick and acidotic, increase the dextrose in the infusate to 7.5–10%. **Do not turn down insulin infusion.**

Bicarbonate

Bicarbonate is usually not necessary if shock has been adequately corrected and should not be required in most cases. You must remember that treatment of the dehydration will correct the acid-base disturbance. In extremely sick children (with pH $<7.0 \pm HCO_3 <5\,mmol\,l^{-1}$), small amounts of sodium bicarbonate can be given after discussion with the consultant endocrinologist. It should be given over 30 minutes with cardiac monitoring.

$$\text{Bicarbonate dose (mmol)} = 0.15 \times \text{body weight (kg)} \times \text{base deficit}$$

The acid base status must then be reassessed.

Note:
• Remember the risk of hypokalemia.
• Continuing acidosis usually means insufficient resuscitation.

Insulin

The insulin should be prepared by adding 50 units of clear/rapid-acting insulin (Actrapid HM or Humulin R) to 49.5 ml 0.9% NaCl (1 unit per ml solution). The insulin infusion may be run as a sideline with the rehydrating fluid via a 3-way tap, provided a syringe pump is used. Ensure that the insulin is clearly labelled.

You should start at 0.1 units kg^{-1} per hour in newly diagnosed children, and in those already on insulin who have glucose levels > 15 mmol l^{-1}. Children who have had their usual insulin and whose blood sugars are < 15 mmol l^{-1} should receive 0.05 units kg^{-1} per hour. Adjust the concentration of dextrose to keep the blood glucose at 10–12 mmol l^{-1}. Adequate insulin must be continued to clear acidosis (ketonemia).

The insulin infusion can be discontinued when the child is alert and metabolically stable (blood glucose < 10–12 mmol l^{-1}, pH > 7.30 and $HCO_3 > 15$). The best time to change to subcutaneous insulin is just before meal time. The insulin infusion should only be stopped 30 minutes after the first subcutaneous injection of insulin.

Potassium

Potassium chloride should be added to each bag of i.v. fluid once the patient has urinated. Add this at a rate of 40 mmol l^{-1} if the body weight < 30 kg, or 60 mmol l^{-1} if > 30 kg. You should measure the levels 2 hours after starting therapy and 2–4 hourly thereafter. Specimens should in general be arterial or venous. Give no potassium if the serum level is > 5.5 mmol l^{-1} or if the patient is anuric.

Admission to ICU

Consider admission to the ICU if the patient is under 2 years of age at onset or if in coma, cardiovascular compromise or is having seizures.

Strict monitoring must continue while the child is transferred to ward or to the ICU (*Box 8.3*).

Added hazards during the management of ketoacidosis include:

Hypernatremia. Measured serum sodium is depressed by the dilutional effect of the hyperglycemia. To 'adjust' sodium concentration, use the following formula:

$$\text{adjusted (i.e. actual) sodium} = \text{measured sodium} + 0.3 \,(\text{glucose} - 5.5) \text{ mmol } l^{-1}$$

> **Box 8.3** Monitoring during transport
>
> - Strict fluid balance; check all urine for ketones
> - Hourly observations: pulse, BP, respiratory rate, level of consciousness and pupils
> - Hourly glucose (Glucometer) during insulin infusion; other biochemistry as clinically indicated
> - 4 hourly temperature measurements

i.e. 3 mmol l^{-1} of sodium to be added to the measured result for every 10 mmol l^{-1} of glucose above 5.5 mmol l^{-1}. If Na is > 160 mmol l^{-1}, the case should be discussed with the consultant. The sodium should rise as the glucose falls during treatment. If this does not happen or if hyponatremia develops, it usually indicates overzealous volume correction and insufficient electrolyte replacement. This may place the patient at risk of cerebral edema.

Hypoglycemia. Hypoglycemia can occur during correction of the hyperglycemia. If the blood glucose is < 2.2 mol l^{-1} give i.v. 10% dextrose 5 ml kg^{-1}. Do not discontinue the insulin infusion. Continue with a 10% dextrose infusion until stable.

Cerebral edema. Some degree of subclinical brain swelling is present during most episodes of diabetic ketoacidosis. Clinical cerebral edema occurs suddenly, usually between 6 and 12 hours after starting therapy (range 2–24 hours). Mortality or severe morbidity is very high without early treatment.

Occurrence of cerebral edema is reduced by slow correction of the fluid and biochemical abnormalities. Optimally, the rate of fall of blood glucose and serum osmolality should not exceed 5 mmol l^{-1} h^{-1}, but in children there is often a quicker initial fall in glucose. Patients should be nursed head up.

The warning signs are given in *Box 8.4*.

Treatment consists of:
- Mannitol 20% 0.5 g kg^{-1} i.v. stat if hemodynamically stable. Give immediately when the clinical diagnosis is made – do not delay for confirmatory brain scan.
- Reduce fluid input to 2/3 and replace deficit over 72 hours rather than 24 hours.

> **Box 8.4** Warning signs of cerebral edema
>
> - First presentation, long history of poor control, young age (< 5 years)
> - No sodium rise as glucose falls, hyponatremia during therapy, initial adjusted hypernatremia
> - Headache, irritability, lethargy, depressed consciousness, incontinence, thermal instability
> - Very late – bradycardia, increased BP and respiratory impairment

- Nurse head up.
- Transfer immediately to ICU.

8.3.6 New presentation of diabetes in a mildly ill child

Assessment

Occasionally an astute clinician makes the diagnosis of diabetes mellitus in a mildly ill child, with < 3% dehydration, no acidosis and no vomiting. Baseline investigations should be carried out, as in the child with ketoacidosis. The diagnosis of diabetes mellitus brings with it a lifetime of treatment. The education and care of child and family should be taken over by a team including a pediatrician, nurses and a dietician. However, management can be initiated without admission to hospital.

Management

Initial insulin treatment. Give 0.25 units kg^{-1} of quick-acting insulin s.c. stat. If the child is within 2 hours of a meal, give the meal-time dose only. Halve the dose if he or she is under 4 years old. Before breakfast and lunch (7.30 a.m., 11.30 a.m.) give 0.25 units kg^{-1} of quick-acting insulin. Before the evening meal (5.30 p.m.) give 0.25 units kg^{-1} of quick-acting insulin and 0.25 units kg^{-1} of intermediate-acting insulin. If this is the first insulin dose, give 0.25 units kg^{-1} quick-acting insulin only, followed by a further 0.25 units kg^{-1} quick-acting insulin at midnight followed by a snack.

Ongoing insulin treatment. Once normoglycemia is achieved and ketonuria disappears, you should change the insulin to a twice daily mixture of short and intermediate insulins usually at 1 unit kg^{-1} but this may need modification. It should be given as 2/3 in morning and 1/3 at night; 2/3 of each dose should be intermediate-acting, and 1/3 short-acting. Occasionally older adolescents go onto a basal bolus regimen of 30–40% intermediate acting insulin given at 10 p.m., with the rest given as short-acting insulin in 3 equal doses before meals.

You must inform your consultant about all admissions of children with diabetic ketoacidosis.

8.3.7 Mildly ill hyperglycemic diabetic patients who are already on insulin

Children who have already been diagnosed as having diabetes mellitus and who are already on insulin can present to the Emergency Department with a mild illness and hyperglycemia. They are usually advised to take 10% of total daily dose of insulin as rapid-acting insulin every 2 hours until normoglycemic (in addition to usual insulin). You should notify your consultant if there are any management issues that you want to discuss.

Suggested reading

Glasner, N., Barnett, P., Mcaslin, I. *et al.* (2001) Risk factors for cerebral edema in children with diabetic ketoacidosis. *N. Engl. J. Med.* **344:** 264–269.
Ward, J.C. (1990) Inborn errors of metabolism of acute onset in infancy. *Pediatr. Rev.* **11:** 205–226.

Chapter 9

Renal emergencies

Colin Powell, T. Reade

Contents

9.1 Acute dysuria

Dysuria is the sensation of pain on micturition and it can arise from irritation in the bladder or the urethra. It is a common symptom in children and can represent very mild disease such as irritation of the external genitalia, or serious infection of the kidney. The younger child is more likely to have trauma or irritation as the cause of dysuria whereas the older child is more likely to have an infectious reason for this symptom (see *Table 1*). Diagnosis as always depends on a good history and examination prior to specific investigation.

Table 9.1 Causes of acute dysuria in children

Mechanism	Cause	Notes
Infection	Pyelonephritis	Involves upper renal tract. Often associated with abdominal pain and systemic signs such as fever
	Cystitis	Can be bacterial or viral
	Urethritis	
	Infectious vaginitis	See chapter 10
Irritation	Ammoniacal dermatitis	From prolonged contact with urine (nappy rash). Can be complicated by candidal infection
	Chemical vulvo-vaginitis	Irritation by poor hygiene, bubble baths or soaps
	Chemical cystitis	Medications such as cyclophosphamide
Trauma	Minor trauma	Examples are: straddle injury, zipper injury
	Foreign body in the vagina	
	Childhood sexual abuse	See chapter 27
	Masturbation	Does not usually cause visible injuries but may cause minor irritation
Miscellaneous	Urolithiasis	Rarely hypercaluria and renal stones
	Mucosal disease: • Stevens-Johnson syndrome • Reiter's syndrome • Behcet's syndrome	Other signs of the condition are usually also obvious
	Misinterpreted dysuria (pinworms)	Vulval irritation and dysuria may be the presenting feature

Urinary tract infection is the commonest renal problem presenting to the Emergency Department. However, other conditions do occur and several are serious, warranting urgent diagnosis and management.

9.2 Urinary tract infection (UTI)

The urinary tract is a common site of infection in children. The annual incidence is up to 1% in girls, but less common in boys. Radiological abnormalities are present in about 40% of children with UTIs, the most common being reflux. Asymptomatic bacteriuria in schoolgirls is about 1–2%.

It is often difficult to diagnose a UTI on history or examination alone in children and a high index of suspicion must be held. The consequences of missing a UTI in a child with even minor urinary tract abnormalities may be significant.

Positive dipstick for leucocytes and nitrites in a sick child does not exclude another site of serious infection (e.g. meningitis). Organisms may also spread from the urinary tract to elsewhere including the meninges. Therefore further investigations as part of a septic work-up (e.g. LP) should not be omitted in a sick child who returns a positive dipstick.

9.2.1 History

Symptoms of serious urinary infections are often non-specific and include fever, irritability, poor feeding and vomiting. More specific features may include loin or abdominal pain, frequency and dysuria. These localising signs are often absent in younger patients. Some children with UTIs may look quite well, while others may appear very unwell.

9.2.2 Examination

This is often normal other than the presence of fever. Loin or suprapubic tenderness may be present. Urinary dipstick testing is only a screening test for a UTI. It has poor sensitivity and specificity (see below).

9.2.3 Initial investigations

A UTI cannot be diagnosed on symptoms alone, nor by culture of urine from a bag specimen. A definitive diagnosis can only be made by culture of urine obtained in a sterile fashion from a mid-stream urine (MSU), suprapubic aspiration (SPA), or a catheter specimen of urine (CSU). Prior antibiotic therapy may lead to negative urine culture in patients with UTI. The laboratory will test for antibacterial activity in the urine.

Any child who is unwell or is under 6 months old should also have blood culture and electrolytes tested and should be considered for lumbar puncture.

Dipstick urine tests

Dipsticks can detect urinary protein, blood, nitrites (produced by bacterial reduction of urinary nitrate), and leucocyte esterase (an enzyme present in white blood cells). They are a screening test only. If you really suspect UTI you must send a specimen for microscopy and culture. Blood and protein are unreliable markers of UTI. Not all organisms produce nitrites and nitrites take time to develop in urine and so have poor sensitivity. Nitrites may appear in the urine in the presence of infections in other body systems.

Not all patients with UTI have pyuria. Leucocyte esterase can only be detected with relatively high WBC counts in urine, so the test has low sensitivity. Leucocytes from local sources (vagina, foreskin) may contaminate urine. Leucocytes appear in the urine in many other febrile illnesses, e.g. upper respiratory tract infection, pneumonia, etc. So the specificity is low.

Overall combined sensitivity for both nitrites and leucocytes is around 50%, i.e. **dipsticks may miss 50% of infections.**

Urine specimen collection

There are several ways to collect urine specimens in children, each with its benefits and problems. Practice differs around the world. In the UK, SPA is the method of choice in infants if a clean catch specimen is not possible. However, in North America, SPA is rarely practised. Parents are offered a choice between awaiting bag screening, confirmed by CSU on positive specimens, or immediate catheterisation.

Urine bag. A urine bag is useful for collecting urine for screening purposes in children who cannot void on request (approximately 0–3 years). The genitalia should be washed with water and dried before application of the bag. Urine is tested with a dipstick for leucocytes and nitrites. If it is positive for either, you should obtain a definitive specimen by SPA (or CSU if SPA fails). If clinical suspicion is high, send a definitive specimen for culture regardless of the dipstick result. A negative dipstick result does not exclude a UTI. Do not send bag specimens for culture in acute presentations.

Antibiotics should not be given unless a definitive urine specimen has been obtained.

Suprapubic aspiration (SPA). SPA remains the preferred method in the UK to collect a minimally contaminated specimen. It should be considered in children too young to obtain an MSU, and with a high probability of UTI, or who are unwell and who warrant a more invasive investigation.

The child should be offered fluid to drink. Bedside ultrasound equipment, if available, can improve the success rate of SPA by detecting a full bladder. One author reports 60% success collection rate of SPA and this increases to 80% if bladder ultrasound is used. The specimen should be screened with a dipstick and then sent for culture.

Any growth from SPA urine usually indicates infection (but note possible contamination by skin commensals and fecal flora may occasionally produce a mixed growth).

Catheter specimens. These are useful if SPA fails. The first few drops of the specimen should be discarded and the remaining specimen should always be sent for culture. Any growth of over 10^3 organisms per ml indicates infection.

Mid-stream urine (MSU). A mid-stream urine can be obtained from children who can void on request. The genitalia should be washed with water and dried before the specimen is taken. The first few millilitres should be voided and not collected and then a specimen is obtained. A pure growth of over 10^8 organisms per ml indicates infection. A pure growth of over 10^5 organisms per ml may indicate early infection and requires a repeat specimen.

9.2.4 Treatment of UTI

Antibiotics may be given orally or intravenously for a UTI. Oral medication is appropriate for those over the age of 6 months who are not systemically unwell. Co-trimoxazole (200/40 mg in 5 ml) 0.3 ml kg^{-1} b.d. orally for 1 week is a suitable antibiotic. Alternatives include cephalexin 15 mg kg^{-1} (500 mg) orally three times a day.

Any child who is unwell, and most children under 6 months, should be admitted for i.v. antibiotics. Treatment options vary around the world but suitable regimens include cefuroxime 50 mg kg^{-1} per dose (maximum 2 g) or gentamicin 7.5 mg kg^{-1} (maximum dose 240 mg) i.v. daily and benzylpenicillin 50 mg kg^{-1} (maximum dose 3 g) i.v. 6 hourly for children over 1 month of age. Gentamicin levels should be taken to ensure appropriate time between subsequent doses. All children should have antibiotic sensitivities checked at 24–48 hours and therapy adjusted accordingly. For children who are still in nappies a prophylactic dose of antibiotic, e.g. co-trimoxazole (200/40 mg in 5 ml) 0.15 ml kg^{-1} in a single daily dose, or nitrofurantoin 3 mg kg^{-1} at night should be maintained until the child is seen for follow up. If the child is not settling, repeat the urine culture to determine eradication of organism.

A shocked child will require fluid resuscitation. Any child with underlying urinary tract abnormalities should be discussed with the registrar or consultant.

9.2.5 Follow up investigations

All children with proven UTI should be referred for follow up in the general pediatric clinic, or by the child's own pediatrician. All those with their first UTI should have a renal ultrasound. A micturating cysto-ure-throgram (MCU), abdominal X-ray and DMSA (dimercapto-succino-acetic acid) scan may be necessary, but the decision needs to be considered on an individual basis. They are usually done in children under 1 year of age, and may be necessary for older children according to circumstances. For older children, discussion of the need for MCU should be deferred to the outpatient follow up visit.

One scheme for investigation of UTIs is shown below (*Table 9.2*).

9.3 Nephrotic syndrome

Nephrotic syndrome is a clinical disorder characterised by edema, proteinuria (> 3 g per day), hypoalbuminemia and hypercholesterolemia. Minimal change glomerulonephritis accounts for 80–85% of nephrotic syndrome in childhood. Complications include infections, thrombosis and renal impairment.

9.3.1 History

Edema is the primary feature. This may be subtle or gross and is usually noticed in the peri-orbital region, scrotum or labia. It may include, in addition, peripheral edema of the limbs and sacrum. The history is often of weight gain, poor urine output and sometimes of discomfort as a result of the edema. A history of preceding upper respiratory tract infection or diarrhea may be present.

9.3.2 Examination

Examination should confirm the presence of edema. Ascites and pleural effusions may be present when edema is gross. Peripheral perfusion and

Table 9.2 Scheme for managing and investigating UTIs

Age	Management	Investigation
<2 years	5–7 day course of antibiotics Prophylaxis until child is seen by the specialist Repeat urine culture 2–3 days into prophylaxis	At follow up, 6–8 weeks later: • Abdominal ultrasound • Plain abdominal X-ray • MCU • DMSA scan
2–5 years	5–7 day course of antibiotics Repeat urine culture 2–3 days after end of course	At follow up 6–8 weeks later: • Abdominal ultrasound • Plain abdominal Xray If clinically indicated: • MCU • DMSA scan
>5 years	5–7 day course of antibiotics	At follow up 6–8 weeks later: • Abdominal ultrasound If clinically indicated: • Plain abdominal X-ray • MCU • DMSA scan

blood pressure should be assessed. Examination should include a search for signs suggesting the onset of complications such as infected ascites, renal vein thrombosis (e.g. enlarged renal mass, loin tenderness and marked hematuria) and cerebral vein thrombosis.

Urinalysis should always be included to make the diagnosis as other causes of edema such as protein losing enteropathy or cardiac failure may occur.

9.3.3 Investigation

Urinalysis usually shows +++ or ++++ protein on dipstick. The degree of proteinuria is variable and is usually of the selective type. Microscopic hematuria is present in 15–20% of patients with minimal change nephrotic syndrome. Microscopy of the urine may show red blood cells or granular casts, which suggests the alternative diagnosis of chronic glomerulonephritis as the underlying cause for nephrotic syndrome.

A timed collection of urine for protein excretion is not necessary when the diagnosis is clear. Blood urea and creatinine tests are important to establish the presence or absence of renal impairment. Blood electrolytes, total protein, albumin, globulin and cholesterol should also be measured.

9.3.4 Treatment

All children should be admitted to hospital with their first presentation of nephrotic syndrome. With relapses, they can sometimes be managed as outpatients after consultation with their treating physician. The components of the treatment will be considered individually.

Albumin

In nephrotic syndrome, acute renal impairment is due to renal hypoperfusion. Albumin is the treatment of choice. Intravenous albumin is indicated for:
• anuria
• hypotension
• poor skin perfusion with skin mottling
• poor capillary return.

These are all indicators of a depleted vascular space. Albumin should be given only in consultation with the treating consultant. The dose is 20% albumin $5\,\text{ml}\,\text{kg}^{-1}$ $(1\,\text{g}\,\text{kg}^{-1})$ over 4 hr i.v. **Beware of the possibility of hypertension and pulmonary edema.**

Gross genital edema causing discomfort may also be an indication for albumin.

Frusemide

Frusemide $(1\,\text{mg}\,\text{kg}^{-1}$ i.v.) should be given only if the peripheral perfusion markedly improves following the albumin or there are signs of pulmonary edema or hypertension.

Steroids

Corticosteroids are usually given in the form of prednisolone. Occasionally their use may be delayed until postrenal biopsy at the discretion of the treating physician. The usual dose of prednisolone is $60\,\text{mg}\,\text{m}^{-2}$ per day as single dose up to a maximum of $80\,\text{mg}$ per day until remission of proteinuria (to trace or negative on urinalysis) for 4 days, then in reducing doses. There are various regimens for dose reduction. One example is:
• prednisolone $45\,\text{mg}\,\text{m}^{-2}$ per day for 8 days then
• $60\,\text{mg}\,\text{m}^{-2}$ per alternate day for 8 days (four doses) then
• $45\,\text{mg}\,\text{m}^{-2}$ per alternate day for 8 days then
• $30\,\text{mg}\,\text{m}^{-2}$ per alternate day for 8 days then
• Reduce by $5\,\text{mg}$ every 8 days until finished

Antibiotics

The altered immune system in patients with nephrotic syndrome is responsible for their enhanced risk of infection. Oral penicillin 12.5 mg kg^{-1} per dose b.d. is effective prophylaxis during the edematous phase. If the child is profoundly ill or appears to have sepsis, give cefotaxime 50 mg kg^{-1} per dose 6 hourly to a maximum of 2 g per dose (to cover *Streptococcus pneumoniae*, *Hemophilus influenzae* and *Escherichia coli*).

Anticoagulants

Renal, femoral, cerebral and pulmonary thrombosis can occur in nephrotic patients owing to hypovolemia, high platelet counts and loss of antithrombin III. Thus low-dose aspirin (10 mg kg^{-1} alternate days) is recommended in edematous nephrotic patients.

General measures

Other general measures include:
- Free fluid intake
- Diet with no added salt
- Strict fluid balance
- Daily weight

9.3.5 Relapses

Over 75% of patients will experience at least one relapse. A relapse is defined as proteinuria ++++ or +++ for 4 days. Management should be discussed with a physician. Prednisolone 60 mg m^{-2} per day should be given until the urine is protein-free for 3 days and then the dose should be slowly reduced as above. If edema is absent, these relapses may not require penicillin and aspirin. Infrequent relapses (less than two relapses within a 6-month period) can be managed in the manner outlined above.

9.4 Hematuria/nephritic syndrome

Hematuria is the presence of red blood cells in the urine. The presence of 10 or more RBCs per high-power field is abnormal. Urinary dipsticks are very sensitive and can be positive at less than five RBCs per high-power field. In the emergency department it is important in evaluating a child with hematuria to identify serious, treatable and progressive conditions.

Red or brown urine does not always indicate hematuria. The discoloration may be as a result of hemoglobinuria, myoglobinuria, some medications and some food. Urate crystals are commonly present in the urine of newborn babies. They can produce a red discoloration of the nappy ('brick dust' appearance), which is sometimes mistaken for blood.

Blood in the urine can come from sources other than the urinary tract (e.g. vaginal hemorrhage, rectal fissure).

9.4.1 Causes of hematuria

Common causes for microscopic hematuria include an association with viral infections, UTIs, trauma and Henoch–Schönlein purpura. Common causes for macroscopic hematuria include the above, but macroscopic hematuria is more likely to come from the bladder or urethra.

Symptomless or 'benign hematuria' can occur frequently in children without growth failure, hypertension, edema, proteinuria, urinary casts or renal impairment.

The investigation and management of hematuria is shown in *Figure 9.1*.

9.4.2 Nephritic syndrome

Nephritic syndrome is a syndrome characterised by hematuria, hypertension, edema, oliguria ± proteinuria. The syndrome is seen most commonly in the context of post-streptococcal glomerulonephritis and less commonly in IgA nephropathy, rapidly progressive glomerulonephritis or Goodpasture syndrome.

9.4.3 Treatment

Many children with isolated microscopic hematuria require no immediate investigation and simply need to be checked to see if the problem persists. This should be arranged with the general practitioner or through outpatient clinic if the family do not have a GP. In the setting of an acute febrile illness, exclude UTI by urine culture and arrange for the urine to be tested again after the acute illness has passed.

9.5 Hypertension

Transient hypertension can occur in a child as a result of stress, fear or pain. Blood pressure (BP) measurements repeated on several different occasions (at least three) are required to diagnose hypertension. The cuff bladder should cover at least 3/4 of the child's arm length, and the child should be quiet and calm. In children with measured high BP, it is important to differentiate between those who have immediately dangerous hypertension and those who may have long-standing hypertension. In these patients a search for a possible underlying cause should be made. *Table 9.3* shows the upper 95th centile measurements for blood pressure.

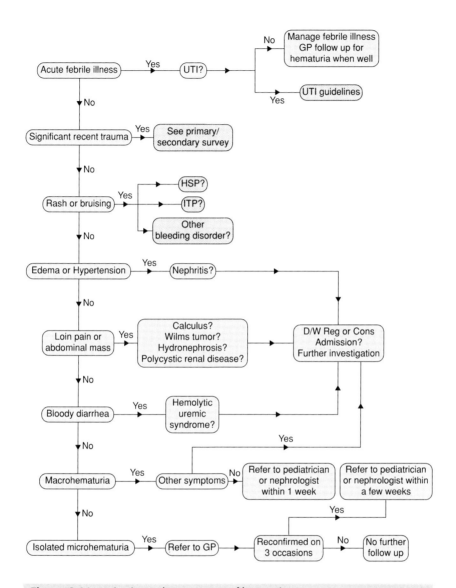

Figure 9.1 Investigation and management of hematuria.

9.5.1 Causes of hypertension

The causes of hypertension break down into essential hypertension and secondary causes.

Secondary causes fall into a few main groups, depending on the system of origin. These include:
- *Renal* (75%): postinfectious glomerulonephritis, chronic glomerulonephritis, obstructive uropathy, reflux nephropathy,

133

Table 9.3 Upper 95th centile for blood pressure

Age (years)	Systolic (mm Hg)	Diastolic (mm Hg)
6	106	64
7	108	72
8	110	76
9	114	80
10	118	82
11	124	82
12	128	84
13	132	84
14	136	86
15	140	88
16	140	90
17	140	92
18	140	92

renovascular, hemolytic uremic syndrome, polycystic kidney disease
- *Cardiovascular* (15%): coarctation of the aorta
- *Endocrine* (5%): pheochromocytoma, hyperthyroidism, congenital adrenal hyperplasia, primary hyperaldosteronism, Cushing syndrome
- *Other* (5%): neuroblastoma, neurofibromatosis, steroid therapy, raised intracranial pressure.

9.5.2 History

The history essentially should contain details of the family history (e.g. pheochromocytoma) and of genitourinary symptoms.

9.5.3 Examination

The examination must include the height and weight, blood pressure measurements of both upper and lower limbs, and a full neurological examination. In addition, *Box 9.1* gives clues to any possible causes of secondary hypertension.

Box 9.1 Causes of secondary hypertension

- *Appearance*: Cushingoid, obese
- *Skin*: café-au-lait spots, neurofibromas, hirsutism, vasculitis
- *Fundoscopy*: hypertensive retinopathy
- *CVS examination*: left ventricular hypertrophy, murmurs (particularly interscapular)
- *Abdomen*: renal/adrenal masses, renal bruits

9.5.4 Investigation

Initial investigations should include:
- urine analysis
- urine microscopy
- blood urea and electrolytes
- creatinine

Further investigations may include:
- urinary catecholamines
- chest X-ray
- ECG
- renal ultrasound
- gluconate scan
- plasma renin pre- and post-captopril
- thyroid function tests
- cortisol/aldosterone levels
- 17-hydroxyprogesterone
- renal angiography.

9.5.5 Management

Asymptomatic hypertension
No urgent treatment is required for asymptomatic hypertension. The child can be investigated and managed as an outpatient and should be referred to the general pediatric outpatient clinic.

Acute severe hypertension
These patients require admission to ICU for urgent treatment. Hypertensive encephalopathy presents as severe headache, visual disturbance and vomiting, progressing to focal neurological deficits, seizures and impaired conscious state, with grossly elevated BP, papilledema and retinal hemorrhages. These patients almost always have chronic renal disease and are on dialysis. The differential diagnosis

includes uremic encephalopathy and metabolic disturbance. BP should be lowered in a controlled fashion, with anticonvulsants given for seizures.

Antihypertensives. The choice includes the drugs listed below, although this is not an exhaustive list:

- *Intravenous labetalol*: 0.2 mg kg^{-1} initially; later by i.v. infusion of labetalol 0.5–3 mg kg^{-1} h^{-1}. It should be avoided if there is heart failure, asthma or bradycardia.
- *Intravenous hydralazine*: 0.1–0.2 mg kg^{-1} (max. 10 mg) stat, then 4–6 micrograms kg^{-1} min^{-1} (max 300 micrograms per min). It may cause tachycardia, nausea and fluid retention.
- *Oral captopril*: 0.1 mg kg^{-1} initially, increasing to a maximum of 1 mg kg^{-1} (max. 50 mg). Thereafter 0.1–1.0 mg kg^{-1} per dose 8-hourly. Captopril is usually effective within 30–60 minutes.

Suggested reading

Chesney, R.W. (1999) The idiopathic nephritic syndrome. *Curr. Opinion Pediatr.* **11**: 158–161.

Gorelick, M.H., Shaw, K.N. (1999) Screening tests for UTIs in children: a meta-analysis. *Pediatrics* **104**: 54.

Chapter 10

Genital problems

Michael Smith and William A. McCallion

Contents

Lower abdominal gynecological pain and menorrhagia are discussed in Chapter 7.

10.1 Penile problems

10.1.1 Phimosis

Phimosis is a tightness of the foreskin so that it cannot be drawn over the glans. It is most logically defined as either physiological or pathological. Physiological phimosis occurs because of the inability to retract infantile foreskin, owing to congenital adhesions between the glans and foreskin. By age 2–3 years, these adhesions break down and retraction becomes possible. However, around 6% of boys still have physiological phimosis at age of 10–11 years. Pathological phimosis occurs when the foreskin cannot be retracted after it has previously been retractable. Clinically this results in ballooning of the foreskin during urination. There may be mild obstruction to urinary flow or recurrent balanitis. Circumcision may be recommended if any of these pathological conditions are present.

10.1.2 Paraphimosis

Paraphimosis is a clinical condition that occurs when the foreskin is retracted and remains proximal to the glans penis. In this position the foreskin becomes progressively swollen due to vascular obstruction and may actually strangulate the glans. This situation will occur after forced retraction of the foreskin (e.g. for catheterization) or vigorous cleaning. If allowed to persist, increasing edema makes reduction progressively more difficult. The usual treatment is manual reduction. A local anesthetic block of the dorsal nerve of the penis is inserted. The foreskin is compressed to reduce the edema and then the foreskin is reduced by pressure on the glans.

Treatment depends on the age and degree of discomfort that the child is experiencing. If the swelling has been present for a prolonged period, then reduction may need to be under conscious sedation. Rarely reduction with accompanying circumcision under general anesthetic is required.

10.1.3 Posthitis/balanitis

Posthitis (inflammation of the prepuce) is more common than balanitis (inflammation of the glans). It is less common in children than in adults. In most cases the cause is infectious in origin although contact irritation, allergy and trauma may also be contributing factors.

The treatment is directed towards the causative organism obtained by swabbing and culture. Mild cases usually respond to twice daily baths with gentle retraction of the foreskin along with a topical antibiotic ointment such as Polysporin. In more severe cases (inflammation involving more than a third of the shaft of the penis), treatment is usually with an oral broad spectrum antibiotic that is effective against uropathogens and staphylococcus (e.g. amoxycillin and clavulinic acid). This is in addition to cleaning and regular baths. These latter simple measures can prevent the recurrence of balanitis.

10.2 Scrotal problems

Acute enlargement or pain in the scrotal area is an important clinical sign as it may signal a surgical emergency. Boys with either of these symptoms need to be seen promptly because of the risk of testicular torsion. Testicular torsion may result in infarction of the testis in 6–12 hours if there is progressive obstruction to the blood supply.

The key questions that direct and inform the management are:
• whether this is a painless or painful problem
• whether it is associated with localized or generalized swelling.

10.2.1 Scrotal pain

Spermatic cord torsion
Torsion is the most important cause of scrotal pain. It is most common in early puberty, but can occur at any age. An unusual attachment of the testis within the tunica vaginalis results in the testis lying transversely and this predisposes to twisting.

Clinically there is an abrupt onset of pain in the testicle often after trauma or exercise. The pain is sharp and is often accompanied by systemic symptoms such as nausea and vomiting. On examination there is a high riding, tender testicle which is made more uncomfortable by elevation. There is a knot of blood vessels at the upper margin, which may be confused with epididymitis. Classically, there is an absent cremasteric reflex on the affected side. If the torsion is allowed to continue, there is increasing scrotal edema and inflammation, which obscure the landmarks.

If there are strong clinical signs of torsion then surgical exploration is indicated. The purpose of surgery is to untwist the affected testicle and anchor the opposite testicle (orchidopexy). Imaging studies are done only when the clinician is sure that torsion does not exist and is seeking supporting evidence. Imaging investigations can be either a nuclear testicular scan or color Doppler sonography. Either is acceptable though sonography is less sensitive.

Torsion of the testicular appendage

There are five vestigial appendages associated with the testis. Torsion can occur of any of them, usually in boys aged 7–12 years. The onset of pain is slow and milder than torsion of the spermatic cord. There are no systemic symptoms but usually only slight swelling of the testis. There may be a bluish discoloration in the upper scrotum ('blue dot sign').

A nuclear scan will show increased blood flow in the upper region, which can be confused with epididymitis. The treatment is usually analgesia, bed rest and scrotal elevation.

Epididymo-orchitis

This condition occurs more commonly in adults and adolescents and is generally rare in children. Inflammation of the epididymi can be viral (adenovirus, mumps or Epstein–Barr virus) or occasionally bacterial in association with anatomical problems of the urinary tract. The possibility of spermatic cord torsion must be considered.

Urinalysis may show mild pyuria. A nuclear scan will show increased blood flow to the epididymis. Treatment is supportive. Antibiotics directed to common urinary pathogens are used when bacterial infection is suspected.

Trauma

Trauma to the scrotum is usually a precisely remembered event in a boy's life. If there is no history, another cause should be sought for scrotal pain. The mechanism of injury is often straddle type such as falling astride a bicycle bar. It is generally rare in prepubertal children because of the small size and mobility of the testes. There is often overlying bruising and, if severe enough, a traumatic hematocele. Surgical evacuation may be required if there is a significant collection of blood. In milder cases, cold compresses and analgesics suffice.

Other causes

The vasculitic process of **Henoch-Schönlein purpura** can involve the spermatic cord and testicle causing acute pain and swelling. Children typically have a purpuric rash on the buttocks and legs, which is diagnostic. Treatment in most circumstances consists of rest and pain relief, although severe testicular swelling may be an indication for steroid treatment.

An **incarcerated inguinal hernia** can also cause acute scrotal pain. There is often a history of intermittent groin swelling, which improves spontaneously. On examination a hernia is detected and cannot be reduced manually. If allowed to persist it can look very much like an acute torsion of the testis with systemic symptoms. Imaging with Doppler sonography or testicular scan can help clarify the cause. Surgical exploration and treatment is required.

10.2.2 Painless scrotal swelling

Hydrocele
Hydrocele is a collection of fluid between the tunica vaginalis and the testicle. In the first year of life the process vaginalis often closes and the hydrocele resolves. It often presents as a clear, bluish swelling in the region of the testicle. If it shrinks with gentle pressure, then there is a hernia component. Surgery is not usually advised before 1 year of age since many spontaneously resolve. If the hydrocele persists, or if there is a hernia component present, then surgery is recommended.

Varicocele
This is a collection of enlarged spermatic cord veins. It is more common in adolescents and on the left side. It is most obvious in the standing position and occasionally causes pain, especially with exertion. In most cases surgery is not required unless there are symptoms of atrophy of the testes (which is rare).

Other causes
An uncomplicated reducible **inguinal hernia** can cause intermittent testicular swelling. This often requires elective surgical repair because of the risk of incarceration.

Acute scrotal edema is a form of urticaria. It starts in the scrotal area and can extend posteriorly. The cause of this is unknown but may include an insect bite allergic reaction, cellulitis or contact dermatitis. Almost all children with this condition are prepubertal. Treatment is symptomatic.

10.3 **Vaginal problems**

10.3.1 Vaginal discharge

Vulvitis
Prepubertal girls have a relative lack of estrogen and are thus prone to vulvitis. It is characterised by an inflamed, irritated vaginal orifice, often with a foul itchy discharge. There can be pain or discomfort on micturition. It can be caused by:

- poor hygiene
- threadworms
- excessive inappropriate washing
- atopic or seborrheic eczema
- specific infections, e.g. streptococcal infection
- rarely candida, only after a course of antibiotics
- sexual abuse

A full history and investigations often provide a few clues to the etiology of the condition. Threadworms are fairly common as a cause of vulval itching, especially at night. Any specific conditions should be treated appropriately and the child and parent should be given advice on appropriate bathing and clothing.

Vulvovaginitis

A girl who has a discharge associated with the vulvitis has vulvovaginitis. The commonest causes vary with the age of the child. Infectious vaginitis is more common in sexually active adolescents and fungal infections are also more common owing to the more acid pH at this age. Children can also acquire infections such as *Chlamydia trachomatis*, gonorrhea and trichomonas via the birth passage or from sexual abuse.

Non-specific vulvovaginitis is most common between the ages of 2 and 6 years, especially in the overweight girl. This has several causes, including:
- infection such as *Staphylococcus aureus*, *Hemophilus influenzae*, *Gardnerella vaginalis*
- sexually transmitted disease
- foreign body (rare)
- non-specific

Child sexual abuse should be borne in mind and excluded if possible (see Chapter 27). Specific infections are treated and general advice given as for vulvitis.

Suggested reading

Brown, M.R., Cartright, P.C., Snow, B.W. (1997) Common office problems in pediatric urology and gynecology. *Pediatr. Clin. N. Am.* **44:** 1091–1115.

Fleisher, G.R., Ludwig, S., Henretig, F.M., Ruddy, R.M., Silverman, B.K. (2000) *Textbook of Pediatric Emergency Medicine* 4th edn. Philadelphia: Lippincott Williams and Wilkins, pp. 1585–1593.

Garden, A.S. (1998) *Pediatric and Adolescent Gynaecology*. London: Arnold.

Kaplan, G.W. (2000) Scrotal swelling in children. *Pediatr. Rev.* **21:** 1–7.

Kass, E.J., Lundak, B. (1997) The acute scrotum. *Pediatr. Clin. N. Am.* **44:** 1251–1265.

Langer, J.C., Coplen, D.E. (1998) Circumcision and pediatric disorders of the penis. *Pediatr. Clin. N. Am.* **45:** 801–812.

Chapter 11

Hematological emergencies

Colin Powell

Contents

11.1 Anemia

11.1.1 Definition

Anemia is defined as hemoglobin less than the lower limit of the reference range for age as shown in *Table 11.1*.

Table 11.1 Lower limits of normal Hb ranges		
Age	**Lower limit of normal range of Hb (g l⁻¹)**	
2 months	90	
2–6 months	95	
6–24 months	105	
2–11 years	115	
> 12 years	Girls – 120	Boys – 130

11.1.2 Symptoms and signs suggestive of anemia

The signs and symptoms of anemia in children are listed in *Box 11.1*.

Box 11.1 Signs and symptoms of anemia
• Pallor • Pale conjunctivae • Flow murmur • Lethargy • Poor growth • Signs of cardiac failure • Weakness • Listlessness • Shortness of breath

11.1.3 Investigation

If anemia is suspected, begin with a full blood examination, blood film and reticulocyte count. Any further investigations will be determined by the blood film appearance. The initial classification is based on the mean corpuscular volume (MCV) (*Table 11.2*).

Table 11.2 Classification of anemia

Cell size	MCV		Classification
Small cells	Low MCV		Iron deficiency anemia Thalassemia
Large cells	High MCV	Megaloblastic	Folate deficiency
		Normoblastic	Hemolysis Liver disease
Normal sized cells	Normal MCV		Acute blood loss Infection Malignancy

11.1.4 Management

You should consider admission with the following factors:
• possible malignancy or infiltrative disorder
• Hb < 6 g l^{-1} (including iron deficiency)
• hemolysis
• child needs transfusion (**where possible defer transfusion until a definitive diagnosis is made**).

11.1.5 Iron deficiency anemia

Iron deficiency is the commonest cause of anemia in children. This microcytic anemia is usually nutritional, owing to insufficient red meat, fish, chicken, green vegetables or pulses, or to excessive cow's milk. It is rarely due to malabsorption or gastrointestinal bleeding. Risk factors include:
• prematurity
• low birth weight
• multiple pregnancy
• exclusive breastfeeding after 6 months of age

Note that iron deficiency can lead to reduced cognitive and psychomotor performance in the absence of anemia.

Treatment of iron deficiency
If the dietary history is strongly suggestive of iron deficiency, the diet should be modified. If Hb is less than 100 g l^{-1}, then iron supplements should be added. Follow up should be arranged to ensure an appropriate response to treatment. If there is a poor response, Hb electrophoresis

should be done to exclude hemoglobinopathies such as thalassemia minor.

Treatment of iron deficiency anemia is shown in *Table 11.3*.

Table 11.3 Treatment of iron deficiency anemia	
Dietary advice	**Iron supplements**
Increase red meat, chicken, fish, pulses, green vegetables	Ferrous gluconate or sulphate according to local guidelines
Limit cow's milk to 500 ml per day	Continue for 3 months after Hb returns to normal to replenish iron stores Add vitamin C to aid absorption
Note: Transfusion rarely required (e.g. cardiac failure, urgent surgery required).	

11.1.6 Hemolytic anemia

Sickle cell disease is a hemolytic anemia associated with crises in homozygous children. Mediterranean, Middle Eastern, Indian, Afro-Caribbean or Afro-American children are mainly affected.

A sickle cell crisis with intra-arterial sickling can cause vasculo-occlusion with infarction of bone and viscera. It presents with pain or other signs of infarction. It is often precipitated by hypoxia or infections, particularly pneumococcal infection. You should search carefully for signs of infection.

Management is with adequate analgesia with intravenous opiates, hydration and bed rest. Transfusion may be required.

Other crises in sickle cell anemia include an **aplastic crisis**, often precipitated by a viral infection, a **hemolytic crisis**, precipitated by viral or bacterial infections, and a **splenic sequestration crisis**, when blood pools in the spleen, especially in younger patients.

Other hemolytic anemias

Hemolytic anemia such as congenital spherocytosis often requires admission and repeat full blood count (FBC) within 6–12 hours to detect continuing hemolysis and the underlying cause.

Investigations should include blood film for red blood cell (RBC) abnormalities (e.g. spherocytosis), Coomb's test, G6PD (glucose-6-phosphate dehydrogenase) deficiency screen, and bilirubin.

11.1.7 Thalassemia minor

Thalassemia minor occurs mainly in South East Asian, Mediterranean and Arabic families. There is often a family history and prepregnancy testing of a partner is important. It is diagnosed on Hb electrophoresis ($HbA_2 > 3.5\%$) and is usually asymptomatic.

Note: *The HbA_2 may not be elevated in the presence of concomitant iron deficiency so a trial of iron therapy should be given before ordering the test.*

11.1.8 Rare causes of microcytic anemia

Rare causes include:
- sideroblastic anemia
- chronic inflammation
- chronic lead poisoning (high blood lead level).

11.1.9 Hypoplastic/aplastic anemia

This occurs in acute leukemia, aplastic anemia and infiltrative disorders but can also be caused by drugs such as cytotoxic agents, chloramphenicol and sulphonamides. It should be considered if the white cells and/or the platelets are depressed. A bone marrow aspirate is usually required to make the diagnosis.

If there is an isolated anemia, you should consider transient erythroblastopenia of childhood (a response to viral infections) or congenital causes such as Diamond–Blackfan syndrome.

11.1.10 Macrocytic anemia

This is very rare in children and is due to vitamin B_{12} or folate deficiency.

11.2 Hemophilia and other bleeding disorders

Bleeding disorders which present to emergency departments include:
- classical hemophilia (hemophilia A), a deficiency of factor VIII inherited as sex-linked recessive disorder
- Christmas disease (hemophilia B), a deficiency of factor IX, inherited as a sex-linked recessive disorder
- von Willebrand disease (hemophilia C), deficiency of von Willebrand factor inherited with both autosomal dominant and recessive patterns.

Hemophilia A and Christmas disease present the same way with easy bruising, bleeding into joints and bleeding from other areas such as mouth, nose and after dental extractions and lacerating wounds.

11.2.1 Management

Many departments have a policy of involving the local hematology department early in the management of any child with hemophilia who presents to the Emergency Department. There are certain important principles in managing patients:

Important general principles
- Individual patient and treatment details may well be held by the patient. Please check them each time the patient presents, as they are liable to change.
- Patients with bleeding disorders have been requested to telephone prior to their arrival. If a telephone call has not been made, triage the patient as promptly as possible.
- Minimise waiting time in Emergency Department.
- Stop bleeding rapidly – it can be dangerous, frightening and painful.
- The arrest of bleeding depends on replacement of the appropriate coagulation factors.

General measures for joint and muscle bleeds
Apply the RICES rules (*Box 11.2*).

Apply these measures to joint bleeds as soon as possible after arrival. They will be continued in the home or hospital.

Analgesia
Paracetamol or a paracetamol/codeine mixture are sufficient in most cases. Aspirin should not be prescribed. If a narcotic is required,

Box 11.2 RICES rules for joint and muscle bleeds
R Rest (in a comfortable position as close to a functional status as possible)
I Ice (cold packs around joints/bleeding sites reduce bleeding and pain)
C (gentle) Compression (bandaging disperses blood and reduces swelling)
E Elevation (of dependant joints to a comfortable position)
S Splint (particularly severe/recurrent bleeds)

morphine or codeine can be given, but the duration of narcotic analgesia should be strictly limited.

Physiotherapy

This commences as soon as pain has subsided and the bleed has been controlled. Direct referral to the physiotherapist for joint and muscle bleeds is essential.

Replacement therapy

Each type of hemophilia has its own specific treatment:

Hemophilia A

- For previously untreated patients and for children who are HCVab negative, treat with recombinant factor VIII 30 IU kg^{-1}. Do not discard any factor VIII – give in multiples of 250 IU. Dosage can be rounded up or down to nearest 250 IU but give the full bottle.
- For all other patients use high purity factor VIII AHF 30 IU kg^{-1}.
- Patients with mild to moderate hemophilia (factor VIII > 3%) may need DDAVP 0.3 µg kg^{-1} (0.5 µg per 20 ml of 0.9% NaCl) i.v. over 20 minutes. Severe bleeds from trauma etc. may require treatment with factor VIII – contact the hematologist.
- Patients with inhibitors to factor VIII and factor IX are treated with recombinant factor VIIa 180 µg kg^{-1}.

Dosage and 'treatable bleed criteria'. Any other bleed possibly requiring treatment should be discussed with the hematologist and confirmed by ultrasound or MRI. Novo VIIa is not effective for hematuria or urinary tract bleeds.

Use universal precautions in the administration of coagulation products. Dispose of all needles, syringes and bottles in a sharps container. Patients who require treatment in the Emergency Department and are then discharged home should be followed up and reviewed within 24 hours or earlier should the need arise. Retreatment may be required.

In children with a joint bleed, use the RICES rules as above. Joint bleeds should be immobilized with a back slab or sling etc., and referred to physiotherapy.

In a case of head injury involving a fall from a height or road traffic accident, treat with a single dose of 60 IU kg^{-1} factor VIII and admit to the hospital if there is any suspicion of concussion or persistent headache or vomiting. For minor knocks to the head, such as contact with furniture or doors, factor VIII might not be needed.

Hemophilia B (Christmas disease). See the comments above for hemophilia A. For patients with Christmas disease, give Monofix 60 IU kg^{-1} i.v. The treatment product comes in bottles of 500 units. Round dose off to nearest 500 and **do not** discard any product. Give second dose, if necessary, 24 hours later.

Note: *Patients with previous allergic reactions or inhibitors are treated with Novo 7a (see above under factor VIII inhibitors).*

von Willebrand disease. See the other comments above. In type I disease, give DDAVP 0.3 μg kg^{-1} i.v. over 20 minutes. Patients with type IIA and IIB disease need plasma-derived factor VIII AHF 30–50 IU kg^{-1}. Patients with pseudo von Willebrand disease (rare) should not be treated with factor VIII concentrate and, if bleeding is severe, they may require platelet transfusion.

Admission
Admission is required for several presentations (*Box 11.3*).

Antifibrinolytic therapy
Patients with oral mucosal bleeds and epistaxes may receive antifibrinolytic therapy for 5–7 days after appropriate factor replacement. Antifibrinolytic therapy such as tranexamic acid (*Table 11.4*) can be used in other situations, for example following dental extraction, but only after discussion with a consultant.

Antifibrinolytic agents are contraindicated for the treatment of hematuria.

Box 11.3 Children needing admission for bleeding disorders

- Suspected intracranial hemorrhage
- Bleeding into the hip or inguinal area
- Persistent mouth bleeding not responding to 60 units kg^{-1} factor VIII and Cyklokapron
- Forearm bleed with persistent hand pain/suspicion of Volkmann ischaemic contracture
- Persistent hematuria
- Bleeding into the neck
- Severe persistent epistaxis
- Tonsillar hemorrhage
- Undiagnosed abdominal pain
- Tight soft tissue bleeds
- Suspected psoas hemorrhage

Table 11.4 Dose table of tranexamic acid

Weight (kg)	Cyklokapron
10–25	250 mg t.d.s.
25–35	500 mg t.d.s.
35–50	750 mg t.d.s.
> 50	1 g t.d.s.

Tranexamic acid: 500 mg tablets, 15–20 mg kg^{-1} per dose t.d.s. orally is used.

11.3 Idiopathic thrombocytopenic purpura (ITP)

11.3.1 Background

ITP is an acquired thrombocytopenia from immune-mediated shortened circulating platelet survival in the absence of other disturbances of hemostasis or coagulation. In most childhood ITP, platelet autoantibodies are absent. Most children present with bruising and petechie alone. In some instances there is oral bleeding, epistaxis, rectal bleeding or hematuria. Morbidity in ITP is usually minimal. The incidence of intracranial hemorrhage is less than 1%.

Patients fall broadly into two categories:
- Acute (about 90%): a self-limiting disease (sometimes preceded by a viral syndrome) with spontaneous resolution within 6 months (usually within 2 months)
- Chronic (about 10%): does not remit within 6 months.

11.3.2 Assessment

The clinical diagnosis of ITP depends on there being manifestations of thrombocytopenia without other abnormal findings, in particular no pallor, lymphadenopathy or hepatosplenomegaly. Confirmation rests on the adequate exclusion of other causes of thrombocytopenia. The most important conditions to exclude are acute leukemia, other marrow infiltrative conditions and aplastic anemia. An FBC and blood film will usually confirm the diagnosis. A bone marrow aspirate is an invasive procedure with some morbidity in children who bruise easily, and is only necessary if the diagnosis is uncertain.

11.3.3 Management

Initial treatment options include no treatment and oral steroids. Without active treatment, most patients' platelet counts will return to a level at which normal activity can be recommended within 4–6 weeks.

Conservative outpatient management

Most patients with a platelet count over $20\,000 \times 10^6 l^{-1}$ and some of those with a platelet count less than $20\,000 \times 10^6 l^{-1}$ can be managed as outpatients with no specific treatment. The following criteria must be met:

- The diagnosis is unequivocal. No pallor, hepatosplenomegaly or lymphadenopathy; isolated thrombocytopenia without anemia, leucopenia or blood film changes.
- There is no active bleeding. Bruising and petechie in isolation, without mucosal, gastrointestinal or renal tract bleeding.
- The child is otherwise well.
- Social circumstances allow confidence about the degree of parental supervision and relative safety of the home environment, particularly for younger children.
- There is ample opportunity for parental reassurance and education in the Emergency Department.
- Follow up is guaranteed within a few days by the on-call general pediatric consultant, who must be contacted and agree with the management plan.

Conservative inpatient management

If the diagnosis of ITP is not certain (e.g. the blood film result is not available) or any other of the above criteria are not met, then admit under the consultant pediatrician following up the child. The decision as to whether to treat patients who do not have active bleeding should be made by the consultant.

Treatment as an inpatient

Any patient with ITP who has active bleeding (oral, aural, nasal, rectal, etc.) even if resolved should be admitted and given oral prednisolone (2–$4\,\mathrm{mg\,kg^{-1}}$ per day for 2 weeks then tapered). Normal human immunoglobulin is also effective but is not usually used for initial treatment. Avoid aspirin and non-steroidal anti-inflammatory drugs.

11.3.4 Acute, relapsing ITP

In some cases, thrombocytopenia will redevelop months or years after the first episode has resolved. These relapses or recurrences are usually precipitated by viral infections. Provided the first episode remitted spontaneously without complication and the patient has been well with a documented normal platelet count between episodes, these cases can be managed as for acute ITP.

11.3.5 Chronic ITP

Ongoing thrombocytopenia after a 6-month period denotes chronic ITP. A history of bruising from infancy should prompt suspicion of one of the rare congenital thrombocytopenias. Careful inspection of the blood film and tests of platelet function will serve to exclude other diagnoses. Bone marrow examination is helpful in confirming chronic ITP. Rarely, splenectomy is required (success rate 70–80%).

11.4 Henoch-Schönlein purpura (HSP)

HSP typically presents with the triad of:
- purpuric rash on the extensor surfaces of limbs (mainly lower) and buttocks
- joint pain/swelling
- abdominal pain.

Abdominal pain or arthralgia sometimes precedes the rash. The commonest age group is 2–8 years. The cause is unknown but there may be a recent history of an upper respiratory tract infection.

11.4.1 Assessment

- **Purpura.** If atypical distribution or the child is unwell, consider meningococcemia, thrombocytopenia, or other rare vasculitides.
- **Joint pain.** Swelling and arthralgia of large joints are often the patient's main complaint. In most situations this pain resolves spontaneously within 24–48 hours.
- **Abdominal pain.** Uncomplicated abdominal pain often resolves spontaneously within 72 hours. However, serious abdominal complications may occur including intussusception, bloody stools, hematemesis, spontaneous bowel perforation, and pancreatitis.
- **Renal disease.** Hematuria is present in 90% of cases, but only 5% are persistent or recurrent. Less common renal manifestations include proteinuria, nephrotic syndrome, isolated hypertension, renal insufficiency and renal failure (< 1%). Renal involvement may only present during the convalescent period.
- **Subcutaneous edema** (scrotum, hands, feet, sacrum). This can be very painful.
- **Rare complications.** Pulmonary and central nervous system involvement.

11.4.2 Investigations

Urine analysis should be performed, and if hematuria is present the sample should be sent for microscopy to quantify the RBC count. Other investigations may include:
• full blood count
• urea, electrolytes with creatinine
• blood culture

11.4.3 Management

All patients presenting with a purpuric rash must be seen by a consultant or registrar, even if the child does not appear unwell.
• Document the child's blood pressure.
• Consider a surgical consult if abdominal features are prominent. Testicular torsion can be hard to differentiate from the pain of vasculitic testicular pain.
• There are some data to support the use of prednisolone. It may prevent the development of long-term renal complications. Consider prednisolone 1 mg kg^{-1} for 2 weeks in all cases (not just those with hematuria). The use of prednisolone will also treat abdominal and joint pain and is particularly helpful for the edema.

11.4.4 Indications for admission

These will include:
• abdominal complication – arrange early surgical consultation.
• renal complication, e.g. nephritis, nephrotic syndrome

Also consider admission for symptomatic treatment of the following:
• severe joint pain – treatment is bed rest and analgesia
• abdominal pain
• painful subcutaneous edema.

11.4.5 Disposition

If the child is discharged from the Emergency Department, then it is imperative that appropriate follow up is arranged to ensure adequate symptom control and resolution of the disease. Short-term support can occur in the Emergency Department but follow up care should soon be transferred to the child's doctor (emphasise the need for ongoing BP and urine review in the letter) or a pediatrician – an appointment can be made in the general medical outpatient clinic. The rash is usually the last manifestation to remit and appears to worsen if the child is very active. As the renal involvement can present up to 6 months after the initial presentation, the urine should be checked regularly for that period. BP should be checked twice during that time. If the child has persistent renal involvement, refer to a pediatrician or pediatric nephrologist for long-term follow up. Some recommend an annual BP and urinalysis for life.

11.5 Febrile neutropenia

11.5.1 Assessment

All febrile hematology and oncology patients attending the Emergency Department should be discussed with the emergency registrar/consultant and the hematology consultant on call.

Note:
- All febrile neutropenic children should be triaged as category 2 or 3. This includes oncology patients who have received chemotherapy in the past 5–14 days and other children with recurrent neutropenia. These children are at increased risk of serious bacterial infection.
- In general, in patients with neutrophil counts of less than $500\,mm^{-3}$, fever more than 38.5°C is an indication for starting empirical antibiotics after taking appropriate cultures.
- The greater the degree of neutropenia and the longer the expected duration of neutropenia, the greater the risk of bacteremia.

Take a history and examine the child, with particular attention to possible sites of infection (*Box 11.4*).

Look for signs associated with anemia and/or thrombocytopenia.

Box 11.4 Possible sites of infection in febrile neutropenia

- Upper Respiratory Tract Infection
- Cuts, abrasions, skin sores
- Dental sepsis
- Inflamed Hickman site
- Mouth ulcers including herpetic
- Anal fissures
- Embolic phenomena of septicemia/bacterial endocarditis (especially if central line is *in situ*)
- Lower Respiratory Tract Infection especially *pneumocystis carinii* pneumonia (fever, cough, tachypnoea, desaturation; chest clear to auscultation; interstitial infiltrate on X-ray)
- Gastrointestinal tract including typhilitis (colonic wall inflammation especially cecum; abdominal tenderness)

11.5.2 Management

All children with a febrile neutropenia should be admitted urgently to the appropriate ward and the hematology consultant should be notified of their admission. Do not delay admission or antibiotics while waiting for results of laboratory investigations unless the consultant advises this. Never administer PR medications. Gain vascular access. If an indwelling central venous line is present, it can be accessed by appropriately trained nursing staff from the Emergency Department or ward for blood sampling and administration of antibiotics.

If there will be a delay of more than 30 minutes before a line can be inserted in the Emergency Department, some hospitals have a policy whereby the child is transferred immediately to the ward.

11.5.3 Investigations

Always do:
• blood cultures – central line and peripheral
• FBC and differential count

If indicated, do:
• urine for microscopy, culture and sensitivities (M/C/S)
• sputum for M/C/S in older children
• chest X-ray (may be no changes while neutropenic)
• cross-match
• stool for M/C/S and viral studies.

Note: *Lumbar puncture is contraindicated as there is often concomitant thrombocytopenia.*

11.5.4 Initial antibiotics

This may vary from unit to unit. All patients should be treated with combination antibiotics. Each department will have its own policy for this.

Note:
• Patients with neutrophil counts of over 1000 mm^{-3} have an increased risk of bacterial infection, principally endogenously acquired from skin, nose and throat or gastrointestinal tract flora.
• Patients with lower grade fevers or higher neutrophil counts, who have evidence of viral infection or a clear localized site such as otitis

media, may be observed carefully or treated with an appropriate oral antibiotic. They should be reviewed over the next 24 hours.

• Patients with persistent fevers may require i.v. antibiotics.

Further reading

Buchanan, G.R. (2000) Idiopathic thrombocytopenic purpura in childhood. *Pediatri. Ann.* **30**(9): 527–533.

Gadner, H. (2001) Management of immune thrombocytopenic purpura in children. *Rev. Clin. Exp. Hematol.* **5**(3): 201–210.

Santagostino, E. Gringeri, A. Mannucci, P. M. (2002) State of care for hemophilia in pediatric patients. *Rev. Pediatr. Drugs* **4**(3): 149–5.

Sadowitz, P.D. Amanullah, S., Souid, A.K. (2002) Hematologic emergencies in the pediatric emergency room. *Emerg. Med. Clin. N. Am.* **20**(1): 177–98.

Chapter 12

Psychiatric emergencies

Patricia O. Brennan

Contents

12.1 Introduction

The Emergency Department is used for psychiatric emergencies in childhood as well as for other emergencies. The patient must be assessed adequately, the emergency aspects of the condition managed and appropriate referral made for more long-term care. The psychiatric emergency situation arises when the adults in the family are no longer able to provide the support and control to help the child with his or her emotions. The fact that this has precipitated an Emergency Department attendance denotes the fact that the child and family have accepted that there is a problem for which help is needed.

The commonest types of emergency psychiatric presentations to a pediatric Emergency Department are:
- conduct disorders
- depression
- suicide attempts and self harm
- somatic presentations of psychological problems
- behavioral problems
  - excessive crying in infants
  - sleep problems
- psychosis
  - organic psychosis
  - psychiatrically based psychoses

12.2 Psychiatric assessment in the Emergency Department

A thorough assessment should be done in every psychiatric emergency presentation (*Box 12.1*). It should seek to determine the following:
- symptoms and type of problem
- impact on the child, e.g. level of distress and impairment of functioning
- risks to child, e.g. of suicide
- strengths of child and family
- beliefs and expectations of child and family

It is important that the child and family are seen together and then the child and family each have time to talk to the doctor on their own.

12.3 Psychosis

This can be organically or psychiatrically based. It presents with alterations in thinking, agitation and confusion, and bizarre distorted thoughts.

Box 12.1 Assessment in psychiatric problems

Relevant history
- history of present crisis, including emotional and behavioral symptoms
- apparent precipitating factors
- past episodes and treatment
- major psychosocial problems, including child abuse
- school performance
- medical history, past and present
- family history, including composition, health of members and interpersonal relationships
- family evaluation, including competences and strengths
- history of drug abuse

Clinical signs
- physical examination and investigations to exclude a medical cause for the presentation
- assessment of mental status
  - behavior
  - orientation
  - memory
  - speech: manner and content
  - affect
  - cognition

Organic psychosis has many causes (*Box 12.2*). If it is suspected, the screening investigations should include the following:
- Blood tests
  - full blood count
  - urea and electrolytes
  - calcium
  - glucose
  - toxicology including alcohol screens
  - lead
  - thyroid function tests
- Urinalysis including toxicology

Adult-type schizophrenia occasionally presents to the Emergency Department in a child with a flat affect, auditory hallucinations, delusions and illogical thinking. The child may be hearing commands to commit suicide or be violent to others.

> **Box 12.2** Types of psychosis
>
> **Organic psychosis**
> - CNS lesions e.g. trauma
> - metabolic causes
>   - hypoglycemia
>   - electrolyte imbalance
> - pharmacological causes
>   - substance abuse
>   - side effects of medication
>   - intentional overdose
>
> **Psychiatrically based psychoses**
> - infantile autism
> - pervasive developmental disorders
> - adult–type schizophrenia
> - manic depressive illness

Emergency management includes treatment for the immediate medical condition, controlling the child's behavior with relief of distress and fear, and referral to the psychiatric services for admission or other longer term care.

12.4 Conduct disorders

These do not often present at the Emergency Department *per se*, but the staff may have to cope with children with these problems. Children with socially unacceptable behavior such as violence and aggression can be a risk to themselves, staff and the general public. Support from security staff may be needed. The behavior often stems from poor adjustment at home when the child has not had adequate or consistent limit setting. It is important for the Emergency Department physician to exclude underlying substance abuse, medical illness or severe psychiatric disorder as a cause of the behavior.

12.5 Depression

Depression does occur in childhood and adolescence. It is different from ordinary sadness in degree, persistence and quality of mood, and may be associated with other symptoms such as low self-esteem, poor concentration, low energy, altered appetite and weight and suicidal thoughts. There may be a genetic predisposition plus the trigger of environmental factors. Its links with hidden factors such as sexual abuse must be remembered.

It can appear in different guises at different ages. Infants may have apathy, poor feeding and weight loss, often as a result of loss of a mother or from poor nurturing. Older children and adolescents can experience mood change or somatic symptoms such as abdominal pain, headache, school avoidance or underachievement, and even alcohol and substance abuse. There is a rising incidence with puberty. Many affected young people also have at least one other psychiatric disorder, such as an anxiety or conduct disorder. Assessment in older children must involve assessment of suicidal potential; direct questioning is not likely to precipitate an event but rather give the child relief by bringing the topic out into the open. Psychiatric help should be sought urgently for those with suicidal intent and less urgently for those without.

12.6 Specific problems

12.6.1 Self-harm

Suicide attempts and episodes of self-harm are relatively common and increasing causes of Emergency Department presentation. In the USA the suicide rate amongst adolescents aged 15–19 years has risen by 44% since 1970. This trend has also occurred in the UK and it is reported that the incidence of child attempts is five times more common than meningitis. Young children imagine death as reversible.

Suicide attempts are usually by ingestion of tablets and are three times more common in girls, although boys succeed twice as often as girls. Boys more often use the more violent and more lethal means such as shooting and hanging.

Characteristics associated with childhood suicide attempts include low self esteem, depression, other psychiatric disorders and hopelessness. Family problems such as alcohol and substance abuse, depressive illness and suicide attempts and disrupted home circumstances are also predisposing factors. Particularly high risk times for the child are just after a suicide threat or attempt, after aggressive or violent behavior, after an argument or rift with friends and after a disciplinary episode with parents or police. Serious suicide intent is characterized by premeditation with proper preparation including a suicide note, timed to prevent discovery and carried out in isolation so that intervention is unlikely.

Any child who presents with self-harm needs an assessment by both the emergency physician and the psychiatrist. Admission may be necessary, particularly if the attempt was serious, if the child still feels suicidal, if there is difficulty in getting cooperation from child or family, or if the child has an underlying chronic disorder.

Roughly 10% of young people who deliberately self-harm will do it again within 1 year and roughly 1% will subsequently kill themselves. The previously well-adjusted child has a good prognosis, while those with pre-existing or on-going psychiatric disorders and family psychopathology have a poor prognosis.

12.6.2 Substance abuse

This is widespread, particularly in adolescence and includes the use of substances such as tobacco, alcohol, solvent inhalation, cannabis and heroin.

- *Tobacco* use leads to dependence. Its use is common in the young.
- *Alcohol*, sanctioned for adults in society, is commonly taken by older children and adolescents, often in excess and is associated with antisocial behavior. These cases are brought unconscious into the Emergency Department.
- *Cannabis* may be used as an occasional recreational drug when it rarely causes dependence. Some users may become chronic users, however.
- *Inhaled solvents* used regularly can cause brain and liver damage. Aerosol propellants can also be harmful and can lead to death from respiratory or cardiac arrest.
- *Other drugs* such as heroin and cocaine are used much more rarely in adolescence and their use is often associated with pre-existing major psychological and social problems.

After emergency treatment the child should be assessed to find any underlying treatable social or psychiatric cause for the behavior, such as peer pressure, parent–child relationship problems or escaping from pressures of life, including boredom. Psychiatric referral is necessary if there are severe underlying psychiatric problems or if the substance becomes central to the patient's life with social dysfunction and physical damage.

12.6.3 School refusal

School refusal or avoidance is different from truancy (a conduct disorder) and is fairly common. It often occurs at the start of a new school or following a school absence with illness, bereavement or holiday. It is commonest after the summer break. The parents are aware of the child's absences and unfortunately tend to support the child in this.

It can present with recurrent somatic complaints for which no organic cause can be found. Many of the physical symptoms (absent at weekends and during holiday periods) are similar to those in depressed children, such as apathy, insomnia, tension headaches, dizziness and gastrointestinal symptoms with nausea and abdominal pain.

Assessment involves a good medical examination and a minimum of baseline laboratory investigation. Thereafter the physician should firmly tell the child and parent that there is no serious illness and that return to school is the best option. The parents need to be convinced that this is so, as they are the ones who will continue to support the child and maintain the school attendance. The longer the absence from school, the greater number of additional problems such as falling behind with work and loss of contact with friends. Support from teaching staff will also be needed.

12.6.4 Excessive crying in infancy

Infants who cry persistently are brought to the Emergency Department as their exhausted parents are at the end of their tether. These infants also often feed poorly and have a disturbed sleep pattern. The parent feels less and less secure and confident in their own ability to feed and calm the child, and may eventually feel so frustrated that they have ideas of harming the child. Although the child is medically well, this situation is a very real emergency situation for the family and must be managed as such by the physician.

The stress on the parents and the efforts that they have already put in must be acknowledged. The parents need to know that the problem is relatively common and that it is related to the temperament of the child. They should be given simple advice such as not overstimulating the child and how to feed and comfort calmly. For those parents who are not too exhausted and who have family or other social support networks, referral for long-term management by a community team is appropriate. For those who are isolated or exhausted, a short admission may be helpful, to allow the parents to get some rest and then assume the caring role again in a supportive environment (see also Chapter 15).

12.6.5 Sleep disorders

The sleep pattern of infants and young children varies. Most sleep through the night from an early age but some appear to need very little sleep or, particularly from 12–24 months, may wake regularly through the night. The causes (and therefore the remedy) are unclear but are thought to be high activity and increased irritability levels, and it is associated with stress within the family and maternal depression.

Management involves a thorough medical examination to assure the parents that there is nothing medically wrong with the child. They should be reassured that the disturbed sleep pattern settles. Sedatives are rarely effective and referral to a primary care or community team for behavioral management may be needed for severe cases.

12.6.6 Recurrent abdominal pain

Recurrent abdominal pain lasting a few hours and occasionally accompanied by vomiting and headache is common in young children. It has been called periodic syndrome or abdominal migraine. It may be precipitated by stress and relieved by rest and is thought to be more common in children with very anxious mothers.

12.6.7 Hysteria

Hysteria can present as hyperventilation and tetany or as abnormal illness behavior such as a limp or paralysis. After emergency treatment and exclusion of an underlying somatic disorder, there must be an assessment of underlying cause or anxiety.

12.6.8 Tics

Tics are common in primary school children, but most disappear spontaneously. Late onset and multiple tic disorders should be referred for a psychiatric opinion.

12.7 Post-traumatic stress disorder

Only a minimum of children who experience a traumatic event will have a disabling stress reaction. However, it is being increasingly realized that a significant proportion do have some reaction (*Box 12.3*).

Box 12.3 Characteristics of PTSD in children

- Prolonged response (at least 1 month after incident)
- Intrusive memories
- Dreams
- Anxious/altered behavior, e.g. clingy, refusal to go to bed
- Avoidance of reminders of incident
- Psychological regression e.g. return of enuresis, soiling
- Physical symptoms, e.g. headaches, abdominal pain
- Re-experiencing incident through play or drawing

It is important for the emergency physician to recognise this and to make the attendance at the Emergency Department for any child as least traumatic as possible, to prevent this distress being superimposed on the trauma of the event itself. A child's reaction to trauma may be:

- Short term
  - distress, fear, crying
  - a need for comfort and protection
- Medium–long term
  - repetitive intrusive thoughts of the accident either when quiet or when reminded of it
  - sleep disturbance, nightmares, fear of the dark or going to sleep alone
  - separation difficulties, especially from parents
  - anger and irritability
  - survivor guilt
  - difficulty in talking about the event
  - concentration and memory problems
  - depression, panic attacks

Any child suffering from significant problems should be referred for psychiatric help.

12.8 Emergency restraint

12.8.1 Principles

Physical restraint and emergency sedation should be used only when other reasonable methods of calming the patient down are unsuccessful. They are rarely used. If a patient who is acting out does not need acute medical or psychiatric care, she or he should be discharged from the hospital rather than restrained. This guideline is based on guidelines produced by the Royal Children's Hospital, Melbourne.

When restraint is required, a coordinated team approach is essential, with roles clearly defined and swift action taken. Unless contraindicated, sedation should usually accompany physical restraint.

12.8.2 Indications

Aggressive and combative behavior in a patient requires urgent medical or psychiatric care. This behavior might:

- compromise the provision of urgent medical treatment (physical or psychiatric)
- place the patient at risk of self-harm
- place staff at risk.

12.8.3 Alternative means of calming a patient

Alternative means of calming a patient to be considered before restraint and sedation are used are listed in *Box 12.4*).

Box 12.4 Alternative means of calming a patient

- Crisis prevention: anticipate and identify early irritable behavior (plus past history)
- Involve mental health early for assistance (intake worker; after hours on-call psychiatric registrar)
- Provide a safe 'containing' environment. This includes a confident reassuring approach by staff without added stimuli
- Listen and talk
- Offer planned 'collaborative' sedation, e.g. oral

12.8.4 Contraindications to restraint

The contraindications to restraint include:
- safe containment via alternative means
- inadequate staff/setting/equipment
- situation judged to be too dangerous, e.g. patient has a weapon
- known adverse reaction to drugs usually used, e.g. neuroleptic malignant syndrome

If staff do not think that they will be able to safely restrain the patient, or manage the threat, then Police should be called.

12.8.5 Procedure

The roles of personnel present should be established, and the person in charge defined. This will usually be the attending doctor.
1. The person in charge assembles a team of seven people, usually from the Emergency Department, including psychiatric nurse and adolescent unit registrar, patient service assistants and security.
2. The drugs are drawn up. The preferred drugs are midazolam 5 mg, haloperidol 5 mg drawn up together. Benztropine should be available.
3. The patient is secured quickly and calmly. At least five people are required, one for the head and one for each limb to hold the patient prone with hands and feet held flexed behind the back.
4. Midazolam 5 mg (onset rapid) and haloperidol 5 mg (onset 15–20 minutes) are given by i.m. injection into the lateral thigh. Beware the risk of needlestick injury.

5. Further titrated doses of midazolam 0.1 mg kg^{-1} may be required (preferable i.v.).
6. Sedated patients must have:
   - continuous presence of a nurse
   - continuous O$_2$ saturation monitoring
   - close observation of conscious state, heart rate, blood pressure and temperature

Complications of emergency sedation include:
- anaphylactic reactions
- respiratory depression
- cardiovascular complications such as hypotension and tachycardia
- extrapyramidal reaction (dystonia) with major tranquillisers, particularly as the benzodiazepine is wearing off. This is treated with benzotropine 0.02 mg kg^{-1} i.v. or i.m. or by repeated small doses of diazepam.

The procedure should be explained to the parents if possible. After restraint, the patient must have a complete medical and mental health assessment, involving the child psychiatric team, to guide subsequent management. The need for on-going restraint should also be considered.

Further reading

Fleischer, G.R., Ludwig, S. (1996) *Synopsis of Pediatric Emergency Medicine.* Williams and Wilkins, Philadelphia.
Goodman, R., Scott, S. (1997) *Child Psychiatry.* Oxford: Blackwell Science.

Chapter 13

Dermatological emergencies

Patricia O. Brennan

Contents

13.1 Introduction

Many children with rashes are brought to the Emergency Department by their parents. The underlying diagnoses are only occasionally of serious conditions, but rashes do evoke enormous anxiety in parents, often either because they fear a serious illness, particularly meningococcal disease or because the rash, particularly in the parents' eyes, is disfiguring.

13.2 Atopic eczema

Atopic eczema is an inherited tendency associated with other atopic states (of asthma, hay fever and urticaria), with type 1 hypersensitivity reactions and raised IgE in 80% of affected patients. It is chronic and relapsing, often worse in winter and in times of stress and is estimated to occur in approximately 10% of children in the UK.

13.2.1 Clinical presentation

The clinical presentation includes an acute picture with erythema, itching and vesicles which ooze and crust, and a chronic phase with thickened dry skin. The distribution varies with age (*Box 13.1*).

Most cases of atopic eczema are diagnosed and managed in General Practice. However, the eczema can become acutely infected with bacteria, especially staphylococcus or with viruses such as herpes simplex and *molluscum contagiosum*.

13.2.2 Management

Infected eczema must be treated promptly, bacterial infections with oral antibiotics, guided by culture of swabs, and eczema herpeticum with

---

Box 13.1 Common distribution of atopic eczema in children

Young infants
- cheeks
- perioral

Crawling infants
- sites of friction, e.g. dorsum of ankles, extensor aspect of knees

Toddler
- flexural creases of elbows and knees

antiviral treatment such as Acyclovir. Emollients and steroids are useful in acute eczema. Dilute hydrocortisone (1%) is usually adequate and this is the only strength which should be used on the face. Stronger steroid preparations may occasionally be used elsewhere. Management of severe eczema is demanding and these children should be under the long-term care of a dermatologist with a specialist team of nurses.

13.3 Bacterial infections

These are common in childhood, the commonest being impetigo.

13.3.1 Impetigo

This is a very common bacterial infection, almost always due to *Staphylococcus aureus*, but sometimes Group B β hemolytic streptococcus. It consists of annular lesions, often with bullae or honey colored crusts. It usually occurs on the face but can occur anywhere on the body and can spread rapidly. Mild cases can be treated with topical antibiotics such as fucidin, but with more severe or more widespread lesions, oral antistaphylococcal antibiotics such as flucloxacillin are required.

13.3.2 Staphylococcal scalded skin syndrome

This is a severe condition, also caused by staphylococcal disease, requiring urgent treatment. It is due to the generalized effects of the toxin of a coagulase-positive staphylococcus from a focus of infection and is most common in babies. Clinically, the child is systemically unwell, with a pyrexia. The skin becomes tender, red and edematous. The epidermis separates causing superficial, thin-walled vesicles or bullae, which rupture easily, leaving large denuded areas.

Treatment is with systemic antistaphylococcal antibiotics such as flucloxacillin or a cephalosporin together with general supportive treatment such as fluids.

13.3.3 Cellulitis

This is a deeper infection of the skin, often caused by a streptococcus, in an unwell, febrile child. It can occur around an infected wound but the route of infection can be obscure. Treatment with systemic antibiotics is required. (See also sections on orbital and pre-orbital cellulitis in Chapter 24.)

13.3.4 Meningococcal septicemia

This life-threatening illness caused by *Neisseria meningitidis* involves many organs, most commonly the meninges. The illness can present in a relatively well child with small purpuric papules. The child can then rapidly become severely ill. Disseminated intravascular coagulation and adrenal hemorrhage are both serious complications.

Immediate systemic high dose antibiotics (penicillin or a cephalosporin) are needed. (See also Chapter 6 section on meningitis).

13.4 Infestations

13.4.1 Scabies

This is a common infestation caused by the human mite, *Sarcoptes scabeii*. The pregnant female burrows through the stratum corneum leaving linear burrows. She then lays her eggs, which hatch after 10–14 days. Itching and rash do not appear for up to 3 weeks after the patient has been affected. The mite can be spread during this time. The linear burrows occur on wrist, interdigital webs of hands and feet, elbows, scrotum and on the palms and soles. In addition, there is a widespread itchy dermatosis with erythematous papules and pustules.

The treatment regimen means simultaneous treatment of all family members and close contacts. Some scabicides are irritant or toxic. However, permethrin 5% cream and malathion 0.5% are well tolerated. They kill the mite immediately but the itching persists. Topical lubricants may be necessary for some weeks as the antiscabetic treatment dries the skin and can increase the itching. Clothes and bedding must be washed on a hot machine wash to kill the mites.

13.4.2 Head lice

Infestation with *Pediculus humanus capitis* is especially common in white schoolchildren in the UK and is spread by head–head contact. The child experiences itching of the scalp and the nape of the neck. In mild infestations, the lice are often not found, but the white empty egg cases (nits) attached near the base of the hairs are visible.

Treatment involves removal of the lice and the nits with a fine-toothed comb. Malathion 0.5%, carbamyl 0.5%, permethrin lotion or shampoo can be used but resistance has been reported. Repeat treatment in 7 days may be needed. Clothes and bedding should be put through a hot machine wash to kill any lice.

13.5 Viral infections

13.5.1 Herpes simplex infections

Most infections in children are due to the herpes hominis virus (HSV) type 1, but a few, resulting from sexual abuse may be caused by herpes simplex virus type 2.

Primary infections
Primary infections in infants and young children can occur as:
• herpetic gingivostomatitis, a self limiting illness of 7–14 days with fever, irritability, vesicles and shallow painful ulcers over the gums, tongue, lips and buccal mucosa
• herpetic whitlow with groups of tense blisters
• clusters of vesicles which rupture and crust over 5–7 days and heal over 10–14 days on any cutaneous or mucous membrane.

Recurrent infections
The virus can persist in nerve ganglia and become reactivated by a number of triggers such as ultraviolet light, stress or surgery. Common sites are lips, cheeks and around the eyes. These lesions are contagious. The corneal infection is serious and can lead to blindness.

Oral Acyclovir or fancyclovir are effective for gingivostomatitis. Topical Acyclovir may prevent spread of the virus. Herpes keratitis should be referred for ophthalmological opinion.

13.5.2 Herpes zoster

Herpes zoster is caused by the DNA virus human herpes virus 3 (HHV-3), in children who have previously had varicella. It is more common in immunocompromised children and may be the presenting complaint in acquired immune deficiency syndrome and rarely in childhood cancer.

Clinical presentation
After an incubation period of 10–27 days, groups of vesicles develop along two to three adjacent dermatomes, most commonly in the thoracic area, sometimes with intense pruritis. Prodromal dermatomal pain and post-zoster neuralgia are both rare in children. Herpes zoster keratitis occasionally occurs in ophthalmic herpes zoster and motor paralysis may also occur, particularly with involvement of the geniculate ganglion (Ramsay–Hunt syndrome). Most children have a mild illness lasting 7–10 days, but immunocompromised children may develop disseminated disease 1–5 days after the dermatome infection.

Herpes zoster can be confused with other infections (*Table 13.1*).

Table 13.1 Differential diagnosis of a bullous rash

Differential diagnosis	Differentiating features
Varicella	More generalized
Hand foot and mouth disease	On palms, soles, and buccal mucosa
Vesicular reaction to insect bites	History of bites
Dermatitis herpetiformis	Generalized
Herpes simplex virus	Usually single cluster of vesicles
Impetigo	Honey-colored crusts

Treatment

In healthy children, no specific treatment is needed. General measures such as cool baths and oral antihistamines give relief from pruritis. Oral analgesics are required if pain is a feature and antibiotics if lesions become secondarily infected. Indications for systemic antiviral agents such as Acyclovir are listed in *Box 13.2*.

Box 13.2 Indications for systemic antiviral agents

- Pulmonary disease
- Chronic salicylate therapy
- Immunosuppressed children
- Ophthalmic herpes zoster infection
- Ramsay–Hunt syndrome
- Adolescents

13.5.3 Other viral infections

These common viral infections are mainly associated with acute erythematous skin eruptions (*Table 13.2*). There is no specific treatment, but general supportive measures such as antipyretics and analgesics are helpful. Rubella and measles are usually prevented by immunizations.

13.6 **Erythema nodosum**

This is a reactive panniculitis, an inflammatory condition involving the fat lobules and/or the intervening fat septe. It occurs especially in adolescents and has been associated with many conditions (*Box 13.3*). It requires no specific treatment.

Table 13.2 Common viral causes of an acute erythematous eruption

Disease	Agent	Clinical disease	Complications
Measles	Measles virus	Systemic illness with prodrome of high fever, cough, rhinitis, conjunctivitis. Blotchy rash and erythema of mucosa.	Bacterial otitis media, pneumonia, encephalitis
Rubella	Rubella virus	Usually mild illness with little or no prodrome. Pink macular eruption first on face, spreading to trunk and then distally	Monoarthritis, especially in adolescent girls. Congenital rubella may give an embryopathy
Slapped cheek disease	Human parvovirus B19	Confluent redness over both cheeks spreading to limbs and occasionally trunk, lasting 3–5 days	Symmetrical arthritis of hands, wrists and knees
Infectious mononucleosis	Human HV	Fatigue, lymphadeno-pathy, exudative tonsillitis, headache, splenomegaly, especially in adolescents. Rash, especially with ampicillin	Thrombocyto-penia, agranulo-cytosis, hemolytic anemia, neuro-logical symptoms, splenic enlarge-ment and rupture

Box 13.3 Precipitating causes of erythema nodosum

Infections
• tuberculosis
• streptococcal infections
• histoplasma
• coccidioidomycosis
Drugs
• oral contraceptives
Other conditions
• sarcoidosis
• inflammatory bowel disease
• lupus erythematosus

13.7 Erythema multiforme

This reactive eruption most commonly occurs after a herpes simplex infection in the UK. Other causes include those listed in *Box 13.4*.

Box 13.4 Causes of erythema multiforme
Drugs
• sulphonamides
• salicylates
• penicillin
• barbiturates
Infection
• herpes simplex
• infectious mononucleosis
• mycoplasma
Systemic illness
• connective tissue disorder
• malignancy

It presents with symmetrical red macules or edematous papules, which evolve into target lesions with concentric color change around a dusky central zone. They occur mainly on the dorsum of the hands and feet and extensor surface of limbs. They can occur in crops lasting 1–3 weeks.

Stevens–Johnson syndrome and toxic epidermal necrosis are the very severe forms of erythema multiforme with constitutional symptoms. The child develops multisystem involvement in Stevens–Johnson syndrome. The skin lesions become extensive and may be hemorrhagic. Mucous membrane involvement can involve the eyes, nose, urethra and rectum. In toxic epidermal necrosis, large areas of skin slough leaving large denuded areas. Intensive support is needed for both these conditions.

13.8 Henoch–Schönlein purpura

This is an immune complex mediated vasculitic disease in young children, often associated with infections, especially with the β hemolytic streptococcus.

It most commonly presents with small raised purpuric lesions, especially of the extensor surface of the lower limbs and buttocks. However, urticaria or joint swelling of knees and ankles can precede the purpura.

The lesions crop over 1–3 weeks. Other organs can be affected (see *Box 13.5*), renal involvement being potentially the most serious as it can progress to nephritic syndrome and renal failure.

Most affected children can usually be managed with rest at home, but the urine should be routinely checked for blood or protein. Other clinical complications include those listed in *Box 13.5*.

Box 13.5 Clinical complications of Henoch–Schönlein purpura

- Arthritis or arthralgia, especially of knees and ankles
- Gastrointestinal involvement with pain, vomiting and occasional melaena
- Scrotal oedema and erythema
- Rarely central nervous system involvement with seizures

Further reading

Cohen, B.A. (1999) *Pediatric Dermatology*. London; Moseby.

Harper, J., Oranje, A. Prose, N. (2000) *Textbook of Pediatric Dermatology*, London: Blackwell Sciences.

Verbov, J.L. (2000) *Handbook of Pediatric Dermatology* London: Martin Dunitz Ltd.

Chapter 14

Poisoning in children

Sarah Denniston, Mike Riordan,
Kathleen Berry and Kathy Lendrum

Contents

14.1 Introduction

A working knowledge of the management of poisoning in children is essential for all those involved in acute pediatric care. An estimated 52 000 people attended Emergency Departments in the UK because of poisoning in 1997, the majority of whom were children. This chapter deals with the general principles of the management of poisoning and offers guidelines for some of the more common or serious toxins.

A B C – The initial management of any child is to assess and stabilise their airway, breathing and circulation irrespective of any poison they have ingested. Only after this has been achieved need one be concerned about the toxin involved.

14.2 History

Ask **what** was ingested and the formulation (it is important to know whether it is in a long-acting form), **how much** (calculate amount per kg body weight) and **when**. Parents should be told to bring the remaining tablets or medicine and the container when they attend with the child. If berries or toadstools have been eaten, then they should bring a good-sized, unchewed bit of the plant where possible. Information on how the child managed to get hold of a medicine may lead to an opportunity to give advice on storage of medicines. Occasionally poisoning may be the presenting symptom of a Munchausen by proxy syndrome.

In young children the ingestion is usually accidental: calculate the maximum possible amount ingested assuming an initially full container and no toxin wasted. In older children ingestion is more likely due to deliberate self-harm or substance abuse, and a careful history of all medications available in the house is required. After the medical treatment for the ingestion, patients in this group will need further assessment for self harm.

14.3 Examination and recognizable poison syndromes

A detailed physical examination, including a full neurological assessment, is essential in establishing the baseline condition of the child, and may provide important clues as to the substance ingested. *Table 14.1* details some recognizable poison syndromes.

Table 14.1 Recognisable poison syndromes

Poison syndrome	Associated signs	Possible toxins
Increased sympathetic nervous system activity (these features are common in disease generally)	Pyrexia Flushing Tachycardia Hypertension Pupillary constriction Sweating	Cough and decongestant preparations Amphetamines Cocaine Ecstasy Theophylline
Anticholinergic activity	Similar clinical picture to sympathomimetics Clinical differences include: pupillary dilation dry mouth hot dry skin	Tricyclic antidepressants Antiparkinson's drugs Antihistamines Atropine and nightshade Antispasmodics Phenothiazines Mushroom poisoning (amanita species) Cyclopentolate eye drops
Increased parasympathetic nervous system activity	Pupillary constriction Diarrhea Urinary incontinence Sweating Excessive salivation Muscle weakness* Fasciculation* Paralysis*	Organophosphate insecticides Drugs for myasthenia gravis, e.g. pyridostigmine

continued

Table 14.1 Recognisable poison syndromes – *continued*

Poison syndrome	Associated signs	Possible toxins	
Metabolic acidosis	Tachypnoea Kussmaul breathing (sighing respiration)	Ethanol Carbon monoxide Antifreeze Iron	Diabetic medication Tricyclic antidepressants Salicylates
Chemical pneumonitis	Cough Respiratory distress Central nervous system depression	White spirit Turpentine Essential oils	
Acute ataxia or nystagmus		Antihistamines Alcohol Anticonvulsants Piperazine Diphenylhydantoin	Barbiturates Carbon monoxide Organic solvents Bromides
Methemoglobinemia	Cyanosis resistant to oxygen therapy	Alanine dyes Nitrates Benzocaine Phenacetin Nitrobenzene	Chlorates Sulphonamides and metoclopramide (in neonates)
Violent emesis		Aspirin Theophylline Iron	

* Owing to excessive cholinergic stimulation at the motor endplate.

14.4 General principles of management

14.4.1 Laboratory investigations

Blood tests may not be required if the dose established in the history is below treatment level. In the unwell or older child, routine drug levels and the collection of serum and urine for toxicology may be indicated. Note that toxicology results will not be available for planning immediate management. The child's blood glucose, hepatic and renal function should be monitored, and the urine regularly tested for blood, hemoglobin, myoglobin, protein and glucose.

14.4.2 Preventing absorption

None of the techniques available to prevent absorption are recommended for routine use, as their efficacy has not been proven and iatrogenic damage may ensue. Activated charcoal (1 g kg^{-1} for infants; 25–50 g for children) may be used if a potentially toxic dose of a drug adsorbed by charcoal has been ingested within the hour. It does not adsorb alcohols, oils, petrochemicals, bleach, iron or lithium [1]. Induction of emesis is not recommended [2]. Gastric lavage [3] or whole bowel irrigation [4] can be used to physically eliminate highly toxic substances such as iron or enteric-coated preparations that are not adsorbed by activated charcoal and have a long gastrointestinal transit time. Large volumes (30 ml kg^{-1} per hour) of osmotically balanced polyethylene glycol electrolyte solution are given enterally to induce a liquid stool. Treatment is continued until rectal effluent clears. Lavage is contraindicated if corrosive or volatile substances have been ingested and the airway must be protected.

14.4.3 Enhancing excretion

The use of active elimination techniques should be restricted to situations in which there are severe ongoing (or predicted) adverse effects as a result of continued exposure to the toxin.

The use of repeated doses of **activated charcoal** (25–50 g 4–6 hourly) to remove toxins undergoing enterohepatic circulation is one of the simplest active elimination techniques (see *Box 14.1*). It carries a risk of bowel obstruction and perforation: careful monitoring of bowel sounds is essential.

Urinary alkalinization can be used to enhance the excretion of weakly acidic drugs such as salicylate, isoniazid, phenobarbitone and dichlorophenoxyacetic acid. It increases the ionised form of the drug in

---

Box 14.1 Substances where repeat doses of activated charcoal may prove useful in enhancing clearance(6).

- Carbamazepine*
- Barbiturates*
- Dapsone*
- Quinine*
- Theophylline*
- Salicylates†
- *Amanita phalloides* (Death Cap Mushroom)†
- Slow release preparations
- Digoxin† and digitoxin‡
- Phenylbutazone†
- Phenytoin†
- Sotalol†
- Piroxicam†

* Experimental and clinical studies
† Volunteer studies
‡ Little firm evidence

---

the urine, which cannot be reabsorbed. Forced diuresis and urinary acidification are not recommended as the risks outweigh potential benefit.

Hemodialysis may be used in salicylate, methanol, ethylene glycol, vancomycin, lithium and isopropanol poisoning. **Hemoperfusion** may be used for carbamazepine, barbiturates and theophylline, and **hemofiltration** is of use in aminoglycoside and theophylline overdose, and may be beneficial in iron and lithium poisoning.

Substances not amenable to significant extracorporeal removal include benzodiazepines, tricyclic compounds, phenothiazines, chlordiazepoxide and dextropropoxyphene.

14.4.4 Supportive management

Most poisoned children are asymptomatic and require only observation. Any symptoms beyond mild gastrointestinal disturbance indicate a need for admission.

Initial management involves the assessment and stabilization of the airway, breathing and circulation. The airway may be compromised by depression of the central nervous system, which may also reduce respiratory drive and increase the risk of aspiration. The circulation can be compromised by excessive fluid loss in vomiting, diarrhea or diuresis, and should be supported with appropriate fluid replacement. Some toxins cause vasodilatation and hypotension. If fluid replacement is insufficient, the child may need inotropic support with a dopamine or dobutamine infusion.

Arrhythmias are relatively uncommon in pediatric poisoning. Initial management involves adequate resuscitation and correction of any hypoxia, hypercarbia, acid-base or electrolyte imbalance. Specific therapy need only be considered if supportive measures are inadequate.

Metabolic acidosis is frequent but only needs correction with fluids and bicarbonate boluses if severe, as correction of mild acidosis may reduce renal clearance of toxin.

14.5 Carbon monoxide poisoning

Carbon monoxide is a colorless, tasteless and odorless gas. It is 'the forgotten killer' according to the Department of Health. Every year in the UK carbon monoxide kills over 50 people and causes significant morbidity in 200 people. Poisoning often goes unrecognized. Accidental poisoning peaks in the autumn and winter. Modern houses and heating systems are not exempt from causing harm – houses often share heating flues that can easily become blocked. Operation of car engines in integral garages can also cause problems. Children and pregnant women are at increased risk of harm from carbon monoxide. Carbon monoxide is formed from the incomplete combustion of hydrocarbons (*Box 14.2*).

14.5.1 Pathophysiology

Carboxyhemoglobin causes tissue hypoxia. Carbon monoxide binds reversibly to hemoglobin with an affinity 210 times that of oxygen. This is a natural scavenging system for the potentially lethal carbon monoxide. The oxygen–hemoglobin dissociation curve shifts to the left and the

---

Box 14.2 Sources of carbon monoxide

- Incomplete combustion of hydrocarbons
- Tobacco smoke
- Motor vehicle exhaust fumes
- House fires
- Inadequately ventilated/functioning heating systems
- Methylene chloride – paint stripper, solvents used in enclosed spaces

oxygen carrying ability of blood is reduced resulting in tissue and cellular hypoxia. The half-life of carboxyhemoglobin is 4–5 hours when air is being breathed. However, the clinical effects of the carbon monoxide may not become apparent until long after any measurable carboxyhemoglobin has disappeared.

The affinity of carbon monoxide to fetal hemoglobin is even greater. In the fetus a steady-state level of carboxyhemoglobin may not be achieved until 40 hours after a maternal steady-state is reached, and the final level may greatly exceed that of the mother. Tissue hypoxia will be more severe because of the exaggerated left shift of the fetal hemoglobin curve. In experimental animal models, carboxyhemoglobin-saturated blood alone does not reproduce all symptoms. Other mechanisms are therefore implicated in its pathophysiology.

Direct carbon monoxide tissue mediated injury
There is a small fraction of carbon monoxide that remains free and dissolved in the plasma. It may enter cells and bind to many intracellular proteins including myoglobin and cytochrome enzymes. Carbon monoxide is thought to cause neutrophil activation and subsequent degradation of unsaturated fatty acids (lipid peroxygenation) which causes demyelinisation of central nervous system lipids. Carbon monoxide may share properties with nitric oxide such as promotion of platelet aggregation and smooth muscle relaxation. 'Free' carbon monoxide may result in the formation of oxygen radicals and cellular death.

14.5.2 Clinical features of poisoning

The clinical features of chronic low level carbon monoxide poisoning are non-specific and often falsely attributed to viral illness. In contrast, severe acute poisoning, such as from a house fire, can cause sudden collapse. The classic cherry red appearance of skin and mucous membranes is normally a postmortem finding. *Table 14.2* and *Box 14.3* describe clues to the diagnosis and the range of acute symptoms.

Tissue hypoxia may cause tachypnea and tachycardia. Cerebral injury can result in headaches, syncope, confusion or seizures. Adults with ischemic heart disease may present with worsening angina. It is important to note that carboxyhemoglobin levels do not correlate well with acute or ongoing symptoms.

Delayed neuropsychiatric syndrome
Ten to thirty per cent of victims show some signs of the delayed neuropsychiatric syndrome 3–240 days after acute carbon monoxide

Table 14.2 Acute symptoms reported after exposure to carbon monoxide

Symptom	Percentage of patients
Headache	91
Dizziness	77
Weakness	53
Nausea	47
Confusion or lack of concentration	43
Shortness of breath	40
Visual changes	25
Chest pain	9
Loss of consciousness	6
Abdominal pain	5
Muscle cramps	5

Box 14.3 Clues to carbon monoxide poisoning

- Maintain a high level of suspicion
- More than one household member (including pets) affected
- Symptoms improve away from source and deteriorate on return
- Symptoms worse after particular activity – cooking, winter heating, starting car in garage
- Sooty deposits on gas fires, boilers, walls
- Smoke accumulating in rooms with faulty flues
- Yellow flames instead of blue

exposure. Symptoms include personality changes, cognitive difficulties, parkinsonism, dementia and psychosis. Clinical and laboratory findings cannot be used to predict who will develop this syndrome. Increasing age does appear to be a risk factor.

Reperfusion injury following tissue hypoxia and oxygen radical mediated lipid peroxygenation have been implicated in the etiology of this syndrome. Abnormalities have been shown on CT and MRI scans which correlate well with neurological signs.

14.5.3 Diagnosis

Maintaining a high index of suspicion must be the keystone to diagnosis in what is typically a non-specific presentation. It is important to remember that carboxyhemoglobin levels fall rapidly once the patient is removed from the source into clean air and the levels may have been much higher than when measured. Therefore, early measurement of carboxyhemoglobin is to be encouraged. The advent of expired breath activated carbon monoxide measuring instruments may make the diagnosis easier in children when doctors are reluctant to take blood gas samples for carboxyhemoglobin. The advantage of an arterial sample over a venous blood sample is that co-existing acidosis can be identified. A normal carboxyhemoglobin level in a non-smoker is 1–3% and rises to 5–10% in a smoker. Pulse oximetry falsely records a high oxygen saturation in the presence of carbon monoxide poisoning and should not be relied upon.

It is important to examine the neurological system carefully and to include tests of balance and coordination (gait, heel to toe, Romberg's test, finger nose), short-term memory and, if appropriate, a mini-mental state examination. Other investigations may include serum electrolytes, liver function tests and creatinine kinase, an electrocardiogram and chest radiography.

14.5.4 Management

Removing the patient from the source of poisoning into clean air as quickly as possible should be the first action. Supplemental 100% oxygen should be applied through a well-fitting mask until carboxyhemoglobin levels reach normal or the patient is asymptomatic. Breathing 100% oxygen promotes carbon monoxide dissociation from hemoglobin and reduces the half-life of carboxyhemoglobin to 40–80 minutes.

The use of hyperbaric oxygen is controversial. Theoretically the level of carboxyhemoglobin falls faster with hyperbaric oxygen, and it is thought that a reduction in cellular hypoxia will reduce lipid peroxygenation. Hyperbaric oxygen is therefore reported to reduce the neurological sequele of poisoning. However, the risks of hyperbaric oxygen include barotrauma to the ears, seizure activity and the potential risks related to transfer of the patient to a unit some distance away from the receiving hospital. An acceptable list of criteria for referral is described in *Box 14.4*.

> **Box 14.4** Indications for consideration of hyperbaric oxygen
>
> - Carboxyhemoglobin level > 20%
> - Loss of consciousness at any time
> - Neurological symptoms and signs (except mild headache)
> - Myocardial ischemia or arrhythmia
> - Pregnancy

A recent Cochrane systematic review on hyperbaric oxygen looked at six randomised controlled trials of hyperbaric oxygen in acute poisoning in non-pregnant adults. Only three were considered of high enough quality to analyse further, all of which used different doses of hyperbaric and normobaric oxygen. Only one study was double blind. At 1 month of follow up, persistent symptoms possibly from carbon monoxide were present in 34.2% of patients treated with hyperbaric oxygen and 37.2% treated with normobaric oxygen. The review concludes that there is no evidence that the unselected use of hyperbaric oxygen reduces the frequency of neurological sequele. Further randomised double blind studies are required before accurate guidelines can be produced.

New animal and human studies have considered the use of hyperventilation while maintaining normal carbon dioxide levels to accelerate carbon monoxide elimination.

14.5.5 Prevention

Carbon monoxide detectors are inexpensive but underused. Regular maintenance of heating and cooking appliances should be encouraged. Counselling and education (e.g. through the child health surveillance scheme) have only a modest effect on the ownership of smoke alarms and an unknown effect on fire-related injuries. Free alarms have a significant effect on the number of functioning alarms and resultant injuries.

14.6 Notes on other specific poisons

14.6.1 Bleach and other corrosives

- Rarely ingested in large volumes
- Charcoal not helpful, lavage contraindicated
- < 100 ml ingested: encourage milky drinks, nausea and vomiting common

- \> 100 ml or industrial bleach: risk of esophageal damage so admit. Monitor fluid balance and airway. Drooling or dysphagia beyond 12–24 hours is a good predictor of esophageal scars – endoscopy is indicated.

14.6.2 White Spirit and petrochemicals

- Causes cough and respiratory distress from aspiration and chemical pneumonitis
- May develop symptoms up to 24 hours postingestion
- If asymptomatic, observe for 6 hours or discharge with advice
- If symptomatic, arrange chest X-ray, consider bronchodilators and continue careful observation – further ventilatory support may be needed.

14.6.3 Paracetamol (acetaminophen)

- Most common accidental overdose in children, rarely serious if liquid preparation
- If certain that $< 150\,mg\,kg^{-1}$ ingested, discharge home
- If < 1 hour from ingestion, consider activated charcoal
- If < 8 hours from ingestion, take timed levels after 4 hours. If level above treatment line on normogram, start treatment with *N*-acetylcysteine [use the high-risk normogram if underweight, pre-existing liver disease, enzyme-inducing drugs]
- If > 8 hours from ingestion, take levels and start *N*-acetylcysteine immediately
- If > 24 hours from ingestion, discuss with poisons advice centre
- If *N*-acetylcysteine is required, take blood for baseline international normalized ratio (INR), liver function tests, electrolytes and creatinine levels. Repeat at 24 and 48 hours.

14.6.4 Ibuprofen and NSAIDs

- Cause headache, tinnitus, gastrointestinal and visual disturbance; might cause hypotension, acidosis, respiratory depression
- Ibuprofen: if $< 100\,mg\,kg^{-1}$, observe 4 hours. If $> 100\,mg\,kg^{-1}$, give activated charcoal and observe for 12 hours
- Mefenamic acid: if $> 25\,mg\,kg^{-1}$, give activated charcoal and observe for 12 hours
- If symptomatic, admit, avoid dehydration, monitor electrolytes, prothrombin and acid base.

14.6.5 Iron

- Causes gastrointestinal disturbance, and delayed multi-organ failure
- If iron level is $< 30\,mg\,kg^{-1}$, discharge home
- If iron level is $> 30\,mg\,kg^{-1}$, perform abdominal X-ray and undertake careful gastric lavage or whole bowel irrigation as indicated by tablet position on imaging
- Iron levels at 4 hours: if $< 55\,\mu mol\,l^{-1}$, discharge home (unless sustained release); if > 55 but $< 90\,\mu mol\,l^{-1}$, observe for 24 hours. If $>90\,\mu mol\,l^{-1}$, treat with i.v. desferrioxamine.

14.6.6 Tricyclic antidepressants

- Cause anticholinergic symptoms, drowsiness, ataxia, agitation, convulsions, hypotension and arrhythmias
- If ingestion exceeds maximum daily dose:
  - if < 1 hour give activated charcoal
  - 12-lead ECG – best indicator of risk of cardiac toxicity is QRS $> 0.1\,sec$
  - asymptomatic with normal ECG: observe for 6 hours
  - asymptomatic with abnormal ECG: observe until normal
  - arrhythmia with compromise: bolus $1\,ml\,kg^{-1}$ 8.4% sodium bicarbonate. Maintain slight alkalosis. Further treatment may include phenytoin, atenolol or propranolol.
  - hypotension: treat with fluids and then sodium bicarbonate or glucagon

14.6.7 Beta blockers

- Cause bradycardia and hypotension – but tachycardia and hypertension if partial agonist; CNS effects and hypoglycemia
- Give activated charcoal if < 1 hour
- If asymptomatic, observe for 12 hours
- Hypotension: treat with i.v. fluid, and i.v. glucagon ($50–150\,\mu g\,kg^{-1}$ in 5% dextrose), isoprenaline or cardiac pacing as required
- Monitor blood glucose

14.7 Admission criteria

Most children require no more than a period of observation. Factors to consider in deciding admission include the adequacy of parental supervision and parental confidence, the availability of emergency care, if the child should deteriorate, and the need for psychosocial assessment in cases of deliberate self-harm.

14.8 Seeking further advice

Specific, expert advice on all aspects of poisoning is available to medical professionals. You should ensure that you are aware of your local (or national) poisons information service and know how to contact them.

A wide range of easily accessible and highly practical advice is available through the National Poisons Information Service (NPIS) website. This free service is restricted to medical professionals. On line registration is available at http://www.spib.axl.co.uk/toxbase/

References

1. Chyka, P.A., Seger, D. (1997) Position statement: single-dose activated charcoal. American Academy of Clinical Toxicology; European Association of Poisons Centres and Clinical Toxicologists. *J. Toxicol. Clin. Toxicol.* **35**: 721–741.
2. Krenzelok, E.P., McGuigan, M., Lheur, P. (1997) Position statement: ipecac syrup. American Academy of Clinical Toxicology; European Association of Poisons Centres and Clinical Toxicologists. *J. Toxicol. Clin. Toxicol.* **35**: 699–709.
3. Vale, J.A. (1997) Position statement: gastric lavage. American Academy of Clinical Toxicology; European Association of Poisons Centres and Clinical Toxicologists [see comments]. *J. Toxicol. Clin. Toxicol.* **35**: 711–719.
4. Tenenbein, M. (1997) Position statement: whole bowel irrigation. American Academy of Clinical Toxicology; European Association of Poisons Centres and Clinical Toxicologists. *J. Toxicol. Clin. Toxicol.* **35**: 753–762.

Recommended reading

Bates, N., Edwards, N., Roper, J., Volans, G. (1997) *Pediatric Toxicology: Handbook of Poisoning in Children*. London: Macmillan Reference Limited.

Ernst, A., Zibrak, J.D. (1998) Carbon monoxide poisoning. *New Engl. J. Med.* **339**: 1603–1608.

Vale, A., Meredith, T., Buckley, B. (1984) *ABC of poisoning. Eliminating poisons*. *B.M.J.* **289**: 366–369.

Chapter 15

The crying baby and infant distress

Colin Powell

Contents

15.1 Introduction

Crying is normal physiological behavior in young infants. The average baby of 6–8 weeks cries or fusses for up to 3 out of 24 hours. Excessive crying (colic) is defined as >3 hours per day for 3 days per week. However, many babies come to the Emergency Department with lesser amounts of crying, as the parents perceive it as excessive.

Infants with 'colic' are well and thriving. There is usually no identifiable medical problem. The parents are often distressed, exhausted and confused, having received conflicting advice from various health professionals and lay sources.

15.2 Assessment

15.2.1 Clinical characteristics

- Crying develops in the early weeks of life and peaks around 6–8 weeks of age.
- It is usually worse in late afternoon or evening.
- It may last several hours.
- The infant may draw up his or her legs as if in pain, but there is no evidence that colic is attributable to an intestinal problem or wind.
- It usually improves by 3–4 months of age.

A thorough history and examination must be conducted to exclude any significant illness. More acute onset of irritability and crying should not be diagnosed as colic. A specific diagnosis is usually present in these cases. Remember, maternal depression may be a factor in presentation. Diagnoses to consider are listed in *Box 15.1*.

15.3 Investigations

If the history is typical and examination negative no investigations are required.

Consider:
- urine microscopy and culture
- stool examination for reducing substances (if watery)
- fluorescein staining of eyes.

15.4 Management

The parents require careful explanation and reassurance that their infant is not unwell or in pain, and that the unsettled behavior will improve

---

Box 15.1 Causes of crying in infants

Longstanding crying
- Reflux oesophagitis
- Cow's milk protein or lactose intolerance
- Raised intracranial pressure
- Shaken infant syndrome

Acute onset of crying
- Otitis media
- Incarcerated hernia
- Testicular torsion
- Anal fissure
- Intermittent intestinal obstruction (e.g. volvulus, intussusception)
- Pneumonia with chest pain
- Corneal abrasion
- Herpangina
- Myocarditis
- Fractured limb
- Shaken baby syndrome
- Hair-tourniquet syndrome

---

with time. However, parents do need empathic acknowledgment of their anxiety and stress, and ongoing support from within and outside the family.

Suggestions that may be helpful are listed in *Box 15.2*.

Medication is rarely indicated. Colic mixtures, gripe water, etc. are of no proven benefit. Formula changes are usually not helpful unless there is proven cow's milk allergy or lactose intolerance. Weaning from breast milk has no benefit.

Provide printed information if possible, as parents are unlikely to remember much given their state of mind at the time.

15.5 Disposition

Referral for early (within days) ongoing support is essential. Options include:
- maternal and child health nurse
- local medical officer/family doctor
- general pediatrician – hospital outpatients

Box 15.2 Management of the well, crying child

- Establish pattern to feeding/settling
- Avoid excessive stimulation – noise, light, handling
- Excessive quiet should also be avoided – most babies find a low level of background noise soothing
- Carry baby in a papoose in front of the chest
- Baby massage/rocking/patting
- Gentle music tapes
- Respond before baby is too worked up
- Have somebody else care for the baby for brief periods to give the parents a break

---

- mother and baby day unit or inpatient unit; for severe cases admission to hospital, if child considered at risk of non-accidental injury or parental exhaustion.

Chapter 16

Febrile child under 3 years of age

Colin Powell

Contents

16.1 Assessment and management

Although the majority of febrile illnesses in young children are caused by viruses, up to 5% of young children with a significant fever without an obvious focus will have bacteremia, usually pneumococcal. Infants usually present with non-specific symptoms and signs of illness, and localising signs of organ–system disease are often lacking. General aspects of the child's behavior and appearance provide the best indication of whether a serious infection is likely. Neither the degree of the fever, its rapidity of onset nor its response to antipyretics are good predictors of serious illness by themselves.

It is imperative to consider the following approach to investigation in the light of local epidemiological data if it is available. There is variation of the prevalence of invasive bacterial infection from population to population. Local guidelines and organism sensitivities should guide administration of antibiotics.

Any febrile child under 3 who appears unwell should be investigated and admitted, irrespective of the degree of fever. *Table 16.1* shows the assessment and management of these children.

16.1.1 Urine culture

Bag urine specimens should never be sent for culture. If the bag specimen is positive for nitrites and/or leucocytes on reagent strip testing, then, according to local practice, a suprapubic aspirate or clean catch urine or catheter urine should be performed and the sample sent for culture. (Practice differs between Australia, the UK and North America, see Chapter 9). Note children with negative urine strip testing could still have UTI, so, if this is suspected, a urine culture should be done regardless of strip test result.

16.1.2 Positive blood culture

Contact the family immediately and arrange clinical review (*Box 16.1*).

Table 16.1 Assessment and management of the febrile infant

Age	Description	Management
<1 month (or <3.5 kg)	Rectal temperature >38°C	Full sepsis work-up and admission for empirical antibiotics
1–3 months	Rectal temperature >38°C	Discuss with registrar/consultant Full sepsis work-up: FBC/film, blood culture, urine culture±CXR (only if respiratory symptoms or signs)+LP If child previously healthy, looks well, WBC 5000–15 000, urine microscopy normal, CXR (if taken) clear, and negative CSF (if taken), discharge home **Review within 12 hours** or sooner if deterioration If child unwell or above criteria are not all satisfied, admit to hospital for observation±empirical i.v. antibiotics
3 months to 3 years	Temperature >38.9°C and clear focus of infection	Treat as clinically indicated
		Discuss with registrar/consultant Investigate as appropriate for clinical focus and admit for treatment
	Temperature >38.9°C and no clear focus of infection	Urine culture if <6 months Discharge home on symptomatic treatment Arrange medical review within 24 hours, or sooner if child deteriorates
	Child looks well	
	Child looks unwell	
	Child looks well	
	Child looks miserable but is still relatively alert, interactive and responsive	Discuss with senior doctor prior to any investigations (at least culture urine if <6 months) Consider full septic work-up in worrisome cases. For cases where the urine is normal but WBC is >15 000, some centers advocate expectant outpatient treatment with parenteral ceftriaxone (50 mg kg⁻¹ per 24 h) until culture results are available
	Child looks unwell (i.e. lethargic, poorly interactive, difficult to rouse, inconsol-, able, tachycardia, tachypnea, poor peripheral perfusion)	Full sepsis work-up: FBC, blood culture, urine culture, CXR (if respiratory symptoms or signs), lumbar puncture *Note:* LP should not be performed in a child with impaired conscious state or focal neurological signs (see Meningitis guideline, section 6.4) Admit to hospital for observation±i.v. antibiotics

> **Box 16.1** Management of positive blood culture in febrile infant
>
> ***Streptococcus pneumoniae***
> - *Child well and afebrile*
>   - If the child is on antibiotic therapy, a 7-day course should be completed
>   - If the child has not received antibiotics, there is no need for investigation or treatment as the infection will have been cleared naturally. Review if clinical deterioration occurs.
> - *Child unwell or febrile*
>   - Sepsis work-up and admission for i.v. antibiotics
>
> **Any other organism (regardless of clinical condition of child)**
> - Sepsis work-up and admission for i.v. antibiotics.

Suggested reading

Haddon, R.A., Barnett, P.L., Grimwood, K., Hogg, G.G. (1999) Bacteraemia in febrile children presenting to a paediatric emergency department. *Med. J. Austr.* **170:** 475–478.

Chapter 17

Major trauma – general

Martin Pusic

Contents

17.1 Introduction

Death from trauma accounts for half of all pediatric deaths. This proportion has persisted despite advances in motor vehicle safety and injury-prevention programmes such as helmet use. Proper emergency medical services management of traumatic injury should be able to prevent up to a fifth of these deaths and proportionately decrease morbidity. What constitutes 'major' trauma is difficult to define even retrospectively, let alone when the patient is coming through the Emergency Department (ED) doors. For the purposes of this chapter, we will consider major trauma to be apparent *traumatic* injury to multiple organ systems. The following principles will help the practitioner to manage these challenging patients as effectively as possible.

- The trauma patient should arrive into a well-rehearsed trauma system made up of a multidisciplinary trauma team, supported by the necessary infrastructure. Responses to predictable contingencies should be planned out ahead of time and, where possible, protocols should be in place.
- Centers that do not have a pediatric trauma programme should nonetheless have pre-arranged transfer agreements with a trauma center with access to appropriate telephone support.
- Life-threatening traumatic injuries allow only a brief window of opportunity for successful intervention. A systematic protocol-led approach, such as the one advocated by the American College of Surgeons, will lead to the most effective use of this 'golden' period.
- After initial stabilization, timely triage to either the operating room or an intensive care setting will result in the best patient outcome.

In this chapter, we will present an overview of trauma management. The emphasis will be on problems specific to children.

17.2 Organization

For a given community, the outcomes for traumatic injury will be best if a well-functioning trauma system is in place. From the ambulance attendants at the scene of the injury through to the rehabilitation specialists to those devising strategies for injury prevention, trauma requires a continuum of care across the medical system.

In the ED, proper management of a child with major trauma requires the various individual talents of a team of professionals all working from the same script. Team members include nurses with pre-assigned responsibilities (e.g. intravenous access, medication preparation and administration, handling the family), the ED physician, pediatric surgeons, surgical sub-specialists as needed (orthopedics, neurosurgery, genitourinary), intensive care physicians, anesthetists and ancillary personnel such as social workers and clergy. The make-up of the team usually reflects local needs and traditions. A single person should be designated the team leader in the emergency situation. Whether this should be a surgeon or emergency physician is left to local preference.

The American College of Surgeons has suggested that trauma management be divided into four main phases:
- *the primary survey* during which immediately life-threatening conditions are identified;
- the resuscitation phase when underlying pathophysiological derangements are addressed;
- the secondary survey where a more detailed examination catalogues all injuries to the patient, and
- finally triage where a decision is made as to the most appropriate site for definitive care for the patient.

The succeeding sections deal with each of these phases in turn.

17.3 Major trauma management

Major trauma is managed along the following lines (*Figure 17.1*) with:
- Primary survey
- Resuscitation
- Secondary survey
- Triage
- Referral for further management

17.3.1 Primary survey

The primary survey (*Figure 17.2*) is a 2–5 minute process in which the clinician looks to exclude or treat immediately life-threatening conditions. This is done according to the mnemonic:

- A – Airway and cervical spine precautions
- B – Breathing
- C – Circulation
- D – Disability (neurological impairment)
- E – Exposure (removal of clothing)

Each element of this mnemonic should be assessed in sequence since Airway takes precedence over Circulation etc.

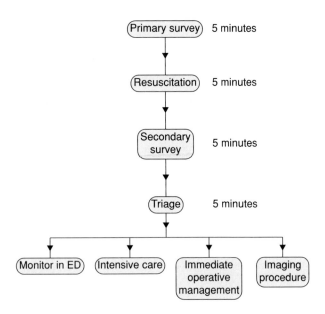

Figure 17.1 Stages of management of major trauma (the first 20 minutes).

A–Airway and cervical spine precautions

All major trauma patients should be assumed to have a cervical spine injury until proven otherwise. Therefore, at the same time as the clinician is assessing the airway, an assistant should be ensuring that the cervical spine is immobilized with a rigid collar or other such system. Air should pass noiselessly through the upper airway. Stridor, gurgling sounds or signs of respiratory distress may indicate airway obstruction. Simple maneuvers, such as oropharyngeal suctioning or the chin-lift/jaw-thrust, may be sufficient to relieve the obstruction. If the maneuvers are not successful, initial bag-valve-mask ventilation followed by rapid sequence intubation while in-line traction is maintained might be required. Severe head and neck trauma or burns can make intubation difficult, although surgical options such as needle cricothyrotomy are only rarely required (< 1%). Increasingly, expiratory capnography is used as a sensitive indicator of correct airway placement.

B–Breathing

Airway and breathing maneuvers should be titrated to achieving adequate chest motion and consequently oxygenation as evidenced by pulse oximetry. All patients should receive 100% oxygen by non-rebreathing facemask at least initially. If careful auscultation reveals asymmetrical breath sounds, life-threatening though reversible causes should be excluded on the primary survey (*Table 17.1*).

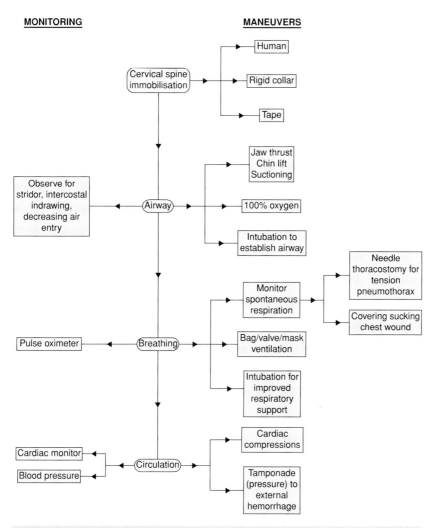

MONITORING   MANEUVERS

Figure 17.2 The primary survey

C–Circulation

Circulation is assessed by measuring the heart rate and quality of pulses, blood pressure, and the skin and CNS perfusion. A heart rate <60 may be a preterminal event; it mandates cardiac compressions. Sites of external hemorrhage should be tamponaded. Large-bore i.v. access should be started as soon as possible, even if the major trauma patient shows no immediate signs of hypovolemia since children can lose up to 15% of their blood volume without showing signs. Except in extreme cases of threatened exsanguination where universal donor blood is started, normal saline or Ringer's lactate is the resuscitation fluid of choice.

Table 17.1 Causes and treatment of poor ventilation

Cause of poor ventilation	Treatment
1. Malpositioned endotracheal tube	Reposition tube, usually by withdrawing it, usually from the right main bronchus
2. Tension pneumothorax	Needle thoracotomy
3. Sucking chest wound	Airtight bandage
4. Gaseous distension of the stomach (crying infant/ overzealous bag and mask ventilation)	Pass nasogastric tube

D–Disability

In the primary survey, the neurological assessment is geared towards life-threatening reversible causes. Cerebral herniation can be ameliorated if promptly identified. Children typically do not develop uncal herniation with its classic findings of ipsilateral dilated pupil and contralateral weakness. Instead, they are more likely to suffer from more generalized brain edema, which results in central herniation. Signs of this include bilateral dilated, poorly responsive pupils and Cushing's response (bradycardia in the face of hypertension). Gentle hyperventilation and mannitol may help decrease the intracranial pressure until definitive neurosurgical intervention. The AVPU method for assessing level of consciousness is useful for documenting the patient's initial neurological state (*Box 17.1*).

E–Exposure

Clothing may hide important signs and therapeutic procedures and should be removed. However, the patient's thermal equilibrium should be monitored frequently and radiant warmers and blankets used when necessary.

Box 17.1 AVPU method for quickly assessing level of consciousness

A   Alert
V   Verbal – responds to verbal stimuli
P   Pain – responds to painful stimuli
U   Unresponsive

17.3.2 Resuscitation

Whereas the primary survey is meant to deal with conditions that are potentially immediately catastrophic, the resuscitation phase is meant to redress general physiologic derangements owing to hypovolemia and possible cerebral herniation (*Figure 17.3*). The overarching principle is that the clinician should stay one step ahead of the pathophysiology – e.g. fluid and blood replacement must ideally be initiated before the patient becomes overtly hypovolemic.

Resuscitation begins with the establishment of intravenous access. Initial attempts should be made at the antecubital fosse and at the site of the

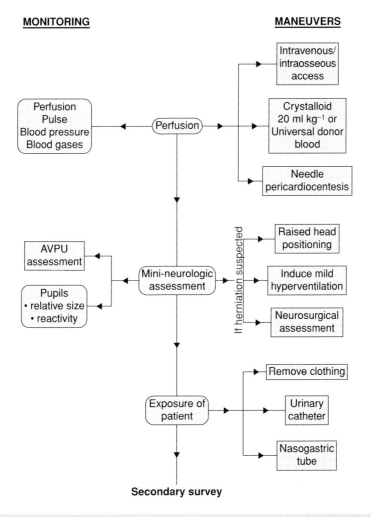

Figure 17.3 Resuscitation

saphenous vein. Catheter sizes depend on the size of the child: ideally 22 g for children < 2 years of age; 20 g for 2–6 years; 18 g for 6–12 years, and 16 g for > 12 years. Failed attempts should be abandoned in favor of a different technique within a set period of time (we suggest 90 s), determined and timed by the team leader. The back-up technique will have been determined ahead of time depending on the experience of the personnel. Intraosseous catheter placement has a high success rate even in inexperienced hands. Femoral vein cannulation using a guide-wire technique or saphenous vein cut-downs are other options.

Once intravenous access is established, fluid resuscitation is begun. Various categories of shock have been defined. All depend on careful assessment of the following:
• Heart rate
• Tissue perfusion
  • brain – AVPU determination
  • skin – capillary refill, temperature of extremities, quality of pulses
  • kidney – urine output
• Blood pressure
• Respiratory rate – in the absence of respiratory pathology, rate reflects degree of lactic acidosis due to lack of tissue perfusion

However, instead of trying to remember a classification of shock in major trauma, the clinician is better off remembering the points in *Table 17.5*.

During the resuscitation phase, again consider the possibility of herniation. If the signs of Cushing's response (bradycardia and hypertension) are worsening or the pupils are more dilated, consider:
• increasing the ventilatory rate
• giving mannitol
• that, in the hemodynamically stable patient, aggressive fluid resuscitation may aggravate cerebral edema
• performing, in refractory cases, neurosurgical intervention such as burr holes (rarely) or craniotomy.

The final task of the resuscitation phase is to intubate 'all orifices' with specific caveats listed in the following table (*Table 17.2*).

17.3.3 Secondary survey

The goals of the primary survey and resuscitation phases are to stabilise the ventilatory and circulatory status of the patient with due consideration of the possibility of cerebral herniation. In under 5–10 minutes, the

Table 17.2 Intubations of 'all orifices' – warnings

Site	Reason for intubation	Warning
Tracheal intubation	Support ventilation	According to airway and ventilatory status
Nasopharyngeal tube	Decrease stomach distension	Avoid this in cases of blunt trauma to the face as there is a risk of the tube passing through a cribriform plate fracture into the brain
Orogastric tube	Decrease stomach distension	Preferred to nasogastric tube in cases of blunt facial trauma
Bladder (Foley) catheterization	Monitor urine output	Contraindicated if blood present at the meatus – in which case a retrograde urethrogram is done Contraindicated if high-riding prostate in post-pubertal boys – may indicate internal urethral disruption
Rectal examination	To assess rectal tone in cases of possible spinal cord injury Blood may suggest intestinal injury To assess prostate	Utility questionable in cases of mild trauma in pre-pubertal children

trauma team will have instituted assisted ventilation, intravascular fluid resuscitation, neuroprotective maneuvers and attached all monitors. They will have considered a nasogastric tube and/or Foley catheter.

After this first pass, they will have made considerable progress in stabilising the patient's physiological status by rapidly instituting treatment for life-threatening, reversible conditions. The next phase is the secondary survey (*Figure 17.4*), where the team proceeds to a more time-intensive detailed assessment of the whole patient while never losing sight of the patient's hemodynamic status. The secondary survey is a complete head-to-toe assessment of the patient. The examination is made more

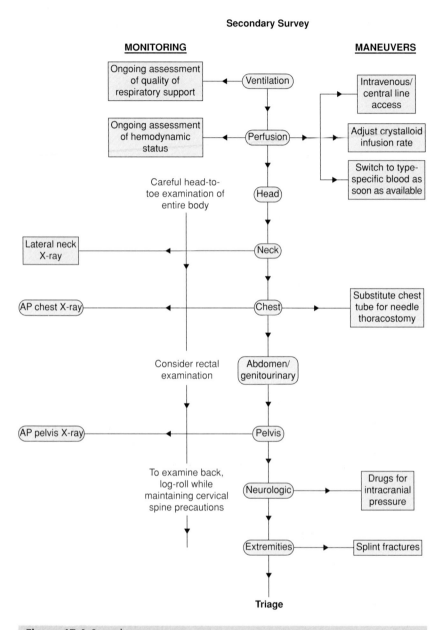

Figure 17.4 Secondary survey

difficult by the need to maintain in-line immobilization of the spine until spinal cord injury is ruled out. Typically, the assessor will examine the patient from the front and then, with several assistants, 'log-roll' the patient on to his or her side to assess the back.

Specific considerations are listed in *Box 17.2.*

Box 17.2 Specific considerations in the secondary survey

History
- AMPLE
  - A – Allergies
  - M – Medications
  - P – Past history
  - L – Last meal
  - E – Environment at time of injury

Head
- Depressed skull fractures
- Tamponade scalp lacerations
- Tongue lacerations
- Hemotympanum

Neck
- Cervical spine X-rays if:
  - neurological signs
  - any neck pain
  - any neck tenderness
  - distracting painful injury elsewhere
  - impaired consciousness
  - penetrating injury

Chest
- Flail chest
- Sucking chest wound
- Hemo/pneumothorax
- Major vessel injury – widened mediastinum on upright chest film

Abdomen
- Contusion
- Distension
- Peritoneal signs
- Rectal examination
  [See indications for diagnostic peritoneal lavage under ancillary studies]

Pelvis
- Palpate iliac spines and pubis

Extremities
- Fractures – splint, reduce
- Neurovascular compromise

Neurology
- Level of consciousness (GCS)
- Deep tendon reflexes
- Rectal tone
- Priapism (suggests spinal cord injury)

Abbreviations: GCS, Glasgow Coma Scale.

Trauma may result from a mechanism that has its own specific set of considerations. References to some of these are listed in *Box 17.3*.

Investigations should be ordered in the ED. A summary of possible investigations is shown below in *Table 17.3*.

Table 17.3 Possible investigations

Study	Indication
Blood tests	
Full blood count	Blood loss
Type and cross match	
Electrolytes, blood urea, creatinine	Renal function
AST, ALT, amylase	Liver contusion, pancreatic contusion
Arterial blood gases	Cardiorespiratory injury
ECG	Myocardial contusion
Plain X-rays	
Cervical spine	See indications listed in secondary survey
	If inadequate, consider CT neck
Chest X-ray	Any abnormality of respiration or any significant injury to chest.
	Note: not to delay diagnosis and treatment of hemopneumothorax
Abdominal series	Upright film in penetrating abdominal
AP	injury
lateral	Verification of NG-tube placement
upright or decubitus	Better than CT to detect hollow-viscus injury with free air
Pelvis	Trauma to torso
	Pain/tenderness in pelvis
	Obtunded patient
Thoracolumbar	Pain or tenderness of spine
	Lap-belt injury
Extremities	As indicated
Computerized tomography	
Head	Altered level of consciousness
without contrast	Hemophilia
Abdomen	Hemodynamically stable blunt trauma
i.v. and GI contrast	of abdomen, especially:
	hematuria
	lap-belt injury
	significant mechanism of injury
	concomitant head injury
IVP	Hematuria
	Supplanted by CT with i.v. contrast except in cases where patient unstable
Retrograde urethrogram	Blood at meatus
	Displaced prostate
Abdominal ultrasound	Can give quick diagnostic information in the ED
	Same indications as for abdominal CT
Diagnostic peritoneal lavage	Used to diagnose need for laparotomy in cases too unstable for CT
	Unstable hemodynamically without clear cause
	Penetrating trauma of chest (not clearly involving abdomen)
	Needs urgent surgery

Abbreviations: ALT, alanine aminotransferase; AP, anteroposterior; AST, aspartate aminotransferase; CT, computerised tomography; ED, Emergency Department; GI, gastrointestinal; IVP, intravenous pyelogram; NG, nasogastric.

> **Box 17.3** Conditions with specific considerations referred to in specific chapters
>
> Burns – Chapter 20
> Child abuse – Chapter 27
> Hypothermia – Chapter 3
> Near-drowning – Chapter 3
> Convulsions – Chapter 6

17.3.4 Triage

Trauma patients do best in a trauma system designed to mobilise appropriate resources in a timely fashion. These resources are typically **expertise** in the form of people, and **locations** in the form of specialized collections of monitoring and surgical equipment. The trauma leader must make complex disposition decisions based on the patient's condition and the local resources. What follows is a list of possible triage decisions. Each boils down to the following question: is this patient in the best possible environment for the level of severity, taking into account the risks associated with transfers between locations?

Level of facility

One of the great advances in trauma care has been the development of trauma systems where resources for trauma care are concentrated in accredited 'Trauma Centers'. A center that sees relatively few trauma patients may prudently elect to transfer the patient to a specialized center after initial stabilization.

Admission versus discharge

Many trauma patients can be safely discharged with comprehensive discharge instructions *after* an appropriate observation period (typically 6 hours) in the ED during which vital signs and neurocognitive status remain normal. Any significant abnormalities in vital sign or worrying symptoms should mandate admission for monitoring. Significant mechanisms such as a fall from a great height or high speed motor vehicle collisions should also prompt consideration for admission.

Admission to Intensive Care Unit (ICU) versus regular inpatient ward

Patients with significant potential for cardiorespiratory instability should be admitted to a monitored setting such as the ICU. These decisions are generally made on a case-by-case basis since no criteria or scoring systems are sufficiently sensitive and specific.

Operating room versus ED stabilization

Proper ED stabilization of a hemodynamically compromised patient will decrease operative mortality. However, some cases require emergency transfer to the operating room as listed in *Table 17.4*.

Table 17.4 Indications for emergency transfer to operating room

Diagnosis	Indication
Head injury – herniation	Relief of raised intracranial pressure • poorly responsive, dilated pupils; asymmetric pupils • rising blood pressure with bradycardia • CT evidence of malignant intracranial bleed
Neck injury	Airway compromise → surgical airway Major vessel injury
Chest/abdomen – blunt	Ongoing hemodynamic instability
Chest/abdomen – penetrating	Ongoing hemodynamic instability Hemothorax drainage Wound exploration
Extremity trauma	Limb threatening vascular compromise

In conclusion, *Table 17.5* lists key points to remember in major trauma.

Table 17.5 Key points to remember in major trauma

Problem	Consideration
The patient can have lost up to 8–9% of blood volume and show *no* changes in vital signs	Establish i.v. access automatically and have a very low threshold for administering a 20 ml kg^{-1} crystalloid bolus
The first assessment of circulatory status is only a start The ongoing trend is as important	Do not get locked into a fluid recipe based only on the initial assessment Insert a Foley catheter to monitor urine output. Reassess all vital signs frequently and adjust the fluid therapy
Be ready to give blood	It always takes longer to get blood than you would think Lack of response to two 20 ml kg^{-1} crystalloid boluses is an indication for blood transfusion Order blood at the first indication that you might need it – this may be before the patient arrives
Hypotension is a very late sign. Unlike adults, children can lose up to 40% of their blood volume with a *normal* blood pressure	Heart rate and perfusion are more sensitive indicators Hypotension in the child should be considered 'pre-arrest' and treated aggressively
Always keep cardiogenic shock in the back of your mind	Cardiac tamponade will get *worse* with aggressive fluid resuscitation Look for muffled heart sounds and distended neck veins
Do not rely on drugs to maintain circulatory status	Hypovolemic shock responds to volume Squeezing an empty pipe even harder with vasopressor will not help Give fluids

Further reading

Advanced Life Support Group (2000) *Advanced Pediatric Life Support – The Practical Approach*, 3rd Edn. London: BMJ Publishing Group.

Chapter 18

Specific major trauma

Stephen Gordon and Martin Pusic

Contents

18.1 Blunt trauma

18.1.1 Blunt spinal cord injury

Spinal cord injury is a rare but devastating complication of trauma. The spine must be kept immobilized in all traumatized children until neurological (in a fully alert child) and radiological examinations can be carried out. Worrisome historical features include a high-risk mechanism (e.g. diving) and limb paresthesias or paralysis, even if only present transiently.

Examination of a spinal cord injured patient can reveal various combinations of motor weakness or sensory impairment while priapism or poor anal tone are ominous signs. To exclude spinal cord injury, a full neurological examination in an alert child must be performed (therefore a child with altered level of consciousness or a painful distracting injury cannot be cleared).

At least anteroposterior and lateral X-rays of possibly affected regions of the spine should be obtained (see indications for cervical spine X-ray on p. 264). Because of the possibility of SCIWORA (spinal cord injury without radiological abnormality), normal X-rays are insufficient to allow discontinuation of immobilization in the child who cannot be fully examined. Computed tomography (CT) or magnetic resonance imaging (MRI) can be helpful in some of these cases.

Children with demonstrated spinal cord injury require ongoing immobilization and specialist consultation. Some consider steroid therapy appropriate, given within 8 hours of the injury (methylprednisolone 20–40 mg kg^{-1} bolus followed by 5.4 mg kg^{-1} per hour × 24 hours). Opinion varies, and it is advisable to check with the local spinal injuries unit for advice.

18.1.2 Pulmonary contusion and hemopneumothorax

Blunt trauma to the chest can result in various lung injuries. Probably the most common is the lung contusion. This can present with ranges of respiratory difficulty from minimally decreased oxygen saturation to frank respiratory failure. Localized findings such as injuries to the chest wall and crackles on auscultation can be important clues. X-ray may reveal nothing initially and then progress to hazy infiltrates, consolidation and accompanying effusion.

Important points to consider in the treatment of pulmonary contusion are listed in *Box 18.1*.

Box 18.1 Considerations in the treatment of pulmonary contusion

- Monitor closely, especially oxygen saturation and respiratory rate
- Provide supportive care with oxygen, CPAP or full intubation and ventilation
- Avoid over-hydration as this worsens pulmonary edema
- Analgesia is too often overlooked – pain results in hypoventilation and worsening atelectasis

---

Pneumothorax is a collection of air outside the lung within the pleural space. It suggests a disruption of an air passage. Physical signs include respiratory difficulty, asymmetrical chest wall motion, decreased air entry and hyper-resonance on percussion. Its importance lies in the possibility that it will progress to a tension pneumothorax where the trapped air exerts enough pressure on the lungs and heart to cause impaired ventilation and circulation. This can be rapidly fatal unless treated with a 14–16 gauge intravenous catheter inserted in the 2nd intercostal space at the mid-clavicular line. After the stylet is removed, a gratifying rush of air should be heard. This is a temporizing measure – a chest tube should be inserted, ideally within 10–15 minutes. Hemothorax can have the same implications as a tension pneumothorax with the added complication of circulatory embarrassment. Treatment is with proper circulatory support and drainage of the hemothorax with a chest tube.

18.1.3 Myocardial contusion and pericardial tamponade

Chest wall injury, especially that which leads to a sternal fracture, can cause a myocardial contusion or traumatic pericardial effusion. Both present with chest pain and tachycardia out of keeping with the degree of hypovolemia.

The danger of a myocardial contusion lies in the possibility of a malignant dysrhythmia. Sentinel changes on the ECG can include ventricular ectopy and ST segment abnormalities. Cardiac enzymes may be useful in documenting the injury. Management is with close monitoring and anti-dysrhythmic medication.

Pericardial tamponade can be rapidly fatal. Chest pain, tachycardia and dyspnea are accompanied by more specific signs such as muffled heart sounds, jugular venous distension and pulsus paradoxus. While echocardiography can be confirmatory and guide pericardiocentesis, it should not delay this procedure in the decompensating patient.

18.1.4 Intestinal injuries

Blunt abdominal trauma can cause a wide variety of injuries depending on the nature and direction of the traumatic force. *Table 18.1* is a partial list of conditions to look out for.

Table 18.1 Injuries associated with intestinal trauma	
Injury	**Look out for:**
Bowel perforation	May not be apparent initially Serial abdominal examinations reveal increasing peritoneal irritability X-ray eventually shows free air Water-soluble contrast studies may be helpful
Duodenal hematoma	Presents with delayed onset of bilious vomiting Upper GI contrast study may be diagnostic Look for associated injuries
Lap-belt injury	Triad composed of: • intestinal contusion or perforation • chance fracture of a thoracolumbar vertebrum • abdominal wall contusion
Handlebar injury	The end of a bicycle handlebar 'spears' the child May cause a traumatic pancreatitis, duodenal hematoma or linear laceration

18.1.5 Hepatic and splenic injuries

Blunt trauma can cause lacerations, contusions or outright fractures of the liver or spleen. Presenting signs include localized abdominal pain, abdominal distension and referred shoulder tip pain that may be aggravated by the recumbent position. Considerable occult bleeding can occur as a result of these injuries. The unstable patient may require urgent surgery. Stable patients can be investigated with abdominal CT or ultrasound. Diagnostic peritoneal lavage is reserved for patients who might have intra-abdominal bleeding who will be unavailable for serial examinations or CT because of the urgent need for a non-abdominal operation. Patients with significant hepatic or splenic injuries should be monitored in an intensive care unit.

18.1.6 Renal injuries

While blunt trauma to the kidney usually causes a simple contusion, more serious injuries such as vascular and collecting system disruptions can occur. These latter conditions must be identified and corrected within hours to assure a good outcome.

Physical examination
These clues are a poor guide to degree of injury except in very severe cases where flank ecchymoses or masses may be detected.

Investigation
The presence of hematuria can help determine which patients require radiological investigation. Gross hematuria from trauma should always have prompt investigation. Microscopic hematuria from minor trauma does not require investigation. Major trauma (severe force or multiple organ systems injured) that involves the abdomen or lower thorax should prompt investigation of the renal system regardless of the presence or absence of hematuria. CT with intravenous contrast is the preferred investigation since it images multiple abdominal organ systems concurrently. The intravenous pyelogram also gives both morphologic and functional (rate of contrast excretion) information. Some centers use renal ultrasound for selected indications.

Management
The majority of renal contusions and hematomas are treated non-operatively with medical support that includes monitoring of urine output with a Foley catheter and serial blood urea and creatinine measurement. Disruption of the renal vasculature may require further delineation with angiography or immediate surgical repair. Collecting system injuries usually require operative repair as well.

18.2 Penetrating injuries

18.2.1 General principles

The general approach for penetrating trauma is similar to that for blunt trauma. The assessment of any patient with potentially significant trauma begins with a rapid evaluation of airway, breathing and circulation, and treatment of immediately life-threatening conditions as they are identified. All patients should receive high-concentration oxygen during the initial evaluation. Intravascular access should be obtained with large-bore catheters and blood should be sent to the laboratory for cross-matching and other studies. A focused physical examination includes removal of all clothing, rolling the patient (while protecting the cervical spine) and quickly testing mental status and movement in all four extremities. After this phase has been completed, the physician can proceed to the more specific evaluation of individual injuries. A team approach with rapid surgical consultation is vital in the appropriate management of these patients.

As part of the initial stabilization of the victim of penetrating trauma, it may be necessary to control ongoing external blood loss. Usually this can be accomplished best by local pressure or packing. The physician should avoid trying to clamp vessels blindly as this carries the risk of further damaging traumatized tissues. Foreign bodies that are still present in wounds (e.g. knives or projectiles) should not be removed but rather stabilized in place, unless their presence interferes with other aspects of management. They may be tamponading bleeding or a clot may have formed around them. Efforts to remove them prematurely may trigger further bleeding.

Physicians need to be aware that bullets can travel unpredictably within the body. Distinguishing entrance and exit wounds is notoriously difficult. While the locations of the wounds may suggest a trajectory and raise concerns about specific organs, bullets may have ricocheted off bone or turned within the body and thus come to lie far from the visible wounds.

18.2.2 Head injuries

The management of head trauma is generally the same for penetrating as for blunt injuries. Scalp wounds of unclear depth in neurologically intact patients may be explored in the ED to determine whether the skull has been breached. In addition to the various lesions found in blunt head trauma, patients with penetrating skull trauma are at risk for vascular lacerations with later formation of arteriovenous fistulas and pseudo-aneurysms. Thus they may require cerebral angiography in addition to CT scan or MRI. Penetrating injuries are also at risk of infection with subsequent meningitis or brain abscess from material introduced at the time of injury, especially if the injuring object violated the sinuses, oral cavity or mastoid air cells. A first-generation cephalosporin is appropriate as initial antibiotic prophylaxis.

18.2.3 Spinal cord injuries

Penetrating spinal cord injury is rare in pediatrics. Stab wounds can lead to partial transections of the cord. These injuries have the potential for significant neurological recovery. In gunshot wounds, the damage is usually more severe due to the higher energy of the bullet and the possibility for secondary injury from associated fractures and bone fragments. All cases of suspected penetrating spinal injury require meticulous immobilization and early neurosurgical consultation. MRI, which is generally the preferred imaging modality for cord lesions, cannot be used when retained metallic foreign bodies are present. Corticosteroids are not indicated in penetrating spinal cord injury.

18.2.4 Neck injuries

Neck injuries can present treacherous clinical problems because of the many vital structures clustered together in a small space. The first priority of assessment and management is to ensure a patent airway. The airway may be compromised either by direct injury to the larynx and trachea or by compression from an expanding hematoma. Patients with progressive neck swelling, stridor, altered mental status or any degree of respiratory difficulty should have a definitive airway established as quickly as possible. Intubation is likely to be difficult in these patients because of anatomic distortion and bleeding. Therefore personnel and equipment must be immediately available for cricothyroidotomy, tracheostomy or transtracheal jet ventilation, in case intubation is not possible. Patients with penetrating neck injuries are also at risk for coexistent pneumothorax. Bleeding can generally be controlled by external pressure. If vital signs are unstable, emergency surgery is indicated.

If the patient is stable and it appears that the neck wound may be superficial, it is appropriate to explore the wound sufficiently to determine whether it has passed through the platysma. Wounds that do not violate the platysma may be sutured and treated as simple lacerations. Any wound that does violate the platysma requires surgical consultation and evaluation. Further probing below the level of the platysma should be avoided, since it can provoke uncontrolled bleeding.

Physical examination should specifically look for signs of injury to the various vulnerable organ systems. Airway injury may be manifest by hemoptysis, hoarseness, pain with coughing or swallowing, or subcutaneous emphysema. Damage to the esophagus may produce drooling, painful swallowing or hematemesis. Vascular injuries can present with a visible hematoma, a pulsatile mass, neck bruits, loss of brachial, carotid or temporal pulses, or with signs of localized or general cerebral ischemia. Hoarseness may also result from localized damage to the laryngeal nerve. The phrenic, facial or hypoglossal nerves, the stellate ganglion or the brachial plexus may also be involved, and their function should be specifically assessed. Patients with clear evidence of injury to respiratory, vascular or digestive structures on physical examination or plain radiographs require surgery, with or without other preoperative studies as determined by the consulting surgeon.

When there is not clear evidence of injury to significant structures as outlined above, the necessity to further evaluate neck injuries is controversial. At a minimum, all such patients with penetrating neck injury beyond the platysma require admission and frequent thorough clinical assessments.

The neck is divided into three zones for the purpose of wound description and management. Zone I extends from the clavicle to the cricoid, zone II from the cricoid to the angle of the mandible, and zone III is above the angle of the mandible. In the past, routine surgical exploration was advocated for all zone II injuries. Zone I and III injuries generally were evaluated with angiography, bronchoscopy, laryngoscopy and esophagoscopy and/or esophagography. Some authorities now advocate more selective operation and work-up for these various groups of patients based on clinical findings, but practice varies among various surgical services and institutions.

18.2.5 Chest injuries

The basic principles of management with a primary survey focusing on controlling the airway, obtaining vascular access and quickly finding treatable conditions that pose an immediate threat to life are the same as for blunt trauma. Most wounds that penetrate the chest wall will have created pneumothoraces. If a **tension pneumothorax** is suggested by physical examination, needle decompression followed by thoracostomy must be performed without awaiting X-ray confirmation. If the chest wound creates a continuing open passage for air to enter the chest cavity, an **open pneumothorax**, the wound must be covered with an occlusive dressing, which is initially taped down on three sides. The fourth side is left free to act as a flutter valve that allows air to leave the chest on expiration, but is pulled against the chest wall by the negative pleural pressure of inspiration and prevents air entry. Once a chest tube is placed, the fourth side of the dressing can be taped down as well. Simple pneumothorax or hemothorax is usually identified by chest X-ray. Chest tube placement is generally required, but careful observation with serial examinations and X-rays is also acceptable for some small pneumothoraces and hemothoraces in otherwise stable patients.

Any gunshot wound to the torso and any stab wound to the chest located between the midclavicular lines threatens the heart and other mediastinal structures. If the patient is stable, an echocardiogram can be performed at the bedside to evaluate for pericardial blood. In a hemodynamically unstable patient, pericardial tamponade should be considered even without classic signs of muffled heart sounds and jugular venous distension. If the unstable patient does not respond to fluid administration and chest tubes, pericardiocentesis should be performed to diagnose and treat the suspected tamponade, followed by a pericardial window procedure in the operating room. Release of pericardial tamponade is also the primary objective of Emergency Department thoracotomy. This approach is indicated for victims of penetrating chest trauma who become pulseless either during transport or after arrival in the Emergency Department or for those who are rapidly deteriorating despite initial stabilization maneuvers. Emergency thoracotomy in these patients will also sometimes allow direct control of massive intrathoracic hemorrhage or maintenance of central blood volume by clamping the descending aorta long enough for transport to the operating room and eventual survival. ED thoracotomy is not beneficial in patients with absent signs of life both at the scene and on arrival to the hospital.

Those patients with potential mediastinal injuries who do not require immediate operation must be evaluated for damage to the great vessels, the central airways and the esophagus. This evaluation might include various combinations of CT scanning, ultrasound, angiography, bronchoscopy, esophagoscopy and esophagography based on the specific clinical findings, the mechanism of injury and local practice.

Patients with stab wounds lateral to the midclavicular line and above the diaphragm who are clinically stable with a normal initial chest X-ray can be observed in the Emergency Department. If, after 4 hours, they remain clinically stable with a normal lung and heart examination, a normal oxygen saturation, and a normal repeat chest X-ray, they may be discharged, provided that they have access to good follow up and can return to the Emergency Department immediately if new symptoms develop.

Injury to the abdomen must be considered in any torso gunshot wound. At full expiration, the diaphragm rises to the level of the fourth intercostal space anteriorly and the inferior scapular tip posteriorly, and a stab wound below these landmarks may have entered the abdomen as well. Careful serial examinations of the abdomen must be performed, possibly with CT imaging. Imaging studies and examination are frequently normal in the case of small diaphragmatic lacerations, yet these tears can grow over time and present months to years later with herniation and even strangulation of abdominal viscera. For this reason, some authorities recommend routine evaluation of these wounds with either laparoscopy or peritoneal lavage (using a cut-off of 5000 red blood cells mm^{-3} for a positive test).

18.2.6 Abdominal injuries

The vast majority of patients with gunshot wounds to the abdomen, even if stable on presentation, will ultimately be found to have injuries requiring surgical intervention. Therefore most authorities recommend routine laparotomy for all abdominal gunshot wounds as soon as possible after initial stabilization in the Emergency Department.

On the other hand, many stab wounds do not breach the peritoneum. Even among those that have entered the abdominal cavity, approximately one-third may be able to be managed conservatively without ever needing surgery. Therefore a more individualized approach is appropriate for stab wounds. Patients with hypotension, peritoneal signs, GI bleeding or protruding bowel should go to the operating room without further diagnostic work-up of their abdomens. If it is not clear whether the peritoneum has been violated, a thorough local wound exploration may be performed. Wound exploration should not include any portion of the injury in the lower chest, as this can precipitate bleeding or pneumothorax. If the wound is clearly superficial, it can be treated with routine wound care and the patient can be discharged. When peritoneal penetration cannot be excluded, the patient must be admitted for 24 hours, at a minimum, for serial examinations. Abdominal CT scans can identify injuries in many such patients, but are poor for diagnosing bowel and diaphragm injuries. Some authorities would recommend either laparoscopy or peritoneal lavage in these patients with possible peritoneal penetration but no immediate indications for full laparotomy. If lavage is performed for penetrating trauma, an RBC count above 100 000 mm^{-3} is considered positive, while a count of 20 000–100 000 is equivocal. As noted above, if diaphragmatic injury is a possibility based on the location of the wound, this cut-off is lowered to 5000. All patients with possible peritoneal penetration should receive broad-spectrum antibiotics.

Patients with penetrating injuries to the lumbar back or flank who are hemodynamically stable require imaging of the kidneys and ureters by either IVP or CT scan. The CT scan is usually preferable as it also gives information regarding possible intraperitoneal injury. If the patient is unstable or has other indications for immediate laparotomy, a 'one-shot IVP' in the Emergency Department or on the operating table can give helpful information about renal function.

Recommended reading

Ferrera, C., Colucciello, S. *et al.* (2001) *Trauma Management: an Emergency Medicine Approach.* St Louis, MI: Mosby Inc.

Fleisher, G., Ludwig, S. *et al.* (2000) *Textbook of Pediatric Emergency Medicine.* Philadelphia: Lippincott, Williams & Wilkins.

Chapter 19

Head injury

Samina Ali and Martin Pusic

Contents

19.1 Epidemiology

Head injury is one of the most common childhood injuries. Annually in the USA, it accounts for more than 500 000 emergency visits, 95 000 hospital admissions, 7000 deaths, and 29 000 permanent disabilities. Head trauma is the leading cause of death among injured children, and is responsible for 80% of all trauma deaths.

Falls account for 37% of pediatric head injuries. Motor vehicle collisions (MVCs) are responsible for 18%, pedestrian injuries for 17% and bicycles, 10%. Infants and toddlers are most likely to fall from their own height. School-aged children tend to be involved in MVCs and sports-related accidents. Abuse can cause head injury in any age group.

Children with significant head injury need to be assessed and stabilized promptly, with the goal of preventing further neurological insult, and minimising the time to necessary neurosurgical intervention or transfer to the intensive care unit (ICU).

19.2 Pathophysiology

19.2.1 Primary brain injury

Brain injury is classified as either primary or secondary. Primary brain injury is the damage that occurs at the moment of impact. It may be due to the penetration of a foreign body, direct blunt injury to the brain, or to non-impact shear forces during an acceleration/deceleration event (most common). We are not able to treat primary brain injury.

19.2.2 Secondary brain injury

Secondary injury occurs some time after the initial insult as a result of impaired substrate delivery (hypoxia, hypoglycemia) or impaired perfusion (ischemia, hypotension) or maladaptive cellular responses to brain injury. These processes can cause both loss of neurones and cerebral edema. Unlike for primary brain injury, many of these processes can be ameliorated with timely supportive medical care.

19.3 Approach to the patient

Figure 19.1 shows the general management of a head injury.

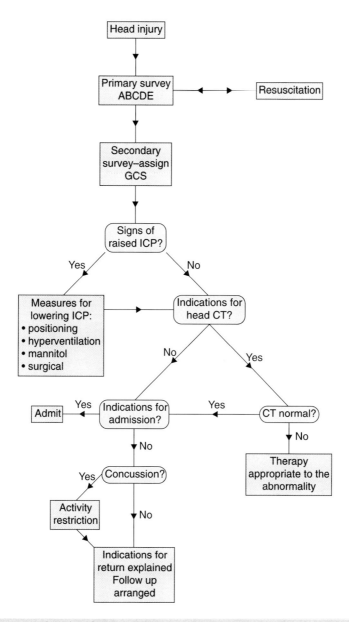

Figure 19.1 Flow chart for general management of head injury.

19.3.1 Primary survey

The first priority in a patient with traumatic brain injury is to rule out the presence of an acute, life-threatening disturbance. The process of identifying and addressing life-threatening injuries should be geared towards maintaining the brain's vital nutrients by correcting hypoxia and hypovolemia. The initial assessment and resuscitation, known as the

235

primary survey, should occur simultaneously and within the first few minutes of the patient's arrival (see Chapter 18).

Resuscitation

The approach to the head-injured patient begins in the same manner as the approach to any trauma patient: airway, breathing and then circulation.

Airway. It is of utmost importance to maintain adequate oxygenation and ventilation for the head-injured patient. Hypoxia and hypercarbia (hypercapnia) can ultimately result in increased intracranial pressure (ICP), which will cause secondary brain injury. Definitive airway management may require endotracheal intubation.

Intubating a head-injured patient should always be done in the safest, quickest manner possible (*Box 19.1*). The act of intubation has been shown to aggravate raised ICP. This rise in ICP with intubation can be blunted using a neuroprotective rapid sequence intubation technique (*Table 19.1*).

During intubation, a second individual should immobilize the cervical spine, in the neutral position. Nasotracheal intubation of the head-injured patient is discouraged since there may be an increased need to flex a potentially injured cervical spine, as well as the increased length of time required for this somewhat more difficult maneuver. Nasotracheal intubation is contraindicated in the patient with facial fractures or apnea.

Breathing. After the head-injured patient is intubated, placement of the tube confirmed and the tube secured, ventilation should be adjusted to maintain **normal** levels of oxygen and carbon dioxide. Decreasing blood carbon dioxide by hyperventilating the patient causes cerebral vasoconstriction and decreased intracranial pressure; however, hyperventilation should be performed only in patients with evidence of increased intracranial pressure.

Box 19.1 Indications for intubation of head injury patients

- GCS ≤ 8
- Acute increase in ICP, necessitating hyperventilation
- Hypoxia
- Hypercarbia
- Inability of patient to protect airway
- Severe thoracic or airway trauma
- Prior to transport of patient (for imaging or transfer of care)

Table 19.1 Neuroprotective technique for intubation of the potentially head injured patient (other methods exist)

Time	Action
5 min before intubation	100% oxygen Lidocaine 1 mg kg^{-1} i.v. Atropine 0.01 mg kg^{-1} i.v. (minimum 0.15 mg) Fentanyl 2 μg kg^{-1} i.v. Defasciculating dose of vecuronium 0.01 mg kg^{-1}
1 min before intubation	Thiopental 5 mg kg^{-1} i.v. (lower dose in potentially hypotensive patients or use midazolam instead) Succinylcholine 2 mg kg^{-1} i.v. (alternatively give vecuronium 0.1 mg kg^{-1} i.v.) Intubate and confirm tube placement
1 min *after* intubation	Continue sedation with either thiopental or midazolam (barbiturate preferred for possible neuroprotective effects) Consider whether to continue muscle blockade with vecuronium

Circulation. Ensuring adequate perfusion is also of great importance. Isotonic fluids should be used for fluid resuscitation. Boluses of 10–20 ml kg^{-1} should be given, with re-evaluation of the patient after every bolus. Some centres advocate the use of *hypertonic* saline (see local protocols). *Hypotonic* solutions should never be used, as they may exacerbate cerebral edema. Blood products should be used for significant hemorrhage, and vasopressors might be required if fluids alone are insufficient to maintain the patient's blood pressure.

Preventing hypotension can prevent secondary brain injury. While overhydration can worsen cerebral edema, this concern should never keep the clinician from repleting a hypotensive patient's intravascular fluid aggressively. Put simply, the ABCs of resuscitation have first priority in the care of a patient with traumatic brain injury.

Disability (neurological considerations)

There are many tools available to assess a child's neurologic status rapidly. The Glasgow Coma Scale (GCS) (*Table 19.2*) and the AVPU (*Box 19.2*) method are two widely known and used tools. The GCS, in its original form, is useful for older children and adolescents (*Table 19.2*). There is a modified version available for infants and toddlers (*Table 19.3*).

Table 19.2 The Glasgow Coma Scale (4–15 years)

Activity	Score	Effect
Eye opening		
Spontaneously	4	Reticular activating system intact
To verbal command	3	Opens eyes on command
To pain	2	Opens eyes in response to pain
None	1	Does not open eyes to any stimuli
Verbal response		
Oriented	5	Aware of self and environment
Disoriented	4	Organized speech, but patient disoriented
Inappropriate words	3	Random words
Incomprehensible	2	Moaning, no recognisable words
No response	1	No response or intubated
Motor response		
Obeys verbal commands	6	Moves limbs when told to
Localises to painful stimuli	5	Moves limb in an effort to avoid painful stimuli
Withdrawal	4	Pulls away from pain in flexion
Abnormal flexion	3	Decorticate rigidity
Extension	2	Decerebrate rigidity
No response	1	Hypotonia, flaccid

Box 19.2 The AVPU system

A Alert
V Responds to **V**erbal stimuli
P Responds to **P**ainful stimuli
U Unresponsive

Assessment of disability should also include a rapid assessment of the pupil size and reactivity.

Exposure

The final component of the primary survey is exposure of the patient. This involves fully undressing the patient, in order to allow for identification of other injuries. It is important to remember that infants are highly susceptible to hypothermia, and care should be taken in order to avoid this by controlling the temperature of the resuscitation room and using heating lamps.

Table 19.3 Modified coma score for infants and children

Activity	Score	Infants best response	Children (< 4 years)
Eyes opening	4	Spontaneous	Spontaneous
	3	To speech	To speech
	2	To pain	To pain
	1	No response	No response
Verbal response	5	Coos, babbles	Oriented – social, smiles, follows objects, converses
	4	Irritable cry	Confused, disoriented, aware of environment, consolable cries
	3	Cries to pain	Inappropriate words, persistent cries, inconsolable
	2	Moans to pain	Incomprehensible sounds, agitated, restless, inconsolable
	1	No response	No response
Motor response	6	Normal spontaneous movements	Normal spontaneous movements
	5	Withdraws to touch	Localises pain
	4	Withdraws to pain	Withdraws to pain
	3	Abnormal flexion	Abnormal flexion
	2	Abnormal extension	Abnormal extension
	1	No response	No response

19.3.2 Secondary survey

Neurological evaluation

Head examination should include pupillary size and reactivity, fundoscopy and skull palpation. Assessment of the cervical spine should be done with great caution. If the patient is not fully alert, has a distracting injury, or is intoxicated, then the rigid collar should be left on and the examination of the cervical spine should be deferred.

A complete neurological examination should be part of the evaluation of a child with traumatic brain injury, but may be complicated by sedatives in use for maintaining ventilation. Motor and cranial nerves should be tested in a cooperative patient. Motor strength can be graded from 0 to 5 (*Box 19.3*).

Cranial nerve examination should include eye movements, gag reflex, corneal reflex and facial symmetry. Level of consciousness, mental status, GCS score reassessment, brain stem function, and respiratory rate

Box 19.3 Muscle strength grading

0	No muscle movement/contraction
1	Trace muscle contraction
2	Muscle contracts, cannot overcome gravity
3	Antigravity movement only
4	Active movement against resistance
5	Normal muscle strength

and pattern should be measured. Deep tendon reflexes, symmetry of movement, Babinski response, signs of basilar skull fractures (*Box 19.4*), signs of increased intracranial pressure (*Box 19.5*), and step-off deformities of the cervical and thoracolumbar spine should also be noted.

Box 19.4 Clinical signs of basilar skull fracture

- Battle's sign (retroauricular hematoma)
- Blood in the ear canal
- Cranial nerve deficits
- Decreased auditory acuity
- Dizziness
- Facial paralysis
- Hemotympanum
- Nystagmus
- Otorrhea
- Racoon's sign (periorbital ecchymosis)
- Rhinorrhea
- Tinnitus

Box 19.5 Symptoms and signs of increased intracranial pressure

- Abnormal pupillary responses – unilateral or bilateral dilation
- Cushing's triad: slow pulse, raised blood pressure and breathing pattern abnormalities
- Decreased level of consciousness
- Full fontanelle
- Headache
- Irritability
- Papilloedema
- Persistent emesis
- Photophobia
- Posturing, decerebrate or decorticate
- 'Setting sun' sign
- Splitting of sutures
- Stiff neck

In infants, the neurological examination may have to be modified for age, owing to inability to cooperate with the examination.

19.4 General management

If increased intracranial pressure is suspected, this should be treated promptly within the emergency department (*Box 19.6*).

Box 19.6 Emergency management of increased ICP

- Head elevation to 30°
- Mid-line positioning of head (not looking to either side)
- Hyperventilation (acute intervention)
- Mannitol or glycerol, 0.5–1 g kg^{-1} i.v.
- Pentobarbital 1–3 mg kg^{-1} loading dose
- Controlled hypothermia 27–31° (controversial)

Early recognition of herniation is of great importance. Uncal herniation (*Figure 19.2*) can cause unilateral dilatation of a pupil, contralateral hemiplegia and spontaneous hyperventilation. If untreated, it will lead to brainstem (central) herniation. Brainstem herniation can also occur independent of uncal herniation. Signs of early uncal herniation include small sluggish pupils, decorticate posturing (abnormal flexion) and Cheyne–Stokes respiration. Late presentation includes fixed and dilated pupils, flaccid muscle tone and apnea. Herniation requires the immediate attention of the neurosurgeon for surgical decompression. Intervention can be carried out in the ED or the operating theatre.

Radiological evaluation should be obtained, as soon as the cardiorespiratory status of the patient is as stable as possible. Guidelines for the most appropriate investigation in a given situation is ongoing in many countries. At present, plain films are useful in particular circumstances, usually when the patient is stable and alert at presentation (*Box 19.7*).

CT scanning has become an increasingly popular mode of imaging for head-injured patients. There has been much debate over what the indi-

---
Box 19.7 Indications for plain films

- Child abuse evaluation (as a part of the skeletal survey)
- Evaluation of the functioning of a ventriculoperitoneal shunt
- Penetrating wounds of the scalp
- Age < 12 months
- Suspicion of foreign body underlying the scalp

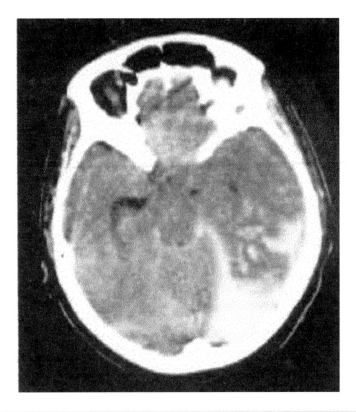

Figure 19.2 CT scan showing uncal herniation with interhemispheric bleed (reprinted from Rosen's *Textbook of Emergency Medicine* Fourth Edition 1997, with permission from Elsevier Science).

cations for CT scanning are. *Box 19.8* outlines the current recommendations from the USA.

Disposition of the patient should be decided based on the clinical appearance of the child. A child with a head injury can be nursed at home, only if there are reliable caretakers to monitor the child's neuro-

Box 19.8 Recommendations for CT scanning
• Presence of neurologic deficit
• GCS < 14
• History of forceful mechanism of injury
• Penetrating injury
• Suspicion of abuse
• If < 1 year, then protracted vomiting, irritability, or poor feeding

logical status. If this is not possible, then an admission might be warranted for social reasons.

19.4.1 Indications for admission

Box 19.9 shows the indications for admission of head-injury patients.

Box 19.9 Indications for admission

- Abnormal CT
- Child abuse
- Fluctuating consciousness
- Focal deficits
- Lengthy loss of consciousness (> 2–5 minutes)
- Persisting signs such as vomiting
- Seizures
- Severe/worsening headache
- Significant amnesia
- Somnolence/irritability in a young infant
- Unreliable caretakers

19.5 Intracranial lesions

19.5.1 Epidural (extradural) hematoma

An epidural hematoma is the result of an arterial bleed, commonly from the middle meningeal artery in the lateral temporal fossa, with an overlying fracture. The diagnosis of an epidural hemorrhage is challenging, as it may be accompanied by a story of only trivial injury. The classic picture of a brief loss of consciousness (LOC), followed by a lucid interval, and then rapid clinical deterioration is inconsistently seen in children. Children will often complain of headache, which will be followed by an altered level of consciousness.

CT scan is the most appropriate investigation. Epidural hemorrhage appears as a lens-shaped hyperdense lesion on the CT scan (*Figure 19.3*). The lesion is usually drained in a neurosurgical procedure, and the patient is given supportive care.

19.5.2 Subarachnoid hemorrhage

Subarachnoid hemorrhages are the most common intracranial bleed associated with birth trauma. The bleed tends to be venous, rather than

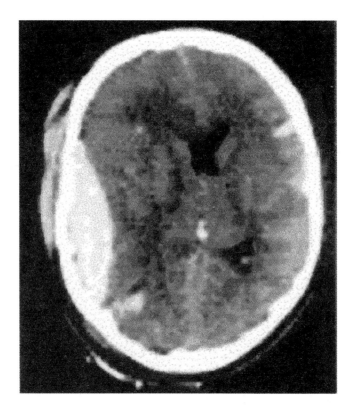

Figure 19.3 CT scan showing acute epidural hematoma (reprinted from Rosen's *Textbook of Emergency Medicine* Fourth Edition 1997, with permission from Elsevier Science).

arterial. The infant is frequently asymptomatic at the onset. The most common symptom is a seizure, at 48 hours of life or later. Treatment is supportive and symptomatic.

19.5.3 Subdural hematoma

A subdural hemorrhage can occur from severe head injury and is the classical intracranial bleed associated with shaken baby syndrome. In this subgroup of children there may be bilateral lesions and there may be an associated skull fracture in the shaken baby impact syndrome. Subdural hemorrhage is a result of venous bleeds, usually of the bridging veins between the layers of the dura. It tends to expand slowly and is usually associated with underlying brain lacerations or contusions.

Physical findings include those of increased intracranial pressure. On CT scan, the hematoma is often crescent shaped, with the concavity in the same direction as the concavity of the skull, spreading diffusely along the inner table of the skull (*Figure 19.4*). If the injury was sustained more than 1 week prior to the imaging, then contrast may be needed in order to identify the lesion. Over time, the blood changes from hyperdense, to isodense as the blood clot liquefies.

Subdural hemorrhages are treated neurosurgically. Symptomatic lesions require drainage of the blood via a burr hole.

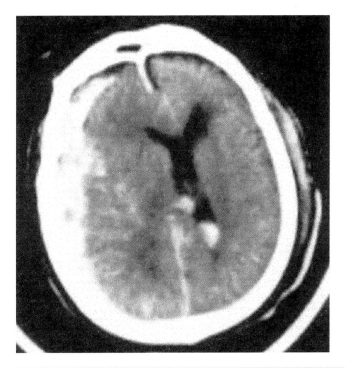

Figure 19.4 CT scan showing subdural hematoma with hydrocephalus (reprinted from Rosen's *Textbook of Emergency Medicine* Fourth Edition 1997, with permission from Elsevier Science).

19.6 **Other head injuries**

19.6.1 Concussion

Concussion is a common injury in children. The hallmark of concussion is amnesia, which may be temporary or permanent. Clinical symptoms that may be found with concussion include dizziness, vomiting, headache, confusion, difficulty concentrating and memory deficits. Concussion can occur, with or without LOC. If LOC does occur, it is rarely for more than 5 minutes.

Most children with concussion require analgesia for pain (e.g. paracetamol), and careful observation by a responsible parent, at home. All parents should be given clear instructions as to the indications for return to hospital, as well as information on sports restrictions (*Box 19.10*).

Box 19.10 Advice given to families compared to severity of concussion

Grade 1 Concussion
Definition: transient confusion, no LOC, mental status abnormalities < 15 min
Recommendations: no sports until asymptomatic for 1 week

Grade 2 Concussion
Definition: transient confusion, no LOC, mental status abnormalities ≥ 15 min
Recommendations: no sports until asymptomatic for 2 weeks

Grade 3 Concussion
Definition: any LOC
Recommendations: no sports until asymptomatic for 4 weeks

If any intracranial pathology is identified by imaging, the patient should engage in no sports activities for the remainder of the season. The patient should be strongly discouraged from future return to contact sports as they risk cumulative effects from repeated concussive injuries. Occasionally, patients will later develop **postconcussion syndrome**. This syndrome is characterized by persistent concussion symptoms, as well as memory and concentration difficulties. As a result, these children may have difficulties with school work and socialisation. They should be referred for follow up.

Rarely, patients may develop what is known as **second impact syndrome**. This syndrome has been reported in football players who have suffered more than one concussion in a short period of time. With the second seemingly innocuous concussion, they develop malignant, diffuse cerebral edema. This syndrome has extremely high morbidity and mortality.

19.6.2 Skull fractures

Linear skull fractures are the most common pediatric skull fracture, occurring in nearly 75% of the cases. The parietal bone is the most common fracture site. Accidental linear fractures rarely cross suture lines.

Normal variations of the pediatric skull and suture lines are often misinterpreted as fractures. It is important to look for bilaterality of the line, as this would suggest a suture. Also, suture lines tend to be finely jagged, while linear fractures are more straight-edged.

'Growing fractures' are a variation of linear fractures that are unique to pediatrics. The child initially suffers a fracture, associated with a dural tear. Infants and young children have rapid brain growth, and they can develop extrusion of the brain tissue or a CSF cyst (leptomeningeal cyst) through the dural defect. This complication requires neurosurgical intervention, and should be referred to the appropriate surgeon. It is in order to facilitate early identification of this lesion that all infants and children under the age of 2 years, who have had a linear fracture, are to be followed by neurosurgery for at least 1 year.

Depressed skull fractures are due to direct, forceful impact and may be associated with concomitant underlying brain lacerations. They can be difficult to diagnose with one radiological view, and may require oblique views for diagnosis. Early referral to a neurosurgical team is essential, as the definitive management of a depressed skull fracture may involve operative elevation of the depressed fragment of bone. Routine prophylactic antibiotics are not recommended.

Basilar skull fractures should be suspected in patients with the appropriate clinical signs such as hemotympanum, Battle sign, racoon eyes, nasal blood or nasal CSF leak. CT scan best diagnoses such fractures, although this test is imperfect. Management generally includes neurosurgical consultation and symptomatic care. Often, no intervention is necessary. Antibiotic prophylaxis is not routinely recommended, even with a CSF leak.

19.6.3 Subgaleal hematoma

Subgaleal hematoma, characteristically presenting as a 'boggy' scalp swelling is the most common complication of a linear skull fracture. It may develop within days to weeks of the initial injury. Clinically and radiologically, it may resemble a CSF collection. However, it is a collection of blood associated with a fracture site. Management is non-interventional, and the lesions almost always spontaneously resorb. Aspiration is not recommended.

19.6.4 Brain contusion

Contusion or bruising of the brain parenchyma is found on CT scan. It is commonly caused by the brain tissue striking the irregular, rigid skull. Contusions are described as either coup or contre-coup. A *coup injury* is a contusion at the site of impact, while a *contre-coup injury* occurs at a site that is remote from the impact. Signs and symptoms of contusion include LOC, alterations in strength or sensation, changes in vision, and occasionally, focal neurologic signs related to the site of contusion. Patients with contusions should be hospitalized with close observation, in order to monitor for further deterioration. A neurosurgical consultation should be obtained.

19.6.5 Scalp lacerations

The scalp is a highly vascularized structure and seemingly trivial lacerations may bleed profusely. Careful attention should be paid to the child's hemodynamic status, as blood loss thought to be insignificant in an adult may cause compromise in a smaller patient. When you are examining a scalp laceration, care should be taken to ensure that the underlying skull is intact. The wound should be explored for foreign bodies, then scrubbed and irrigated. The lesion can be closed with a variety of techniques, depending on the type of laceration. A relatively short and linear laceration can be treated by simply plaiting a small tress of hair tightly over the lesion. This is effective only if the bleeding is relatively mild, and the child's hair is long enough! Histoacryl glue is an alternative treatment for small lacerations or sutures may be used.

19.6.6 Minimal head injury

Minimal or trivial head injury describes an injury to the head with no significant clinical signs or symptoms either at the time of the injury or at the time of presentation to the ED. Often, the child will have a superficial laceration or swelling of the forehead or scalp. Treatment might be needed for minor pain, for example with paracetamol. The parents should still be instructed in the signs and symptoms that should prompt return for re-evaluation. The child's presentation to the hospital should be used as an opportunity to counsel the parents about head injury prevention, such as helmet use in sports.

19.7 Non-accidental trauma

The most common cause of death from physical abuse is secondary to head trauma. It is estimated that up to one-third of head injured pediatric patients who are admitted to the ICU are victims of non-accidental trauma. In infants under 1 year of age, this number reaches 95% for severe head injuries. The vast majority of victims are under the age of 2 years. Any child for whom the given history for an injury is not consistent with the actual injury sustained, should alert the physician to the possibility of child abuse (see Chapter 27).

19.8 Conclusion

There is a widespread belief that pediatric patients tend to have better outcomes with head injury, as compared to older patients. In fact, studies do confirm this. An important exception to this generalization is the infant and toddler group. They tend to have a poorer prognosis than their other pediatric counterparts. In all age groups, meticulous supportive medical care and attention to evolving neurological signs can improve outcomes.

Further reading

Mansfield, R.T. (1997) Head injuries in children and adults. *Crit. Care Clin.* **13**: 611–628.

Savitsky, E.A., Votey, S.R. (2000) Current controversies in the management of pediatric minor head injuries. *Am. J. Emerg. Med.* **18**: 96–101.

Fleischer, G. and Ludwig, S. *et al.* (2000) *Textbook of Pediatric Emergency Medicine*. Philadelphia: Lippincott, Williams and Wilkins.

Chapter 20

Emergency burn management including smoke inhalation

Stephen Gordon and Kathy Lendrum

Contents

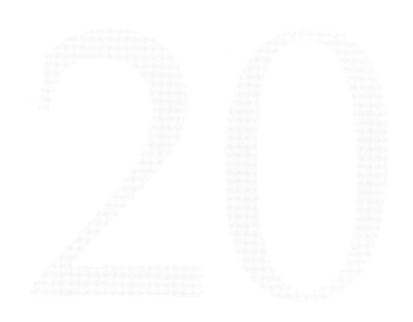

20.1 Burns

20.1.1 Introduction

Burn injuries are common in the pediatric age group and range from trivial local wounds to acutely life-threatening conditions. The emergency physician plays a vital role in stabilizing the patient, preventing secondary injury, and triaging the patient to appropriate specialty care as needed.

20.1.2 Pathophysiology of burns

The skin helps to regulate fluid and heat balance and acts as a barrier to infection. When tissue is injured or destroyed by thermal energy in a burn, all of these functions are jeopardised. Immediately after a major burn, patients are at risk of hypovolemia through several mechanisms. Massive amounts of fluid can be lost to the environment as transudation occurs across the burned area. Intravascular volume depletion is further exacerbated by fluid shifts within the tissues. Edema develops locally as a direct response to injury, while vasoactive mediators released at the burn site also provoke a more diffuse capillary leakage in both the systemic and pulmonary circulations. Mediators released from the burn site can depress cardiac function, hampering the normal compensations for hypovolemia. Circulatory function is also affected by hemolysis, produced both by direct heat injury to red blood cells in the burned area and from a microangiopathic process in damaged vascular beds. Hypothermia is common as the skin loses its ability to shunt blood away from cold-exposed sites. Exposure to cold ambient temperatures during prolonged resuscitation must be avoided as much as possible.

Infection is not generally a threat in the emergency phase of burn management. However, sepsis remains the leading cause of death in burn patients who survive beyond initial resuscitation. Localized infection is a common complication of smaller burns, particularly those which present after 24 hours, and leads to delayed healing and poorer ultimate cosmetic outcome. Proper sterile technique and local wound care is essential in preventing these later sequele.

Physicians must be alert to the possibility of other types of injury often associated with burns. Patients burned by fires in enclosed spaces such as house fires or motor vehicle accidents could have suffered from inhalation of carbon monoxide, cyanide gas or other gaseous toxins. They might have suffered hypoxic insult, when environmental oxygen has been depleted by the fire. Finally other major trauma due to falls or explosions could have occurred.

20.1.3 Classification

Burns are classified by the depth of the damage relative to the various structures of the skin. *Superficial or first-degree burns* damage only the epidermis. The classic example is a sunburn. Clinically these burns are manifested by redness and tenderness without blistering and they generally heal uneventfully in about a week.

Partial-thickness or second-degree burns penetrate into the dermis, but hair follicles and sweat glands remain and provide a source for re-epithelialisation of the wound from within. The clinical hallmark of second-degree burns is blister formation. These burns are characteristically very painful because of the presence of exposed nerve endings. Partial-thickness burns are often further subdivided into superficial and deep types, representing injury to less or more than half of the thickness of the dermis, respectively. In the superficial subgroup, blisters are typically thin-walled and the skin appears pink and moist. In deep partial-thickness burns, blisters are thick-walled. The wound is drier and may have a pale, speckled appearance, owing to the presence of many small thrombosed vessels at the base of the wound. Most superficial second-degree burns will heal without major scarring, while deeper second-degree burns may require skin grafting.

In *full-thickness or third-degree burns*, the entire dermis is destroyed. These wounds appear grey or charred. There is no pain, as nerve endings have been destroyed (although surrounding areas of second-degree burn may make this distinction difficult). Spontaneous healing can occur only from the edges of the wound inwards, since deep dermal structures within the affected area are absent. Skin grafting is usually necessary.

The term *'fourth-degree burn'* is sometimes used for burns that extend beyond the skin into muscle and other tissues.

20.1.4 Initial stabilization

As with any accident victim, the first priorities in managing a burn patient are the 'ABCs' (see Chapter 3). The burn patient's airway is vulnerable to anatomic obstruction from direct heat injury or smoke inhalation, or it may become obstructed as a result of depressed mental status secondary to hypoxia, inhaled toxins or associated head injury. All patients presenting with major burns should be given 100% oxygen. Facial burns, singed nasal hairs, soot in the mouth and nose, or carbonaceous sputum all increase the likelihood of significant airway insult. If any of these signs are present, the airway should be visualized directly to assess pharyngeal or glottic edema. Airway edema can be expected to worsen over the first 24–48 hours after injury. To prevent difficulties with intubation after swelling has progressed to frank obstruction, elective intubation should be performed for all patients with signs of respiratory difficulty such as hoarseness or stridor, and in all patients with edema seen on laryngoscopy. If the possibility of other trauma exists (e.g. if the patient has fallen while escaping from a house fire), proper cervical spine immobilization should be maintained until a cervical spine injury can be excluded. Wheezing due to airway injury may respond to a nebulised beta 2-agonist. Vascular access must be obtained as quickly as possible in all patients with major burns. Ideally i.v. lines should be placed through unburned skin, but this is not always possible. An initial bolus of 20 ml kg^{-1} of normal saline or Ringer's lactate can be given while further assessment is proceeding.

During initial stabilization, any clothing should be removed and burned areas should be covered loosely with clean, dry sheets or wet sheets to prevent sticking as long as the concomitant cooling is not an issue.

20.1.5 Burn assessment

First assess the:
• depth
• size
• site
• infection

Once vital functions have been stabilized, the burns should be examined and assessed with respect to depth and extent. Burn extent is described as the percentage of body surface area suffering second-degree burns or deeper. First-degree burns need to be assessed and described, but are not included in the calculated total percentage body surface area. The 'rule of nines', used to calculate surface area involvement in adults, is inappropriate for children with their relatively larger heads and smaller extremities. Special charts have been developed for use with children (*Table 20.1*).

The extent of smaller burns can be estimated by using the fact that the palmar surface of the patient's own hand, including fingers, is equivalent to 1% of total body surface area. Circumferential burns must be carefully noted, so they can be observed for complications requiring escharotomy, as detailed below under 'wound care'.

Part of the assessment of any burn injury should be to determine the possibility of child abuse. The history of how the injury occurred, as pro-

Table 20.1 Percentage total body area in children

Body region	Percentage of total body surface area		
	Infant (%)	Toddler age 2 years* (%)	> 10 years (%)
Head and neck	20	13	9–10
Upper limb	9	9	9
Torso (anterior)	18	18	18
Torso (entire)	36	36	36
Lower limb	13	16	18

* Values for toddlers are interpolated approximations.

vided by the child's caretaker, should be evaluated for plausibility and consistency with both the child's developmental stage and the physical examination findings. Accidental burns in young children most often result from hot liquids and will have characteristic splash or drip patterns. Deep burns with discrete geometric edges are especially suspicious, particularly those on the buttocks or in a stocking-and-glove distribution. Deliberate burning with cigarettes, curling irons or other objects often leaves distinctive marks. If there is any suspicion of inflicted injury, appropriate reporting and further work-up must be initiated by emergency physicians.

20.1.6 Pain management

Assessment of pain should be part of the emergency burn assessment. Inadequate analgesia can compound the lasting effects of the initial traumatic experience. Generous analgesia should be provided as soon as possible (within the limits of safety in maintaining ventilation and perfusion). In severe cases, pain can be rapidly controlled by giving intravenous morphine at doses up to 0.15 mg kg^{-1} every 15 minutes until the pain is controlled and then approximately every hour thereafter. Sedatives such as diazepam or midazolam can also be helpful. Intramuscular analgesics should not be used as they are held in the tissues when perfusion is inadequate and then may be released as a bolus when perfusion improves. The pain control service should be involved in these cases right from presentation to the ED.

20.1.7 Fluid therapy

As described above, burn victims are at risk for profound hypovolemia and require impressive amounts of fluid to maintain adequate circulation. Several different formule exist for calculating fluid requirements, all of which have their own convinced proponents. The most widely used is the Parkland formula. It calculates the fluid required over the first 24 hours after the time of injury as follows:

$$\text{Fluid requirement in mls for first 24 hours} = 4 \times \% \text{ burn} \times \text{weight(kg)}$$

Note that % burn is the body surface area burned exclusive of first degree burns.

In children under 5 years, this must be adjusted by adding the usual maintenance fluid requirements. Half of the replacement volume should be given in the first 8 hours (counting from the time of the burn, not time of presentation), with the remainder given over the subsequent 16 hours. This fluid is usually given as crystalloid, most often Ringer's lactate. No supplemental potassium is generally required, as destruction in burned tissue leads to release of large amounts of intracellular potassium.

Whichever formula is used in calculating fluid requirements, it should be used only as a rough guide. Adequacy of the fluid replacement must be continuously assessed by monitoring vital signs, perfusion, mental status and urine output. In patients with large burns, a Foley catheter should be placed early to allow quantification of urine output, with the aim of maintaining urine output of at least $1 \, \text{ml} \, \text{kg}^{-1}$ per hour. Occasionally a brisk diuresis despite other signs of intravascular depletion may result from stress-induced hyperglycemia.

20.1.8 Wound care

General measures
There is no role for systemic antibiotics in the initial management of burns. They do not decrease subsequent infection rates, but do promote antibiotic resistance. Instead, wounds require careful surveillance with judicious use of antibiotics for clinical signs of infection.

Tetanus immunization status should be assessed in all burn patients, and booster shots and/or tetanus immunoglobulin should be given as needed.

Minor burn wound management
Parents or care providers in the field should treat localized burns by removing clothing from the affected area and placing the burned skin

under cool running water for 10 minutes, to help dissipate heat and stop the process of tissue destruction. The burn can then be covered with a clean cloth or clingfilm. Care must be taken not to make the patient hypothermic.

In the Emergency Department, burns can be irrigated with cool saline. There is controversy and little evidence as to whether blisters should be debrided or left intact. Small scraps of devitalised skin from bulle which have ruptured spontaneously can be removed. Prompt dressing reduces the pain of the burn. We suggest one of two methods for dressing minor burn wounds.

- A paraffin gauze or Mepital dressing is placed over the wound and then covered with a dry dressing. This dressing is redone twice weekly at first, and then weekly. This method avoids the pain and emotional trauma of frequent dressing changes.
- Topical antibiotic ointments are applied to the wound, most often silver sulfadiazine. Bacitracin is preferred on the face, where sulfadiazine can cause unsightly bleaching of the skin. Note that sulfadiazine is also contraindicated in cases of sulfa allergy or glucose-6-phosphate dehydrogenase (G6PD) deficiency. Loose, dry gauze dressings should be placed over the antibiotic ointment and changed twice daily. These frequent dressing changes may be traumatic for some children.

Major burn wound management

In cases of more extensive burns requiring hospitalization, local wound care should be decided in consultation with the admitting service, as practices differ widely. There has recently been interest in a wide variety of alternative semipermeable and biologic dressings. A simple initial approach is to cover large wounds with clingfilm (e.g. Saran Wrap®) until the child gets to the Burns Unit. This keeps out the air and thus cuts down pain and allows the plastic surgeons to see the wound without taking dressings off. The clingfilm is removed in the Burns Unit to put on the definitive dressing.

Circumferential full-thickness burns of the extremities can lead to distal ischemia, as edema develops over the 24–48 hours following injury and the burn acts as a constricting tourniquet. In such cases, distal perfusion needs to be closely monitored, preferably with Doppler monitoring of pulses. If perfusion is compromised, an escharotomy must be performed down to the level of the fascia. Circumferential full-thickness burns of the chest can similarly cause constriction and impairment of ventilation. Again, emergency escharotomy is indicated if this occurs.

20.1.9 Disposition

Children presenting to the ED with burns and scalds usually require further care. *Box 20.1* lists considerations to help clinicians in making appropriate referral decisions. We admit all children with burns under a plastic surgeon to a Burns Centre in the UK.

If patients are discharged from the ED, their caretakers must be given scrupulous instructions regarding technique of dressing changes and signs of infection, which would require them to seek emergency medical attention. All burns deeper than first degree should be re-examined by a physician. Practice varies, but most change the dressing as little as possible to reduce pain and distress for the child. An initial redressing rate of between 5 and 10 days is advised in most centers. The top layers of the dressing may need changing more frequently, to keep it dry.

Box 20.1 Admission criteria for burns patients

General
- Underlying medical conditions (e.g. immunosuppression, condition affecting wound healing)
- Electrical (risk of dysrhythmia) or chemical burns (risk depends on nature of chemical)
- Inhalation injury (monitor respiratory status)
- Burns that are circumferential or cross major joints (high complication rate)
- Second- or third-degree burn on the face, hands, feet or perineum
- Suspected child abuse
- Concern regarding the ability of the caretakers to comply with medical recommendations and follow up

Under 10 years of age
- Burns totalling > 10% of BSA
- Deep second- or third-degree burns of > 3% BSA
- Burns in the nappy area of young babies

Over 10 years of age
- Burns totalling > 15% of BSA
- Deep second- or third-degree burns of > 5% BSA

Abbreviation: BSA, body surface area

20.2 Smoke inhalation

20.2.1 Pathophysiology

Heat

Flames and dry heat injure the upper airways whereas the inhalation of steam or hot gases can also cause severe injury to lower airways and lung parenchyma. Heat will cause erythema, edema, hemorrhage and ulceration. Respiratory failure will result from gradual swelling and airway obstruction over 48–72 hours. It is important to recognise the potential dangers early before intubation becomes impossible due to edema.

Chemical Injury

Smoke is a mixture of gases in which carbon particles are suspended. These are deposited at different levels of the respiratory tree depending on size. Various toxic substances coat the carbon particles and cause direct damage to mucosa (*Box 20.2*). Mucus production is increased and can obstruct airways; ciliary action and surfactant production are reduced further increasing the work of breathing.

Box 20.2 Toxic substances in smoke

- Hydrochloric acid
- Ammonia
- Ketones
- Organic acids
- Hydrogen cyanide
- Carbon monoxide

Asphyxia

In a fire in an enclosed space, atmospheric oxygen levels are greatly reduced. Hydrogen cyanide has a direct toxic effect at cellular level binding to cytochromes and blocking oxygen utilization. Organs with a high metabolic rate (e.g. heart and brain) are preferentially injured leading to myocardial and central nervous system depression. This results in shock, hypoventilation and coma increasing asphyxia further. Anerobic metabolism produces lactate causing a metabolic acidosis. Concentrations of 180 ppm of cyanide cause death in under 10 minutes.

20.2.2 History and examination

Any history of a child being in a fire and potentially inhaling smoke must be taken seriously, even if the fire is said to have been a minor one. The face, skin and respiratory system must be examined carefully. Signs of potential smoke inhalation are listed in *Box 20.3*. Stridor and drooling, a hoarse voice and signs of respiratory distress suggest impending airway obstruction. A chest X-ray should be taken early.

> **Box 20.3** Signs of potential inhalational injury
>
> - Facial burns
> - Conjunctivitis
> - Rhinorrhea
> - Sooty deposits in nostrils or oropharynx
> - Carbonaceous sputum

20.2.3 Management

Following a major fire or burns injury, the ABC sequence of management should be adopted. Injury to the cervical spine should be considered. Any child in respiratory distress needs urgent tracheal intubation. All children should be given 100% humidified oxygen. Early hypovolemic shock is not attributable to any burn until intra-abdominal, intrathoracic or peripheral sources of bleeding are excluded.

Once impending airway obstruction is suspected, then early intubation is essential since progressive airway edema in the days following injury will make later intubation very difficult. Compared to adults, small tracheal diameter will result in earlier airway compromise. In cases of airway obstruction fibreoptic techniques, and needle and surgical cricothyroidotomy should be considered.

Ongoing care is supportive. Children are at risk of developing pulmonary edema and the adult respiratory distress syndrome. Secondary bacterial infections also occur. Research is looking at adjunctive therapy such as aerosoled 21-aminosteroids, *N*-acetylcysteine and heparin.

Carbon monoxide levels should be measured and managed as above. Cyanide poisoning should be considered in cases of heavy smoke exposure, metabolic acidosis or a high carboxyhemoglobin level. The specific treatment of cyanide poisoning includes sodium nitrite and sodium thiosulphate with regular monitoring of methemoglobin levels.

Further reading

DiGuiseppe, C., Higgins, J.P.T. (2000) Systematic review of controlled trials of interventions to promote smoke alarms. *Arch. Dis. Child.* **82**: 341–348.

Joffe, M. Burns. In Fleisher, G., Ludwig, S. *et al.* (2000) *Textbook of Pediatric Emergency Medicine.* Philadelphia: Lippincott Williams & Wilkins.

Nagel, T., Schunk, J. (1997) Using the hand to estimate the surface area of a burn in children. *Pediatr. Emerg. Care* **13**: 254–255.

Chapter 21

Pediatric skeletal injuries

Karen J.L. Black and Martin Pusic

Contents

21.1 Introduction

Children's bones contain less mineral and are more porous than those of an adult. As a result, they are more likely to bend or buckle than fracture completely. In addition, a child's periosteum is more elastic, stronger and less firmly bound to the cortex. Therefore they are more likely to remain intact when subjected to an external force, so children have fewer comminuted fractures and a lower incidence of non-union. As children grow, their bones are constantly being remodelled. We can often accept greater degrees of angulation in children without aggressive reduction since remodelling will eventually bring the fracture site into alignment. However, some apparently undisplaced epiphyseal injuries lead to increasing limb deformity with growth. The possibility of child abuse is an important consideration in all pediatric fractures, especially in infants.

The key part of this chapter is a table detailing the management considerations for most types of pediatric fractures, organized by bone. In addition we will describe a number of non-traumatic conditions with which the emergency pediatrician needs to be familiar.

21.2 Clinical presentation

Fractures result from a deformational, traumatic force applied to a bony region of the body. The first step in managing these injuries is to take a careful history of the event that led to the injury. While the history may be unclear, the physician might be able to discern whether the injury was due to twisting forces or an axial load, or if it was due to hyperextension versus hyperflexion. Knowing the mechanism allows the physician to look for characteristic fracture patterns. A history of loss of limb function is significant and limb fracture is much less likely in the patient who has been able to walk even a few steps. The physicians should seek to determine whether there has been a previous injury to the affected region and whether the patient suffers from any sort of chronic condition that could affect bone integrity (e.g. osteogenesis imperfecta, hyperparathyroidism). In cases where sedation or anesthesia may be required, the patient should remain fasting and the time of the last meal should be recorded. Finally, in all cases but especially for children under 2 years old, child abuse should be considered. The described mechanism of the injury must be carefully compared with the physical and radiologic abnormalities and the whole child assessed. Any discrepancies must be further investigated.

Examination should be geared to ascertaining the position and likelihood of fracture. The affected region should be inspected for bruising, swelling and deformity. The joint above and below the injury must be fully examined. The vascular status is ascertained by feeling the temperature of the area and checking the capillary-refill time as well as distal pulses. The first available person must immediately reduce a cold, pulseless extremity. The neurological status of affected limbs must also be checked and documented on an ongoing basis, especially before any manipulations.

Fractures are painful. We advocate immediate pain medication, preferably an intravenous opioid analgesic such as intravenous morphine $(0.1–0.15 \, \text{mg kg}^{-1})$. Nitrous oxide is also useful in the older child. This will facilitate temporary splinting (also an excellent comfort measure) and positioning for X-ray.

21.3 Indications for X-ray

X-rays should be obtained whenever a fracture is suspected since the radiographic findings guide therapy (e.g. splint versus no splint, need for reduction) and allow us to predict the course of recovery. We do many unnecessary X-rays in order to avoid missing fractures. This sensitivity/specificity trade-off can be rationally determined by using decision rules. These rules are generally far from perfected, especially in pediatrics, but useful rules have been developed for foot and ankle X-rays (Ottawa Foot and Ankle Rules) (*Box 21.1*), cervical spine X-rays (Nexus Low-Risk Criteria) (*Box 21.2*) and knee X-rays (Ottawa Knee Rules) (see *Box 22.2*).

21.4 Fracture types

21.4.1 Buckle, greenstick and bowing fractures

When a long bone suffers a bending force, one side of the cortex is under tension while the other is compressed. When the force exceeds a

---

Box 21.1 Ottawa Foot and Ankle Rules

Absence of *all* of the following precludes the need for an X-ray:
- Tenderness over posterior 6 cm of the medial malleolus
- Tenderness over posterior 6 cm of the lateral malleolus
- Tenderness over the navicular bone
- Tenderness over the base of the 5th metatarsal bone
- Inability to take 4 steps
  - At the time of the injury
  - At the time of assessment

> **Box 21.2** Nexus low-risk criteria
>
> Absence of *all* of the following precludes need for cervical spine X-ray:
> - Posterior midline cervical spine tenderness
> - Focal neurological deficit
> - Altered level of consciousness
> - Intoxication
> - Distracting painful injury

certain threshold, fracture results. In an adult, it is the side under tension that fails first, followed by a clean separation of the remainder of the bone. In a child, it is the side being compressed that fails first, resulting in buckling of the cortex being compressed. In most cases, this dissipates enough of the force so that this is the only injury. The resulting fracture is termed a *buckle fracture*. In some cases, the side under tension also fails resulting in fracture on one side and buckling on the other – the so-called *greenstick pattern* (*Figure 21.1*). Bowing fractures (*Figure 21.2*) result from the same bending mechanism of injury applied to long bones such as the radius, ulna or fibula; however, instead of resulting in one (buckle) or two (greenstick) areas of complete bony disruption, the forces cause a multitude of microfractures along the side under compression (*Figure 21.3*). The fractures may be missed on X-ray – views in two planes and comparison views can help identify them. Bowing fractures often require reduction despite their innocuous appearance.

In each of these three fracture types, the periosteum remains intact so that healing is likely to proceed well.

21.4.2 Avulsion fractures

In children, ligaments and tendons are stronger than bone, so avulsion at the site of attachment is common. The most frequent sites are:
- Tibial plateau at the site of the attachment of the anterior cruciate ligament
- Proximal 5th metatarsal at the insertion of peroneus brevis
- Anterior superior iliac spine at the insertion of the sartorius muscle
- Lateral epicondyle of the elbow at the common extensor origin

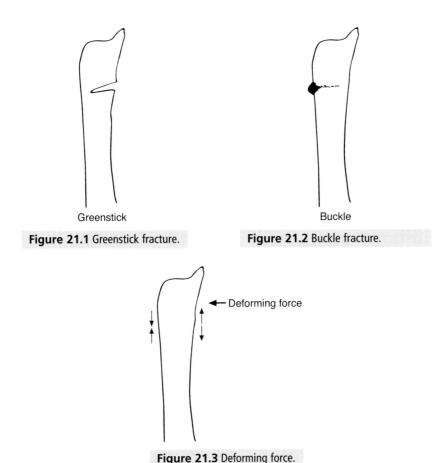

Greenstick

Figure 21.1 Greenstick fracture.

Buckle

Figure 21.2 Buckle fracture.

← Deforming force

Figure 21.3 Deforming force.

21.4.3 Growth plate fractures

The epiphyseal growth plate is a cartilaginous layer that lies between the physis and metaphysis of long bones. In axial and oblique injuries of the ends of the bones, the growth plate can be a 'fault line' for a fracture. These fractures occur in five main patterns first described by Salter and Harris (see *Figure 21.4*)

Besides being a convenient way of describing fractures, the Salter–Harris (SH) classification is also useful for prognosis since increasing Salter–Harris number is correlated with worse prognosis. SHI fractures can be difficult to see on X-ray if undisplaced. This situation arises most commonly in children with lateral malleolus tenderness. If swollen and tender, a short-leg case/cast is indicated until the child is re-evaluated a week later. SHV fractures are rare (0.3%), have high-energy mechanisms of injury, are associated with multiple bony and soft-tissue injuries, and are usually not detectable on radiographs taken at presentation.

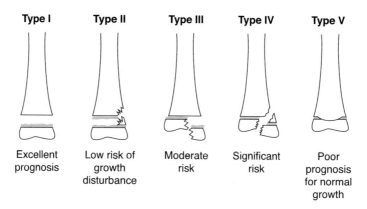

Figure 21.4 Salter–Harris classification of growth plate fractures.

21.4.4 Toddler's fracture

A toddler's fracture is a spiral or oblique fracture of the tibia in a child 1–3 years of age. Distinguishing features include the fact that there is often no history of a fall or other injury. The child presents either limping or refusing to walk. On examination, it may be difficult to localize the lesion. The clinician should work hard to be certain that the hip is not in fact the cause for the child's pain. The fracture may not be visible on the initial X-ray, or may only be visible on one projection; 10 days later, however, at re-X-ray, it may be obvious either as a lucent line or with periosteal reaction. While bone scanning can confirm the diagnosis in these cases, it is usually not necessary since casting is required for pain reduction and protection regardless of the X-ray findings.

The differential diagnosis of the limping toddler includes:
• septic arthritis
• transient synovitis
• osteomyelitis
• another type of fracture including:
  • metaphyseal corner fractures at the knee
  • Salter–Harris type I fractures at the distal fibula
• discitis – inflammation of an intervertebral disc

21.4.5 Child abuse

While child abuse is covered in detail in Chapter 27, a few points bear repeating here. Any fracture, regardless of its appearance, can in fact be due to child abuse. Keep the following in mind:

- The described mechanism should correlate with the observed findings:
  - A spiral fracture is likely the result of twisting – toddler's fractures are rarely due to abuse
  - A transverse fracture is unlikely the result of a twisting mechanism and more likely due to a direct blow
- The younger the child the greater the possibility of child abuse
  - Consider a skeletal survey in children under age 2 years
  - The body mass of a child < 12 months is insufficient to fracture a normal long bone in a fall from the height of a crib
  - Femoral fractures in children < 12 months are due to child abuse in at least 50% of cases
- Look for typical child abuse fracture patterns
  - Any type of rib fracture
  - Metaphyseal corner fractures
  - Fractures in unusual locations: femoral, hand or foot fractures in non-weight-bearing children; scapular fractures; humeral fractures away from the supracondylar area
  - Fractures of multiple ages
  - Skull fractures, particularly complicated ones or ones which cross suture lines.

21.5 Table of fracture management

Table 21.1 presents a management for common fracture seen in children. Local guidelines may vary. It is not meant to be an exhaustive listing but rather an approximate guide to what is done in the majority (> 75%) of cases together with significant possible complications. The table is arranged in a top → down, proximal → distal fashion.

21.5.1 Casts and splints for traumatic injuries to the extremities

The purpose of splints and casts is to immobilize the affected bone to reduce pain in the short term, and allow healing over the following weeks. In some fractures casts prevent deformity, or hold the fracture in place after reduction. Splints offer less protection than casts, but are good for stable fractures, phalangeal fractures and as a temporising measure before definitive treatment (i.e. reduction). Joints should be splinted in a functional position to allow continued use of uninjured digits, and to reduce joint stiffness and contracture after the splint is removed. Commercial splints are available for some areas for example immobilization of the humerus, wrist or knee.

Table 21.1 Common fractures in childhood

Bone	Fracture type/location	Usual management	Potential complications
Clavicle	Middle third (common >2 years and newborn)	No reduction unless severely displaced Supportive sling or figure of eight bandage for 3 weeks, further 3 weeks activity restriction	Normal to have callus bump after healing complete
	Medial third (rare) (epiphyseal separation)	Differentiate from sternoclavicular dislocation – use CT	Can cause pressure on tracheal or great vessels if posteriorly displaced
	Lateral third	Differentiate from acromioclavicular dislocation in adolescent Supportive sling, later physiotherapy	
Scapula	Body or neck	Immobilize with sling and wrap around chest ×3–6 weeks	Associated injuries often significant injuries to chest, head and neck
	Glenoid	Orthopedic referral recommended	
Humerus	Proximal	Immobilize in sling/collar and cuff/Velpeau bandage Reduce (open reduction and internal fixation – ORIF) if >50% displacement or >30% angulation in child with <2 years' growth remaining	
	Mid-shaft 2 peaks (0–3 years and >12 years)	Immobilize with collar and cuff/Velpeau bandage/sugar tong cast or hanging cast. ORIF or external fixation for severely displaced	Look for evidence of child abuse in <3 years Hanging cast improperly applied can increase deformity

continued

	Distal (supracondylar) (common 4–12 years)	Grade 1 – undisplaced and stable	3% have associated ipsilateral forearm fracture
		Collar and cuff ± backslab × 3 weeks	Neurovascular problems rare
		Grade 2 – partially displaced but ends still in contact	Cubitus varus deformity, malunion
		Closed reduction, immobilize in flexion ± wire fixation	
		Grade 3 – complete displacement	Arterial injury (brachial)
		Reduction under general anesthetic	Compartment syndrome
			Nerve palsy (median with extension injury – distal fragment posterior), ulnar with flexion injury (distal fragment anterior – unusual). Volkmann's ischemic contracture <1%
	Epiphyseal (infancy)	Reduce and immobilize	Cubitus varus
			Consider child abuse
	Medial epicondylar avulsion (8–12 years)	If simple, immobilize in posterior splint with forearm in pronation	Ulnar nerve paresis
		If associated with elbow dislocation or if medial epicondyle is incarcerated in joint or if ulnar nerve palsy, need ORIF	Difficult to diagnose in <6 years as ossification incomplete
	Lateral condyle (Salter IV)	If displaced >2 mm require reduction and pinning	Prone to poor functional outcome with slow union and stiffness of joint
Ulna	Olecranon	Extension cast for 2–3 weeks then change to flexion for 2 weeks	Usually occur in conjunction with other elbow injury (fracture or dislocation of radial head)
		ORIF if widely separated	
	Coronoid	Treat associated injuries (usually traumatic elbow dislocation)	
	See forearm fractures		

continued

269

Table 21.1 Common fractures in childhood – *continued*

Bone	Fracture type/location	Usual management	Potential complications
Radius Forearm	Head and neck (Salter I, II and metaphyseal)	Immobilize at 90° flexion, forearm neutral rotation above elbow cast for 4–6 weeks Angulation > 15° need orthopedic consultation	Loss of range of motion Overgrowth of radial head
	Proximal and middle third	Closed reduction and above elbow cast for 6–8 weeks Proximal third – forearm in supination Middle third-forearm neutral rotation If unstable need general anesthesia and often ORIF	Difficult to reduce Prone to losing position in cast
	Monteggia fracture dislocation (fractured ulna with dislocated radial head)	Anterior or lateral dislocation: reduce and immobilize in flexion and supination above elbow cast Posterior dislocation: reduce and immobilize in extension cast Open reduction might be necessary	Look at line through radial shaft and head – should bisect capitellum in any view (AP, lateral, oblique) Palsy of posterior interosseous nerve
	Galeazzi fracture dislocation (radial shaft fracture with dislocation of distal radio-ulnar joint) (rare) Distal (very common)	Reducing fracture will often reduce dislocation also. Might require open reduction	Few with proper orthopedic management
	Buckle	Below elbow cast or removable splint for 3 weeks	Rare
	Greenstick	Non displaced – below elbow cast for 3 weeks	Rare

		Management	Complications
	Epiphyseal (Salter I or II usually)	Reduction if angulation > 15°, cast in above elbow in supination	Remodel well
		Closed reduction for all displaced fractures, cast for 6 weeks. Occasionally need ORIF, especially if associated supracondylar fracture	Can have asymmetrical growth arrest. Higher risk of growth disturbance if late or repeated manipulation
Carpal bones	Scaphoid (rare < 10 years)	Thumb spica splint or cast if clinical exam positive even if X-rays negative. Repeat X-rays in 2 weeks if negative at presentation	Non-union (less risk than adults). Avascular necrosis of proximal pole
Metacarpal	Thumb metacarpal head Salter II or III	Minor angulation – manipulate and below elbow cast in functional position. Can need ORIF	Growth disturbance if Salter III. Contracture if inappropriate immobilization – should have IP extension, MP flexion and thumb abduction
	Distal 5th metacarpal (boxer's fracture)	Closed reduction if > 30° angulation	
	Salter I or II middle metacarpals, or shaft	Immobilize in gutter splint with wrist neutral and metacarpal phalangeal joint at 70°, orthopedic/plastic referral	
Phalanx	Proximal, Salter I, II or III	Reduce if angulated, must assess rotational deformity carefully. Once reduced, buddy tape for support	Growth disturbance and deformity
	Distal crush/physeal fracture or Mallet finger – hyperflexion injury	Manage soft tissue injury. Careful reduction and splinting	Growth disturbance and deformity

continued

Table 21.1 Common fractures in childhood – *continued*

Bone	Fracture type/location	Usual management	Potential complications
Pelvis	Avulsion – ASIS – AIIS	Crutches for 4 weeks with minimal weight bearing, then gradual increased activity	
	Ischial tuberosity	Consider ORIF if widely separated (>2 cm avulsion of ischial tuberosity)	
	Single breaks in pelvic ring	Generally stable, bedrest for 2–4 weeks External fixator if pubic diastasis with disruption of anterior sacroiliac joint	Associated genitourinary and neurovascular injuries
	Double breaks in pelvic ring	Unstable, can need traction, internal or external fixation Stabilize urgently by wrapping sheet around pelvis to compress and tamponade bleeding	Life threatening hemorrhage with pelvic vein disruption Genitourinary, abdominal and vascular injuries common
	Acetabulum (rare)	If dislocation of femur – reduction by orthopedics (open or closed) If major disruption of pelvis treat as above	Osseous necrosis of femoral head, post-traumatic arthritis, instability of joint
Femur	Proximal physeal	Open or closed reduction unless only minimally displaced	Osseous necrosis of femoral head in displaced fractures very common
	Slipped capital femoral epiphysis (8–15 years)	Strict non-weight-bearing and urgent orthopedic referral	Leg length discrepancy 10–25% bilateral
	Neck	Traction and splinting followed by open or closed reduction	Osseous necrosis 40%
	Intertrochanteric (uncommon)	Spica cast 6–8 weeks If significant displacement – ORIF	Osseous necrosis 5%

Shaft		
• Infant <10 kg <8 years	Traction × 3 weeks or hip spica	Overgrowth, leg length discrepancy
• <8 years	Hip spica with 1 cm shortening recommended for 6 weeks. If pathologic – external fixator. If multiple injuries consider internal fixation	Vascular injury
• >8 years	Traction, hip spica, external or internal fixation for 6–12 weeks	Malunion, poor remodelling. Growth arrest of distal growth plate, angular deformity, rotational malunion
• Adolescent	Intramedullary rod	
Knee		
Distal femoral physis Salter II	Splint, closed reduction under general anesthesia, cast × 6–8 weeks	High incidence growth arrest. Peroneal nerve damage with medial displacement. Neurovascular compromise with anterior displacement of distal epiphysis
Avulsion fractures and ligamentous injuries	Incomplete – closed reduction and immobilize in extension in knee splint. Complete – ORIF (arthroscopic possible). Arthrocentesis in ED if large hemarthrosis	Compartment syndrome. Joint instability
Proximal tibia physis (rare) Salter II, III or IV	Closed or open reduction and long-leg cast for 6–8 weeks	Popliteal neurovascular bundle stretch or contusion. Compartment syndrome. Deformity, growth arrest, leg length discrepancy

continued

273

Table 21.1 Common fractures in childhood – *continued*

Bone	Fracture type/location	Usual management	Potential complications
	Patella	Non displaced – long-leg cast for 4 weeks Displaced > 3 mm – ORIF Avulsion of distal pole with extension sleeve of articular cartilage – ORIF Dislocation – reduce and immobilize in knee splint for 4 weeks	Be aware of bipartite patella Knee stiffness, quadriceps atrophy, extensor lag, persistent pain
Tibia/fibula	Proximal metaphysis	Reduction and long-leg cast for 4–6 weeks Orthopedic referral	Compartment syndrome Valgus deformity common Delayed or malunion
	Shaft	Stable – long-leg cast for 4–6 weeks and refer Unstable (both bones) consider ORIF if open fracture, compartment syndrome, concomitant head injury or femur fracture	Compartment syndrome seen in minor tibial fractures – major fractures tear interosseous membrane allowing decompression If spiral and pre ambulatory child, consider child abuse
	Toddler's fracture (< 3 years) common	Non-displaced – long-leg cast for 3–4 weeks Radiographs negative – repeat in 10 days or bone scan	
	Stress fracture (> 8 years)	Look for subperiosteal new bone formation – may need bone scan to diagnose Rest only treatment recommended	
	Distal fibula Salter I	Below knee cast if clinically suspicious and re-examine at 10–14 days with X-rays Immobilize for 3 weeks	

	Distal tibia Salter II	Closed reduction and long-leg cast for 4–6 weeks – often associated with fibular greenstick fracture	Joint stiffness, pain, arthritis
	Tillaux–Salter III (adolescent) Triplane fracture (Tillaux plus Salter II = Salter IV) (uncommon)	Lateral epiphysis displaced – ORIF Need CT scan to delineate joint damage and number of fragments ORIF	Joint stiffness, pain, arthritis
Tarsal	Fracture dislocations (rare)	Reduction, stabilization if >2 mm displacement – non-walking below-knee cast	Difficult to diagnose Osseous necrosis of talus
Metatarsal/ Phalanx	5th metatarsal diaphyseal metaphyseal junction	Orthopedic referral for fixation	Delayed or non-union
	Avulsion fracture base of 5th metatarsal	Distinguish from accessory ossification centre Immobilize in weight-bearing cast for 3–6 weeks	
	Intra-articular fracture 1st proximal phalanx	Often require pinning	
	Undisplaced phalangeal fracture	Buddy strapping of toes and metatarsal pad until comfortable	
Cervical spine	See Neurotrauma		

continued

Table 21.1 Common fractures in childhood – *continued*

Bone	Fracture type/location	Usual management	Potential complications
Thoracolumbar spine	Compression fracture (L1 most common)	Bedrest and symptomatic mobilization, consider orthosis for multiple areas of compression	Associated abdominal injuries common with seat-belt mechanism
	Flexion/distraction Chance fracture (horizontal splitting through body and posterior elements)	Immobilization with well moulded orthosis	

Casts are still usually made of plaster of Paris, although there is increasing use of more recent preparations, such as the colored fibreglass cast. This is more durable in active children and the children often favor the more cheerful, colorful cast. Waterproof liners are now available.

The extent of management of displaced fractures within the ED varies from place to place. Some hospitals have a policy of referral of all displaced fractures to the orthopedic surgeons, while others undertake more active treatment within the ED itself.

21.6 Non-traumatic orthopedic conditions

21.6.1 Osteogenesis imperfecta (OI)

In OI, collagen is not formed properly resulting in osteopenic, fragile bones. The severity depends on the type and can range from subclinical to crippling. The main importance of this condition to ED practitioners is in the differential of child abuse (both cause multiple fractures of different ages) and in simply raising the possibility for further investigation. Initial fracture management should be the same as for other cases.

21.6.2 Osgood–Schlatter disease

This is painful inflammation at the site of insertion of the patellar tendon into the tibial tubercle. It may be due to repeated microfracture, tendinitis, apophysitis or a combination of the three. Physically active boys aged 11–15 years are most often affected. Clinical examination shows an inflamed, tender tibial tubercle. Swelling may be seen. X-ray can be normal or show an irregular, enlarged tibial tubercle. While the disease is self-limited, resolving when the tibial tubercle fuses (usually by age 15 years), the associated chronic pain may require activity modification (jumping sports are worst), strengthening exercises and/or physiotherapy, non-steroidal anti-inflammatory medication and, rarely, long-leg casting.

21.6.3 Osteochondritis dissecans (OD)

OD occurs in adults and children 10–15 years of age. It involves avascular necrosis of a small piece of subchondral bone. It is most frequent at the lateral femoral condyle. The cause is usually not clear. Presenting signs can include pain, swelling of the affected joint and, if the fragment of articular cartilage avulses, locking of the joint. The necrotic segment is usually apparent as a radiolucent area on X-ray, although, in the initial acute phase, the bone may appear radiologically normal. Treatment is usually casting with a long-leg cylindrical cast for 3–5 months.

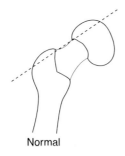

Normal

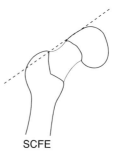

SCFE

Figure 21.5 Normal bone.

Figure 21.6 Slipped capital femoral epiphysis.

21.6.4 Slipped capital femoral epiphysis (SCFE)

Hip pain in children warrants aggressive investigation. Even putting aside infectious conditions such as septic arthritis and osteomyelitis, misdiagnosis of deforming hip conditions can have life-long implications for the patient. In SCFE, the epiphyseal growth plate of the femoral head fractures resulting in displacement of the capital epiphysis (*Figure 21.5* and *Figure 21.6*). The condition is typically seen in obese boys during their adolescent growth spurt, although a case as young as 8 years old has been reported. It is frequently bilateral. Symptoms such as limp and knee or hip pain may be acute or subacute in onset and can often follow a minor injury or a jump from a height. The slip can generally be seen on frog lateral X-ray when the appearances of the right and left hip are compared. A minor slip may not be detectable on an AP view. Early identification allows stabilization of the slip with metal pin fixation. The greater the slippage, the worse the prognosis so it is axiomatic that every child of 8 and over with hip pain be suspected of having this condition and investigated.

21.6.5 Legg–Calve–Perthes (LCP) disease

LCP results from an interruption of the blood supply of the femoral head leading to avascular necrosis. It usually occurs between 5 and 9 years, with boys outnumbering girls considerably. The disease is frequently bilateral. Onset of hip and/or knee pain along with limp is usually gradual, without evident precipitating trauma. X-rays reveal nothing for the first 2 weeks and then develop lucency and gradual deformation of the femoral head. Ultrasound can detect an effusion before X-ray changes in some children. Treatment is usually with traction and immobilization for many weeks, although some centers treat with splints, which allow the child to be mobile.

21.6.6 Transient synovitis of the hip

Transient synovitis of the hip occurs most commonly between the ages of 2 and 7 years, often 2–3 weeks after an upper respiratory tract infection. It is slightly more common in boys than girls and it can be bilateral. It recurs at least once in approximately 10% of children. It is characterised by the onset of hip or knee pain or limp in an afebrile child. Abduction, adduction and rotation of the hip are often reduced. A full blood count, ESR and C-reactive protein (CRP) are usually normal but an ultrasound of the hip shows the effusion.

If all the blood investigations are normal, the child can be managed with rest at home and the effusion can be monitored regularly by ultrasound. Children who have a large effusion or a prolonged effusion should be referred for orthopedic review.

21.6.7 Compartment syndrome

Tight, unyielding, strong fascia envelopes 'compartments' of soft tissue occur in several sites in the upper and lower extremities, most commonly in the forearm. Injured soft tissues such as muscle usually swell. If the swelling occurs within these fascial compartments, the pressure within the compartment can rise above the mean arterial pressure resulting in ischemia and tissue death. The cardinal signs and symptoms of compartment syndrome are pain, pallor, paresthesia, paralysis and loss of pulses. In practice, pain is the most sensitive. The other signs, particularly loss of pulse, are late signs indicating that significant damage has already taken place.

All patients with disproportionate pain after a soft tissue injury or fracture should be suspected of compartment syndrome. Tissues begin to die within 6 hours of ischemia so that expediency is important. In unclear cases, compartment pressure can be measured. Treatment is removal of any constricting dressing and emergency fasciotomy.

Suggested reading

Broughton, N.S. (1997) Chapters 22 (Upper limb) and 23 (Lower limb) in: *A Textbook of Pediatric Orthopedics*. London: WB Saunders.

Swischuk, L.E. (1992) *Emergency Radiology of the Acutely Ill or Injured Child*. Baltimore: Williams & Wilkins.

Chapter 22

Minor trauma

Martin Pusic and Patricia O. Brennan

Contents

22.1 Abrasions and contusions

Direct blows to the skin and underlying muscle result in contusions. Oblique contact of the skin with a rough surface results in frictional damage to the skin and this is termed an abrasion.

History-taking should focus on the nature of the incident – when? how? are there any features suggestive of non-accidental injury? what was the environment (barnyard, possible foreign bodies)? and is the patient immunocompromised or had immunizations? On *physical examination*, document the injuries carefully, especially if non-accidental injury is at all a consideration. Examine the entire body and verify the integrity of any associated bones and joints by checking for bony tenderness and movement of joints. *Investigations* are rarely needed with abrasions and contusions. However, swabs of infected abrasions can determine antibiotic usage and X-rays can help detect the presence of radio-opaque foreign bodies or exclude underlying bony injury.

The *management* of each of these is relatively straightforward. It is orientated towards patient comfort and the prevention of complications. For *contusions*, ice packs four times daily decrease the pain and swelling as do simple analgesics. Contusions of the quadriceps can lead to myositis ossificans (chronically painful calcifications within the contused muscle – early ambulation and physiotherapy can decrease this risk). Calf contusions rarely lead to compartment syndrome, so patients should be warned to return if the pain gets progressively worse or any weakness develops.

Abrasions also respond to ice and analgesics. Infection is a greater risk for abrasions since the epidermal barrier has generally been compromised. They should be cleaned with antiseptic soap and any debris removed. Special techniques such as scrubbing under conscious sedation might be required to remove 'tattooed' material such as road tar. Full thickness abrasions greater than 1–2 cm in diameter require plastic surgery follow up. Dressing protocols vary according to local practice. Some centers dress all abrasions with a thick layer of antibiotic ointment and the parents are instructed to change the dressing at least daily. Others use non-adherent dressings such as paraffin gauze (sometimes impregnated with antiseptic) under a cotton gauze dressing. Tetanus status must be up to date in all open wounds and antibiotic prophylaxis considered in heavily contaminated or infected wounds (cephalexin 20–40 mg kg^{-1} per day in three divided doses).

22.2 **Lacerations**

Minor lacerations are quite common in children. There can be a whole range of severity from minimal nicks through to complex full-thickness lacerations involving vital structures and tissue loss.

The *history* should again include details of the incident causing the injury, such as when, where and how the injury happened. Significant details include lacerations from glass, which may result in glass remaining in the wound, and lacerations on the knuckles, which could be from a punch resulting in teeth penetrating the skin.

The *examination* should be thorough and include the size and depth of the laceration, detection of any foreign bodies and of damage to any underlying structures such as nerves or tendons. Lacerations through some areas such as the red margin of the lip or the edge of the eyelid deserve special consideration.

Management for the successful ED physician includes a full complement of techniques both to repair the laceration and to make the process as painless as possible. One technique will not fit all. Clinicians are especially encouraged to become familiar with new topical anesthetics (e.g. lidocaine–epinephrine (adrenaline)–tetracaine [LET]) and tissue adhesives (e.g. Histoacryl, Dermabond). These advances have done much to decrease the suffering of children with minor lacerations. The management of lacerations is laid out in the flow diagram (*Figure 22.1*).

Keep in mind the following:
- Dirty (e.g. barnyard injuries, bites) or old (> 12–24 hours) lacerations may be better off left open and then closed secondarily at 3–5 days.
- Debridement and irrigation are at least as important as the closure technique.
- Use behavioral and pharmacological calming techniques to improve the outcome on multiple levels.
- Use buffered, warm lidocaine injected with a small-gauge (30 G) needle or, better still, use topical anesthetics.
- Use absorbable sutures or tissue adhesives wherever possible to avoid the trauma of suture removal.
- Laceration repair does not end with the last stitch – have you taken care of the following: antibiotic prophylaxis, tetanus, splinting, dressing, explanation of precautions and a dose of analgesic for when the local anesthetic wears off?

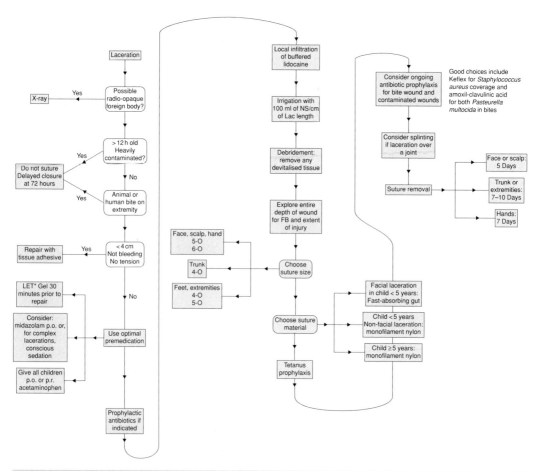

Figure 22.1 Laceration management flow chart.

22.3 Sprains and strains

Injuries to ligaments, tendons and muscles are very common amongst children. While the majority are quite benign, in some, long-term morbidity can result unless the injury is properly managed from the outset.

In children under age 8, it is a truism that their ligaments are generally stronger than their bones. Thus an injury mechanism that might result in a ligament sprain in an adult (e.g. ankle inversion resulting in a talofibular ligament injury) will usually cause a fracture in a child (e.g. Salter–Harris I fracture of the distal fibula).

Similarly, because children's limbs are shorter and their weight is smaller, their muscles are generally subject to less force and therefore are less likely to be strained. As a result, a clinician should be very cautious making a diagnosis of a soft-tissue 'sprain' or 'strain' in a prepubertal child. Some examples of situations where an adult would sprain a ligament but a child is more likely to sustain a fracture are given in *Table 22.1*.

Tendon injuries are also different in children. In several sites (most notably at the base of the 5th metatarsal and at the tibial tuberosity) tendons insert into ossification centers known as apophyses. A deforming force across the tendon is more likely to injure the apophysis than the tendon.

Facts that should be noted on *history* include a description of the mechanism of injury including the position of the affected part when the force was applied to it, and the direction and nature of the force. The treatment since the injury and the level of activity achieved by the child are also significant. Certain lines of questioning not directly concerned with the present injury might be required to exclude the possibility of non-accidental injury (e.g. past history of suspicious injuries, nature of supervision at the time of the injury).

General *management* of true sprains or strains consists of elevation of the affected extremity, ice compresses four times daily while the tissue is inflamed, simple analgesics and initial rest followed by early ambulation. More specific treatments are mentioned in the appropriate section. Because of their excellent flexibility and relative weakness, children are unlikely to sustain severe muscle strains. Any injury that persists beyond 48 hours or that requires more than simple analgesia should be investigated further.

Table 22.1 Injuries from comparative mechanisms in adults and children

Diagnosis in an adult	What to watch out for in children
Ankle sprain	Salter–Harris I fracture of the distal fibula
Knee sprain (e.g. ACL)	Avulsion fracture of the insertion of the ACL into the tibial plateau
Wrist sprain	More likely to be a torus fracture of the distal radius and/or ulna
Elbow sprain	Occult fracture

Abbreviation: ACL, anterior cruciate ligament.

22.3.1 Foot injuries

Toe sprains are common, usually due to stubbing the toe on the floor. As long as a displaced fracture is not suspected, X-ray is usually not required and treatment is cold compresses, buddy taping to the adjoining toe and the use of shoes with a hard, inflexible sole.

Plantar fasciitis is an overuse injury to the plantar fascia, usually at its insertion into the calcaneus. The pain is aggravated by walking and can be elicited on physical examination by hyperextending the toes. Treatment is by elevating the heel with either shoe inserts or, in severe cases, casting. Anti-inflammatory medications can also help.

In *traumatic injuries*, the Ottawa foot rules can help indicate the need for an X-ray (*Box 22.1*). Common sites for fractures include the toes, distal metatarsals and apophysis at the base of the 5th metatarsal. Stress fractures present with a chronic history of, usually, mid-foot pain. The fracture may not be detectable using plain radiography; bone scans are helpful in these situations. See Chapter 21 for specific treatments of traumatic foot injuries. Minor injuries benefit from ice compresses for 10 minutes, up to four times daily, and anti-inflammatories and hard-soled shoes.

Box 22.1 Ottawa foot rules

X-ray if any *one* of the following are present:
- Unable to walk 4 steps at any time (now or at time of injury)
- Tenderness at navicular
- Tenderness at base of 5th metatarsal

Ingrown toenails are common from infancy right through to adulthood. The problem is that one edge or corner of the nail becomes buried in the eponychial fold. Most cases resolve with insertion, after a toe lidocaine block is performed, of cotton underneath the nail corner so that it is lifted away from the skin fold. The care-giver can be instructed on how to keep the nail edge free. In more refractory cases, a wedge of the toenail is removed (*Figure 22.2*).

Avulsed nails can result in cosmetic deformities unless the nail's germinal matrix is preserved. In older children, the key is anatomic repair of any lacerations of the nail bed and eponychium *and* maintenance of the separation of the two sides of the eponychial fold. To maintain the fold, either suture the avulsed nail back into place between the sides of the

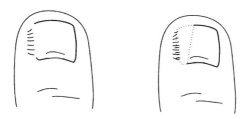

Figure 22.2 Ingrown toenail. Dotted line shows nail resection margins.

fold or pack the fold with vaseline-impregnated gauze. However, in younger children, excellent cosmetic results with regrowth of a normal nail have resulted from conservative management with regular weekly dressings in some centres.

Subungual hematomas can be quite painful. Puncturing the overlying nail with an 18 G needle or heated paperclip will relieve the discomfort.

22.3.2 Ankle

Inversion injuries can lead to *ankle sprains*. As noted above, the younger the child, the more likely that an ankle sprain is actually a growth plate fracture of the distal fibular epiphysis. Careful physical examination will demonstrate tenderness over the lateral malleolus and not over the talofibular ligament. The need for an X-ray can be determined by applying the Ottawa ankle rules (see *Box 21.1*).

22.3.3 Knee

A number of disorders can cause pathology in the knee. Four major knee *ligaments* can each be torn or strained. The younger the child, the more likely that a given force will *not* cause a ligament disruption but rather avulse its insertion into bone. The mechanism of injury may predict which structure is injured. For example, a valgus stress is most likely to damage the medial collateral ligament and medial meniscus. The need for X-rays can be predicted using the Ottawa knee rules (*Box 22.2*). There is increasing evidence that these are valid in children. Regardless of the X-ray findings, children who are unable to weight-bear or have a marked knee effusion will benefit from splinting, usually with a posterior slab.

Patellar pain is common in children. A history of knee pain aggravated by prolonged sitting and going up stairs may be due to *chondromalacia patellae*. Referral for physiotherapy may be helpful.

Box 22.2 Ottawa knee rules

X-ray if any *one* of the following are present:
- Isolated tenderness of the patella (i.e. no bone tenderness of the knee other than the patella)
- Tenderness at the head of the fibula
- Inability to flex to 90°
- Inability to bear weight both immediately and in the ED (4 steps; unable to transfer weight twice onto each lower limb regardless of limping)

Acute patellar pain due to trauma may be due to *patellar dislocation*. If the patella is dislocated, sedation may be required before applying a gentle medial, lifting force to replace it. Immobilization using a posterior slab and crutches is required for some weeks afterwards.

Patellar tendonitis (jumper's knee) is usually an overuse injury that generally responds to conservative therapy. For prognostic reasons, it must be distinguished from Osgood–Schlatter disease, especially if conservative measures fail.

Osteochondritis dissecans, avascular necrosis of a bony fragment in the knee, can present with pain.

22.3.4 Hip

Hip pain is a worrisome symptom for children of all ages. In infants and even toddlers, clinicians should always be alert to the possibility of *congenital hip dislocation*.

Septic arthritis can present in a very non-specific fashion in non-weight-bearing children. This diagnosis should be considered in all febrile children with musculoskeletal complaints. Conversely, a screening musculoskeletal examination should be done on all febrile children. Tests for white blood count and C-reactive protein can help with equivocal cases.

In school-age children, Legg–Calve–Perthes disease is a potentially treatable avascular necrosis of the femoral head. Early identification (usually on plain X-rays) is important to minimize morbidity.

Around the time of puberty, *slipped capital femoral epiphysis* (SCFE) is an important cause of hip pain. It has been reported in children as young as 8 years. This is essentially a fracture through the growth plate separating the femoral capitellum from the femoral neck. Delayed diagnosis can result in increased slippage and a poorer prognosis. Therefore, SCFE must be considered in any pre-teen or adolescent with hip pain. A frog lateral X-ray of the hips is valuable in making the diagnosis.

22.3.5 Shoulder

Trauma to the shoulder of children is more likely to cause fracture than either humeral dislocation or acromioclavicular (AC) joint separation. Nonetheless these injuries can occur, usually in adolescents. *Humeral dislocation* is usually provoked by an awkward fall onto an outstretched arm. Most dislocations find the humeral head displaced anteriorly with respect to the glenoid fossa. On physical examination, the humeral head can be palpated anteriorly and the patient generally refuses to move the arm due to pain. An X-ray (typically the Y-view) will prove the dislocation. There are multiple maneuvers for replacing the humeral head. A key factor is proper analgesia and sedation using, for example, midazolam and fentanyl. A straightforward maneuver is to have the patient, once safely sedated, lie prone on an examining table with the arm dangling towards the floor. Gentle downward traction is usually all that is required of the clinician. Once replaced, the humerus should be supported with a sling or Velpeau dressing for 4–6 weeks following.

Acromioclavicular joint separation is uncommon before adolescence. The joint is markedly tender on examination. X-rays can appear normal unless views are taken with the patient holding weights to pull the acromion downwards. Treatment is generally with simple analgesics and a supportive sling.

22.3.6 Elbow

Trauma to the elbow rarely causes a true sprain of elbow ligaments. Instead, fractures or contusions are far more common. Determining whether the injury was due to a direct blow versus a hyperextension injury can be helpful. For example, hyperextension injuries should prompt a careful search for supracondylar fractures. *Elbow fractures* often are not visible on X-rays taken at the time of injury. Indirect signs on the X-ray (elevated anterior or posterior fat pads) can raise the clinician's suspicion of fracture. However, any child with a painful, swollen elbow is best managed as though there is a fracture regardless of the X-ray findings. Place the limb in a posterior slab splint and arrange for follow up examination and X-rays 10 days later.

The 6 month–3 year old child who presents refusing to use his or her elbow presents an interesting challenge. The *pulled elbow* (nursemaid's elbow) is due to a pulling on the arm that results in subluxation of the radial head. The child often holds the wrist, with the elbow flexed and both parents and doctors suspect wrist rather than elbow problems. In cases where the history is not clearly that of a pulling mechanism (e.g. unwitnessed injury), the clinician should exclude the possibility of fracture before going on to maneuvers designed to replace the radial head. Any elbow swelling (indicated by loss of the dimples normally seen on either side of the olecranon) or bony tenderness should prompt an X-ray.

To replace the radial head:
1. Warn the parent and child that you will perform a brief but painful procedure to replace the radial head.
2. For a pulled right elbow: take the dorsum of the hand of the affected limb into the palm of your left hand. With your right hand, lightly grasp the medial aspect of the distal humerus.
3. Use your left hand to **hyperpronate** the child's forearm until either a click is felt with your right hand or the end point is reached.
4. If this is unsuccessful, a back-up technique is to use a similar positioning of your hands, but in this case, **hypersupinate** the child's forearm and then flex the elbow completely. Again feel for a click or stop when you reach the end point.

These techniques are successful in over 95% of cases. The child may take a few minutes of rest and play to realise that the elbow is no longer painful. In a case where both fail, place the limb in a posterior slab and arrange orthopedic follow up within 24 hours.

22.3.7 Wrist

Wrist sprains are uncommon in children. Suspect a fracture in every case – have a low threshold for taking an X-ray. In particular, remember to consider *scaphoid fractures*, especially in the adolescent age group. If there is any palpable tenderness in the area of the 'anatomic snuffbox', cast the limb in a thumb spica splint, regardless of the X-ray appearance.

In cases where the patient is in significant discomfort without there being a fracture on the X-ray, a volar splint can help decrease the pain. Follow up assessment with repeat X-rays at 10 days can detect fractures not apparent at the initial assessment.

22.3.8 Fingers

Finger sprains and minor undisplaced *buckle fractures* are common. As long as growth plates are not involved, treatment is straightforward with the affected digit being taped to the longest adjacent finger so that the two move in concert. This provides mechanical support in the case of further trauma but allows freedom of movement. Rigid splinting is generally not required.

A special case of digit sprain is the *gamekeeper's thumb*. Here there is a sprain of the ulnar collateral ligament of the metacarpal phalangeal (MCP) joint of the thumb, usually due to severe abduction of the joint. The joint is usually markedly swollen and tender, especially over the ligament. The degree of the sprain dictates management. A complete tear requires a thumb spica cast or surgical repair while incomplete tears can be supported with a simple splint. To determine the degree of injury, the examiner should hyperabduct the first MCP. If the joint opens widely compared to the uninjured thumb, the ligament has been completely disrupted. A solid end point, however, indicates that the ligament is largely intact. A digital nerve block at the level of the metacarpals is often required to perform this otherwise painful maneuvre.

Finger dislocations are also problematic. In these cases, joint ligaments have generally been completely disrupted. Reduction is accomplished by anesthetising the joint using local anesthetic and then applying firm axial traction. At times, conscious sedation may be required. Once the finger is reduced, it should be immobilized in an appropriate plaster splint for 4–6 weeks with follow up by a hand surgeon.

Mallet finger occurs when the flexor digitorum profundus tendon is avulsed at its insertion into the base of the distal phalanx. The patient will be unable to extend the distal phalanx. On X-ray, an avulsion fracture is often seen at the base of the distal phalanx. Treatment is with a splint that keeps the joint continuously in extension for 4–6 weeks. A hand surgeon should be involved in the care of this injury.

22.3.9 Neck

Whiplash injuries occur as a result of sudden unanticipated motions of the neck such as those seen in occupants of a motor vehicle struck from behind. Clearly the important consideration is to exclude the possibility of serious cervical spine injury such as fracture or SCIWORA (spinal cord injury without radiological abnormality). The key distinguishing features are severity of pain and tenderness of the spine as opposed to supporting musculature and the presence of neurological deficits. Appropriate imaging is helpful. When in doubt, leave the patient immobilized in a hard neck collar until cervical spine injury is ruled out.

Simple cases of whiplash can be treated with anti-inflammatory medications such as ibuprofen. Use of soft collars is of unproven utility.

Strain of the sternocleidomastoid muscle can result in *torticollis* where the child holds the head in a tilted fashion with the chin pointing away from the affected muscle. The key is to identify the cause (*Box 22.3*). Torticollis due to simple muscle strains usually responds to hot compresses and sleep to relax the muscle and analgesics to help with the pain.

Box 22.3 Causes of torticollis

- Odontoid or subluxation injuries of the cervical spine
- Pharyngitis with inflammation of the prevertebral tissues
- Lymphadenitis over the belly of the sternocleidomastoid muscle (SCM)
- Congenital torticollis
- Vestibular problems – infection, tumor
- Ocular problems – tumor, strabismus

Chapter 23

Bacterial soft tissue infections

Alison Freeburn and Michael B.H. Smith

Contents

These are a common reason for pediatric attendance in the emergency department, and many can be managed well as an outpatient. The clinical presentation of each infection depends on specific characteristics of the infecting organism and the location and depth of the infection. Characteristics of bacterial skin infections are listed in *Table 23.1*.

Table 23.1 Characteristics of bacterial skin infections

Characteristics	Examples
Affecting superficial areas usually without systemic signs	Impetigo Abscess (can be deep and spread) Felon Paronychia Ingrown toenail
Affecting deeper tissues or with spreading and systemic signs	Lymphadenitis Cellulitis Fasciitis Staphylococcal scalded skin syndrome

23.1 Superficial or localized infections

23.1.1 Impetigo

This is the commonest bacterial skin infection in children. It occurs more frequently in hot, humid weather. The lesions characteristically begin as red macules followed by fragile vesicles, which subsequently rupture to leave a yellow-crusted lesion. Pruritus is a common symptom and systemic symptoms are unusual. It is spread to other areas by inoculation through scratching. Because of its highly contagious nature, affected children should not return to school or day-care before the lesions heal.

The usual causative organism is *Staphylococcus aureus* or group A beta-hemolytic streptococcus.

Treatment is dependent on the extent of the lesions. For small areas of involvement, topical antibiotics, such as fucidin cream are used with gentle cleaning to remove the crusts. Oral antibiotics, such as flucloxacillin or azithromycin, although some would use amoxycillin–clavulinic acid, are required for more extensive lesions. When there is widespread disease or coexisting skin disease, inpatient care with parenteral antibiotic therapy is required.

Complications of treatment are rare, but post-streptococcal glomerulo-nephritis may occur. Most cases show complete resolution in 7–10 days on treatment without scarring.

Bullous impetigo is an unusual variant caused by *Staphylococcus aureus* and is toxin mediated. The toxin appears to act extracellularly and causes separation of the cells of the epidermis. The majority of cases occur in those under 2 years of age. The lesions begin as vesicles that quickly turn to bulle. The bulle rupture leaving a moist erythematous surface, over which light brown crusts form. Systemic symptoms such as pyrexia, lethargy and diarrhea may be present but are uncommon. Treatment is with oral antistaphylococcal antibiotics. Healing occurs without scarring and complications are rare.

23.1.2 Abscess

This is a localized dermal collection of pus within one or more layers of the skin surface. It is formed anywhere on the body following skin trauma. The immediate skin flore are the usual pathogenic agents. There is localized pain, erythema and swelling and, on clinical examination, a firm, fluctuant swelling develops. Systemic symptoms are uncommon, but localized cellulitis or lymphangitis may supervene.

Treatment is by incision, drainage and cleaning of the affected area. Antibiotics are only indicated if there are systemic symptoms or the patient is immunocompromised. The usual antibiotic of choice is an antistaphylococcal agent such as oral flucloxacillin or cephalexin.

23.1.3 Felon

A felon is an infection of the pulp space of a phalanx. An abscess forms as the infection spreads and is limited by the septa within the pulp area. The pulp is red and swollen, and intense, throbbing pain is present. Infection may spread to the underlying bone, joints or tendon. Treatment is prompt surgical drainage in conjunction with oral anti-biotics effective against staphylococcal organisms.

23.1.4 Paronychia

Paronychia is an acute or chronic infection of the periungal tissues. Acute paronychia almost always involves the fingers, and is due to the introduction of pyogenic bacteria through minor trauma. This leads to the formation of an abscess giving pain, swelling and erythema around the affected area. *Staphylococcus aureus*, *Pseudomonas* or *Proteus* species are the most common organisms. Treatment is by separation of the cuticle on the affected side from the nail to allow drainage of pus. Antibiotics are only required if significant cellulitis is present.

Chronic paronychia is associated with conditions such as ingrown toe-nail, and clinically there is inflammation and thickening of the eponychial fold. There may be purulent discharge present. Treatment may be either conservative with wedging of the affected nail and appropriate antibiotic cover, or more aggressive with excision of part of the affected nail and lateral skin fold with careful follow up.

23.1.5 Ingrown toenail

This typically affects the great toenail as a result of poorly fitting shoes or improperly cut nails. Erythema, swelling and pain around the affected nail is common, and infection may be present, giving rise to chronic paronychia.

Treatment may be conservative, with antibiotics and the use of gauze wedges to elevate the affected portion, or surgical – either simple avulsion of part of the nail or surgical excision. Good foot care is essential to prevent recurrence. See also Chapter 22.

23.2 Deep or spreading infections

23.2.1 Lymphadenitis

Inflammation of the lymph nodes may be generalized, as in systemic infection, or localized. It can be caused by a wide variety of pathogens, such as streptococci, mycobacterium or viral infections, and the primary infection is usually apparent. Occasionally biopsy or excision is necessary to make a diagnosis.

Lymph node enlargement may be asymptomatic or may be acutely painful and tender. Rarely the overlying skin may be inflamed. Treatment depends on the underlying cause and, with eradication of the primary infection, the lymphadenitis usually settles. Firm, non-tender lymphadenopathy may persist in some cases.

23.2.2 Cellulitis

This is an acute, spreading infection of the dermis and subcutaneous tissues. Underlying skin lesions and trauma predispose to the development of cellulitis. Group A beta-hemolytic streptococcus or *Staphylococcus aureus* are the most common pathogens. Clinically the affected area is erythematous, hot and tender. It is a spreading lesion with indistinct margins, and not infrequently, with visible tracking within the lymphatic system. Systemic symptoms, such as pyrexia and tachycardia are common. The treatment of cellulitis is dependent on the site of infection and the presence or absence of systemic symptoms.

Neonatal

In the neonate, cellulitis should always be treated with intravenous antibiotics, because of the poor ability of the host to localize and contain infections. Periumbilical flare should be treated aggressively, as omphalitis and necrotising fasciitis may develop. The antibiotics of choice for periumbilical infections are flucloxacillin and an aminoglycoside or third generation cephalosporin.

Facial

Facial cellulitis should almost always be treated with parenteral therapy because of the potential spread to deeper structures posteriorly. The treatment of choice is usually a second generation cephalosporin, even in the absence of any systemic symptoms or elevated white blood counts.

Extremity

Cellulitis of an extremity without systemic symptoms and with a normal white blood count (WBC) should initially be treated in the outpatient department with an oral antibiotic such as flucloxacillin. The following are criteria for intravenous antibiotics:
• no improvement within 24–48 hours
• extensive infection
• infection near a joint
• systemic symptoms
• elevated WBC

Once systemic symptoms have resolved, the 10-day course of antibiotics may be completed on an outpatient basis. Most cases show resolution with adequate antibiotic treatment.

Eye

If a child presents with swelling and inflammation of the eyelids and around the eye, it is important to differentiate between preseptal and orbital cellulitis – see Chapter 24.

Perianal

Perianal streptococcal cellulitis is an unusual but distinct form that occurs mainly in children. Clinically there is marked perianal erythema, pain on defecation and anal fissures. The condition may become chronic if not treated with appropriate antibiotics.

23.2.3 Necrotizing fasciitis

This is a severe infection of the subcutaneous tissues involving the deep layer of superficial fascia. Group A streptococcus causes the most severe infections and, if associated with toxic shock syndrome, has a high case mortality. Other non-group A streptococci, aerobic Gram-negative bacilli and anerobic Gram-positive cocci can also be responsible, but the course is less severe and the mortality rate is much lower, although significant morbidity may result.

There is acute onset of localized swelling, erythema and extreme skin tenderness. The tenderness is much more prominent than that associated with cellulitis. Systemic symptoms are present and out of proportion to the skin signs. Intravascular depletion, with hypotension, is common. The infection spreads along the fascial plane and cutaneous signs do not reliably indicate the extent of tissue necrosis. As the disease progresses, the affected tissues may darken from red to purple to blue. Gangrene of the tissue can develop but is a late and ominous sign. The diagnosis is confirmed by surgical exploration, which should occur as soon as possible after the diagnosis is suspected.

Treatment is initial hemodynamic stabilization followed by parenteral antibiotic treatment with cephalosporins. Surgical debridement should be performed when the patient is hemodynamically stable.

Scarring is inevitable because of the extensive debridement that is required. Amputation of an affected limb is occasionally required. Mortality is associated with presence of the toxic shock syndrome and may approach 30%.

23.2.4 Staphylococcal scalded skin syndrome

A severe form of staphylococcal infection is staphylococcal scalded skin syndrome (SSSS). It usually occurs in younger children. SSSS begins abruptly, with systemic symptoms, such as pyrexia and irritability, associated with an erythematous rash. Bulle develop rapidly with subsequent rupture and exfoliation of the skin, leaving large areas of bright red skin surface. There is rapid progression of the skin lesions.

Treatment is with intravenous antibiotics and careful monitoring of fluids and electrolytes as there may be increased fluid losses through the exposed areas. Topical antibiotics are not useful.

Further reading

American Academy of Pediatrics Committee on Infectious Diseases. (1998) Severe invasive group A streptococcal infections: a subject review. *Pediatrics* 101(1), 136–140.

Darmstadt, G.L. Cutaneous bacterial infections: In: Behrman, R.E., Kliegman, R.M. Jenson, H.B. (Eds) *Nelson Textbook of Pediatrics*, 16th edn, WB Saunders Company, pp. 2029–2031.

Herting, R.L. (2001) Dermatology: skin infections. In: *University of Iowa Family Practice Handbook*. http://www.vh.org/Providers/ClinRef/ FPHandbook/Chapter13/02-13.html

Jain, A., Daum, R.S. (1999) Staphylococcal infections in children: Part 3. *Pediatr. Rev.* **20**: 261–265.

Llera, J.I., Levy, R.C. (1985) Treatment of cutaneous abscesses: a double blind clinical study. *Ann. Emerg. Med.* **14**: 15–19.

Mawn, L.A., Jordan, D.R., Donahue, S.P. (2000) Preseptal and orbital cellulitis. *Ophthalmol. Clin. N. Am.* **13**(4).

Merck & Co, Inc (1995–2001) Bacterial infections of the skin. In: *The Merck Manual of Diagnosis and Therapy*, http://www.merck.com/pub/mmanual/ section10/chapter112/1129.htm

Park, R. (2001) Impetigo from emergency medicine/infectious diseases. *eMedicine*, http://emedicine.com/emerg/topic283.htm

Rounding, C. and Hulm, S. (2001) Surgical treatments for ingrowing toenails. *Cochrane Database Syst Rev*, http://www.cochrane.org/cochrane/revabstr/ ab001541.htm

Swartz, M.N. (2000) Cellulitis and subcutaneous tissue infections. In: Mandell (ed). *Principles and Practice of Infectious Diseases*, 1037–1043.

Chapter 24

Ocular emergencies

Patricia O. Brennan

24.1 Introduction

Ocular emergencies are common in childhood and fall into two main groups, infections and trauma. In both, there is adequate time for careful clinical assessment of the child, and if necessary discussion with or referral to an ophthalmologist. Minor injury may bring to light preexisting conditions such as strabismus or retinoblastoma.

In this chapter we describe emergency systematic history and examination of eyes and the common infective and traumatic conditions of childhood that lead to attendance at Emergency Departments. It should be noted that ophthalmic antibiotic practice varies from country to country and local guidelines should be followed. Chloramphenicol is used commonly in the UK, but very rarely if at all in North America.

24.2 History

A full history should be taken from both the parent and if possible the child. It may be difficult to get an accurate history from the parent if the injury resulted from poor supervision or child abuse or from the child if he or she was doing something forbidden at the time of the injury (*Box 24.1*).

24.3 Examination

It takes time and patience to assess the eyes and eyesight especially in a young or frightened child. It is best to leave any unpleasant parts of the

---

Box 24.1 Essential elements of the history in ocular emergencies

- The injury
  - what was the mechanism [e.g. blunt/penetrating trauma, radiation, chemical, foreign body (size/velocity/nature e.g. steel/copper)]
- Duration and time and onset of condition
- Other symptoms e.g. irritation, discharge, injection, swelling, epiphora, diplopia
- Eyesight now, e.g. diplopia, blurring, floaters, flashes of light
- Eyesight previously, e.g. patching, eye operations, glasses, contact lenses
- Other associated conditions, e.g. head injury
- General health, illnesses, hospital admissions
- Medication
- Allergies
- Immunizations, particularly tetanus prophylaxis

examination until last and perform the non-contact parts of the examination first. Young children may need to be held firmly to facilitate examination. Up to about 18 months, infants will sometimes open their eyes in surprise when held aloft. If you need to separate the eyelids, make certain you only press on the orbital margins so that no pressure is put on the globe.

24.3.1 Visual acuity

The eyes are for seeing. A proper examination has not been performed (for both clinical and medicolegal reasons), unless visual acuity has been checked (*Box 24.2*). This is difficult in a non-compliant child or one who is obtunded or who has severely swollen eyelids or eye pain. Each eye must be tested separately, by occlusion of the opposite eye and the results recorded. Something must be recorded, even if it is 'visual acuity unobtainable'. Test visual acuity in very young children by getting them to fixate on a face or a colorful toy and more formally in older children using Snellen's charts or Allen's pictures. If visual acuity is very poor, carry out gross assessment by counted fingers or light perception. *Box 24.2* shows normal development of eye function.

Box 24.2 Normal development of eye function

- 6 weeks: fixes, beginning to follow
- 10–12 weeks: fixes with accurate following
- 3 years: 20/40 vision
- 4–5 years: 20/30 vision
- 6 years and up: 20/20 vision

24.3.2 Examination of the external eye

The external eye and surrounding tissues should be examined systematically (*Box 24.3*).

The pupils can demonstrate signs of both local eye injuries and also intracranial injuries. A unilateral dilated fixed pupil indicates a focal lesion such as optic nerve damage or an ipsilateral intracranial hemorrhage. Bilateral small pupils may indicate opioid drugs or pontine hemorrhage and large fixed pupils indicate a tectal lesion of the brain.

Other examinations are listed in *Box 24.4*.

> **Box 24.3** Examination of the external eye
>
> - **Lids and periorbital tissue:** symmetry, swelling, bruising, lacerations, ptosis and crepitus
> - **Orbital rim:** step-offs or irregularity, sensory deficits in surrounding tissue
> - **Conjunctiva:** color, hemorrhage, epithelial damage stained in a cobalt blue light after instillation of fluorescein. N.B. Remove contact lenses first
> - **Cornea clarity**
> - **Upper and lower fornices** for foreign matter (after eversion of the upper eyelid)
> - **Exophthalmos/enophthalmos:** suggesting ruptured globe or orbital fracture

> **Box 24.4** Other examinations in ocular emergencies
>
> - **Anterior chamber:** clarity or blood/haziness
> - **Pupils:** shape, size, symmetry and reaction to light and accommodation
> - **If penetrating injury of the globe is suspected at this stage, a large hard shield should be taped to rest on the margins of the orbit and the child referred urgently for ophthalmological assessment**
> - Absence of the **red reflex** may mean corneal scar, cataract or intraocular hemorrhage
> - **Fundoscopy:** difficult and leads to only a very limited examination in most children unless mydriatics are used and the child is cooperative. Referral to an ophthalmologist is often needed for a further examination of the fundus
> - **Visual fields:** tested in the older child by confrontation
> - **Ocular motility:** checked simply with the child's head steady, by moving an attractive toy, testing all cardinal gazes

24.4 Investigations

Useful investigations are shown in *Box 24.5*.

The conditions in *Box 24.6* need urgent referral to an ophthalmologist.

24.5 Ocular trauma

Eye injuries are common in children and are three times more likely in boys than in girls. They are the commonest cause of blindness in children in the USA.

Box 24.5 Investigations in ocular emergencies

- **Viral and bacterial swabs**: for Gram staining and culture (mainly used for detection of chlamydia and gonorrhea)
- **X-rays**: for high velocity radio-opaque foreign bodies such as glass or metal and for fractures of the facial skeleton. Beware, some newer alloys do not show on X-rays
- **CT scans**: axial sections for defining the structural integrity of the eye and coronal sections for extraocular muscles, walls of the orbit, foreign bodies and intracranial and intraorbital hemorrhage
- **Ultrasound**: for radio-opaque and radiolucent orbital foreign bodies, but needs direct contact with the eyelids and globe and is not well tolerated by children

---

Box 24.6 Conditions needing urgent referral for an ophthalmological opinion

- Eyelid wounds
  - crossing lid margins
  - deep, possibly full thickness laceration
  - over the inner canthus near the nasolachrymal duct
- Corneal wounds
  - alkali and other concentrated chemical contamination
  - deep lacerations/abrasions
- Hyphema
- Pupillary irregularity and loss of reflexes
- Penetrating wounds of the globe
- Vitreous hemorrhage
- Retinal detachment

24.5.1 Chemical injury

Chemicals, particularly concentrated acids and alkalis and organic solvents, can cause major injury to the eye. The nature of the chemical should be evident from the history. The patient usually presents with pain and blepharospasm. The damage is proportional to the concentration and pH of the solution, and the duration of exposure and rapidity in instituting treatment.

In general, neutralizing agents to the chemical are contraindicated as the neutralization reaction usually gives out heat and exacerbates the damage to the eye.

Alkalis, such as ammonia and concentrated bleach, are held in the tissues and cause severe eye damage. They saponify the cell membranes, denature collagen and thrombose vessels with disruption, tissue softening and opacity of the cornea. In addition, they can cause a rapid rise in pH in the anterior chamber damaging the iris, ciliary body and the lens. Reflex protective activity closes the eyelids and keeps the burning agent in contact with the eye.

Acids can also cause severe damage. Because they cause precipitation of proteins, a barrier to further penetration, the damage is more often confined to the ocular surface. Hydrofluoric acid is the exception with progressive damage similar to an alkali.

Any chemical contamination of the eye is a painful emergency. Management is listed in *Box 24.7*.

The ophthalmologist may use mydriatics to dilate the pupils to reduce pain from ciliary spasm, topical steroids to reduce inflammation and potassium ascorbate drops in alkali burns to restore levels of potassium ascorbate in the anterior chamber. Occasionally corneal transplantation may be necessary.

Box 24.7 Management in chemical contamination

- Remove contact lenses
- Instil local anesthetic if necessary
- Irrigate the open eye copiously with saline or water through an intravenous infusion giving set for at least 30 minutes until the pH in the lower fornix remains neutral
- Decontaminate surrounding affected skin
- Refer to ophthalmologist

24.5.2 Thermal burns to the eyes

Thermal burns from tobacco ash, cigarette burns or sparks, cause corneal epithelial damage with edema and clouding of the cornea and reduced visual acuity. The epithelial cells slough and regenerate rapidly. Minor lesions are treated as for corneal abrasions. Corneal or deep burns should be referred at once for an ophthalmological opinion.

Occasionally burns of the eyelids and eyes are associated with facial burns. These can cause extensive edema and the globe should be examined before edema closes the eyelids. Deep burns of the lid margins can lead to ectropion or entropion. Smoke and chemical fumes from a fire can cause chemical conjunctivitis.

24.5.3 Irradiation keratoconjunctivitis

This can follow up to 6–10 hours after exposure to ultraviolet light, e.g. from a sun-ray lamp or from sunlight reflected off snow. The child presents with severe pain, photophobia and lachrymation. The injury can lead to stippling of the cornea. Symptomatic treatment consists of oral analgesia and padding of the eye for comfort.

Solar burns of the macula also occur. These burns generally heal spontaneously.

24.5.4 Foreign bodies

Children frequently present with a sensation of a foreign body in the eye. This may be painful and the child will be reluctant to open the eye. It is particularly important to get a good history of the child's activity when the foreign body entered the eye. A high velocity metallic foreign body sustained while the child was hammering suggests that the body may be embedded in the tissues, and an X-ray should be obtained for radio-opaque foreign bodies.

If the child is cooperative, amethocaine eye drops can be instilled and the lid everted to look for a subtarsal foreign body. Care must be taken when you are everting the lids, as pressure on the orbit may convert a small penetrating wound into a large one. A conjunctival foreign body can usually be removed with a damp cotton wool bud but corneal foreign bodies can be more difficult. After removal, the eye should be stained with fluorescein to check for epithelial damage. If this is absent, antibiotic eye drops such as chloramphenicol or gentamicin 0.3% are given for a few days and the child discharged. Referral to an ophthalmologist is needed if there is difficulty in examining the child, or in removing the foreign body, or if there is a rust ring remaining after removal of a metallic foreign body.

24.5.5 Sharp trauma

Lacerations of the eyelid
Superficial horizontal extramarginal lacerations of the upper eyelids can be sutured in the ED. The sutures must not grasp deep eyelid tissue as cicatricial eversion of the eyelid margins can result. Deeper lacerations and particularly any full thickness lacerations that might be associated with injury to the globe and to the nasolachrymal duct, and those through the lid margins should be referred to an ophthalmologist for assessment and closure.

Eye-wall laceration and penetrating injury

All but very minor penetrating injuries of the eyeball are associated with damage to the intraocular contents. Lacerations may be very small and subtle and give little immediate pain or disability. Fluid, iris or choroidal tissue may be seen herniating through the laceration. If the laceration is in the cornea, the pupil can look irregular with a teardrop shape, pointing towards the rupture. Visual acuity may be reduced.

In the ED, any eye with a potential penetrating injury should have minimal assessment and the eye shielded. The shield should rest on the bony margins of the orbit, to avoid pressure on the globe. Any visible penetrating foreign body should be left in situ. An anti-emetic is given as the injury itself can cause vomiting, raising the intraocular pressure. In addition, tetanus prophylaxis must be brought up to date, and the patient will need intravenous antibiotics such as clindamycin or ceftazidime before urgent referral to an ophthalmologist for surgical repair to the eye.

Complications such as disruption of tissues, introduction of infection or scar tissue can lead to loss of the eye and occasionally the opposite eye develops sympathetic ophthalmitis, leading to complete loss of vision. Wounds with a good prognosis include those with:
• good initial visual acuity
• anteriorly located wounds
• small wounds

24.5.6 Blunt eye injury

There are many causes of blunt trauma to the orbit and eyeball including a blow from a punch, a squash ball or a champagne cork. They lead to bruising, swelling, bony tenderness and deformity, numbness of the cheek, surgical emphysema and epistaxis.

Black eye/orbital hematoma

A black eye from a blow to the orbit with bruising and edema to the eyelids is usually benign. It can occasionally be dramatic with discoloration mainly through the loose tissue of the eyelid, surrounding skin and orbit and gravity, giving discoloration below the eyes within a few days. Occasionally bilateral 'black eyes' result from mid-line bruising of the forehead. Icepacks early in the injury help minimize the swelling. The bruising can take up to 2 weeks to resolve and the pigmentation can be left for several weeks or months. Periorbital hemorrhage and scleral hemorrhages can be caused when the blood tracks down from an anterior cranial fossa fracture.

Blow-out orbital fractures

In blunt trauma the eyeball is forced backwards and the walls of the orbit, usually the inferior or medial walls, 'blow-out'. It can present with:
- *enophthalmos*: the contents of the orbit sink into the fracture
- *proptosis*: with hemorrhage into the orbit
- *infraorbital nerve damage*: in inferior fractures, causing numbness of the ipsilateral malar region
- *trapping of the inferior oblique and inferior rectus muscles*: leading to limited ocular motility, particularly loss of upward gaze
- *trapping of the medial rectus muscle* and damage to the nasolachrymal duct in medial fractures: the patient may complain of diplopia.

As 20% of orbital fractures are also associated with eyeball injuries, patients with blow-out fractures need referral to an ophthalmologist. X-rays may show the 'teardrop sign' but have little place in the investigation of orbital fractures. CT scan gives optimal information of both the orbit and the brain. Once the edema has settled, 85% of fractures settle with no treatment. The patient should be managed with rest, analgesia and antibiotics to prevent orbital cellulitis. Valsalva maneuvers such as straining at stool or blowing the nose should be avoided.

Scleral and subconjunctival hemorrhages

These are common and can result from blunt trauma, birth trauma, conjunctivitis or chemical irritation. They can also be associated with raised intrathoracic pressure. They are usually focal, but can be diffuse or multiple. If they are extensive with no posterior border, they may be an indication of significant penetrating orbital trauma. No treatment is needed, but the hemorrhage can take a week or two to resolve.

Corneal and conjunctival abrasions

Conjunctival and corneal abrasions occur from a foreign body in the eye, or from direct trauma, for example when the eye is caught by a twig. They present with the sensation of a foreign body, pain, blepharospasm or photophobia. Corneal abrasions often give reduced visual acuity and are especially painful as the superficial corneal nerves are exposed. Assessment will exclude other eye injury. A drop of fluorescein in the eye, in a cobalt blue light shows a fluorescent green area of epithelial damage. If the abrasion is an isolated injury, prophylactic antibiotic eye drops (e.g. chloramphenicol or gentamicin 0.3%) and an eye-pad for comfort only are needed. The abrasion should be reviewed in 2 days by which time it should be healed. Healing is slowed if there is human, animal or vegetable matter in the wound. Corneal abrasions associated with significant pain, central lesions and those with an irregular pupil should be referred for an ophthalmological opinion.

Hyphema

Hyphema, or a bleed into the anterior chamber of the eye is the commonest cause of admission for eye trauma in the USA. It is caused by rupture of the fine capillaries in the iris or ciliary body after a blow to the eye, and presents with pain and decreased visual acuity and occasionally sleepiness. On examination the red cells floating in the anterior chamber give appearance of a red haze or a settled layer of blood in the anterior chamber. One third of cases have other ocular injuries. The child should be transferred for admission, sitting up at 45° during transport to keep the blood settled at the lowest level. Daily intraocular pressure will be measured and if raised, treatment considered with glycerol or mannitol. The use of systemic antifibrinolytic agents such as tranexamic acid or aminocaproic acid to prevent secondary hemorrhage is controversial.

Blood in the anterior chamber can result in staining of the cornea, decreased visual acuity and even amblyopia (*Box 24.8*).

Box 24.8 Predictors for staining of the cornea in hyphema

- Prolonged hyphema
- Raised intraocular pressure
- Presence of corneal damage
- Rebleeding

Rebleeding during recovery (peak at 3–5 days after the original injury) leads to a particularly high risk of staining and increased risk of secondary glaucoma.

Other anterior segment injuries

Several other conditions can occur in the anterior chamber from blunt trauma (*Box 24.9*).

Fundal hemorrhages

Hemorrhages can occur in all layers of the retina, often at the periphery. These can only be seen by indirect ophthalmoscopy. Fundal hemorrhages occur in severe head trauma, for example following a road traffic accident or in association with any cause of raised intraorbital pressure, in leukemia and in blood dyscrasias. They are seen in approximately 20% of newborns within 24 hours of birth, particularly after forceps and

---

Box 24.9 Other conditions occurring from blunt trauma to anterior chamber

- *Iridodialysis*: separation of the iris base from the ciliary body, associated with hyphema
- *Traumatic miosis/mydriasis*: initial miosis (constriction) followed by mydriasis results from blunt ocular trauma, with minimal or absent pupillary reaction to light
- *Traumatic uveitis*: a mild inflammatory reaction of the iris and/or ciliary body 24–72 hours after blunt trauma giving pain or aching in the eye, photophobia, redness and occasionally pupillary constriction. The ophthalmologist will treat it with dilatation of the pupil and topical steroids
- *Angle recession*: separation or posterior displacement of the tissues at the anterior chamber angle at the site of the trabecular network occurs in 20% of cases of hyphema and may result in secondary glaucoma
- *Contusion cataracts*: occur when the structure of the lens is altered and aqueous enters the lens substance causing it to swell and become cloudy. It can occur within a few days of the injury, but may be delayed for years
- *Lens subluxation or lens dislocation*: can result from blunt eye trauma

---

vacuum extraction deliveries, but these usually resolve within a few days. Few are present 2 weeks after birth. They are rarely if ever caused by cardiopulmonary resuscitation [1].

Bilateral fundal hemorrhages in the postneonatal infant are strongly suggestive of the shaken baby syndrome (see non-accidental injury section). Green [2] suggests that the shaking forces apply to both the brain and the vitreous where they produce subhyaloid and intraretinal hemorrhages. These can occur in front of, within or under the retina [3] (*Box 24.10*).

Retinal detachment

Blunt trauma can exert a traction effect on the retina resulting in retinal detachment more commonly in children than adults, as the vitreous body is more adherent. The child complains of a curtain effect across the visual field or visual disturbance with flashes of light or floaters. All should be referred to an ophthalmologist.

> **Box 24.10** Types of fundal hemorrhage
>
> - *Vitreous hemorrhage*: curved or linear streaks or diffuse hemorrhage
> - *Preretinal hemorrhage*: dark red dome-shaped masses, most dense at the center when fresh and occasionally with a horizontal fluid level as they mature
> - *Intraretinal hemorrhage*: superficial flame-shaped hemorrhages or slightly deeper dot hemorrhages
> - *Subretinal hemorrhage*: between photoreceptors and underlying pigment layer
> - *Choroidal hemorrhage*: at the posterior pole

24.6 Infections

Infections of the eyelids, lachrymal system and orbit present at every age. Most can be diagnosed with minimal investigation and treated as an outpatient.

24.6.1 Eyelid infections

Various structures in the eyelids can become infected, usually causing only minor problems.

Hordeolum (stye)

This is an infection of the eyelash follicle, usually by a staphylococcal species. It presents with mild pain and redness and localized or generalised swelling of an eyelid. Hot spoon bathing with a wooden spoon wrapped in a bandage dipped in warm water and pressed against the lids, is soothing. Removal of the eyelash aids drainage, but is not usually tolerated by the child. In addition, topical antibiotic ointment such as chloramphenicol 1% (UK) or gentamicin 0.3% twice daily aids resolution.

Chalazion

This is a cyst of a meibomian gland, which has become infected. It presents and is treated in the same way as a stye, but it may need to be excised if it fails to resolve. Neither hot spoon bathing nor eyelash removal are helpful.

Blepharitis

Blepharitis is a generalized inflammation of the eyelids caused by staphylococcal infection, seborrheic dermatitis and allergies to soap and shampoo. Irritation and the sensation of a foreign body are associated with redness, itching and crusting of the lid margins. It usually resolves with removal of any allergen, eyelid hygiene and antibiotic drops, such as erythromycin or bacitracin.

24.6.2 Infection of the nasolachrymal sac

A blocked nasolachrymal duct in infants can present with epiphora. It can be associated with a staphylococcal or streptococcal infection of the nasolachrymal sac presenting with pain, swelling and redness in the medial canthal region. The infection usually resolves after massage four times daily of the area together with topical antibiotics. Oral antibiotics, such as Augmentin (amoxicillin/clavulanate) may be needed in moderate and intravenous antibiotics in severe infections. Always refer these cases to an ophthalmologist.

24.6.3 Conjunctivitis

Conjunctivitis is common and presents with a red painful eye. Most causes in children are infective with a purulent discharge with a different range of organisms occurring at different ages. Allergic conjunctivitis also occurs in childhood.

Neonatal conjunctivitis
The commonest causes of neonatal conjunctivitis include:
- *Neisseria gonococcus*
- *Hemophilus influenzae*
- *Streptococcus pneumoniae*
- *Escherichia coli* and
- Viruses

Investigations include swabs for *N. gonococcus* and other pathogens and serological tests on conjunctival secretions for chlamydia.

Gonococcal infection is particularly dangerous as it can cause progressive keratolysis and perforation within 24–36 hours. It usually presents 2–5 days after birth with a severe conjunctivitis and a copious discharge. A prompt diagnosis can be made with microscopic examination of exudates for Gram-negative intracellular diplococci. The eye should be copiously irrigated with saline regularly and the baby given parenteral penicillin or third generation cephalosporin such as Ceftriaxone or Cefotaxime i.v. together with topical erythromycin or bacitracin four times daily.

Chlamydial conjunctivitis, acquired from passage down the birth canal occurs up to 14 days after birth with lid swelling and copious purulent discharge. Diagnosis is made by enzyme-linked immunoassay (EIA) and direct fluorescent antibody (DFA) test using monoclonal antibody. Treatment consists of 14 days oral erythromycin together with tetracycline (not in North America) or erythromycin eye ointment.

Bacterial and viral conjunctivitis in infants and older children

Bacterial conjunctivitis is more common than viral conjunctivitis in children. Conjunctivitis with red, painful, purulent conjunctiva is usually caused by bacterial infection with *Hemophilus influenzae*, *Streptococcus pneumoniae* or *Staphylococcus aureus*. Viruses, especially adenovirus and measles virus can cause conjunctivitis as part of a systemic infection. They usually present with less discharge than bacterial causes. After swabbing for Gram stain and culture, the eyes are cleaned and antibiotic eye drops instilled 2 hourly for 1 day and then 6–8 hourly according to local protocols. Chloramphenicol, tetracycline or erythromycin are commonly used in the UK, and erythromycin, gentamicin and polymyxin-B/bacitracin are used in the USA. Hygiene measures for the patient such as separate towels and flannels will prevent spread of infection.

Allergic conjunctivitis

This is often associated with other allergic symptoms of sneezing and a runny nose, often in an atopic individual in response to specific allergens such as plant pollens or cat dander. Massive swelling of the conjunctiva (chemosis) with a jelly-like appearance can occur, especially after vigorous rubbing. Once the patient is removed from the allergen and refrains from rubbing, the symptoms rapidly settle. Topical lubricants and cool compresses are soothing. Antihistamine, orally and in eye drops, helps. Prophylactic mast cell stabilizing drops on a regular basis help in some patients, often taking up to 10 days to be effective.

24.6.4 Herpes simplex keratitis

Herpes keratitis usually by type I but occasionally type II herpes simplex, is the commonest infectious cause of blindness in developed countries, although trachoma remains the commonest cause worldwide. Type I is often associated with a characteristic vesicular lesion on the face, and results in a corneal dendritic ulcer where the edges are formed by virus infected cells. All layers of the cornea can be infected and corneal opacities can result. All need ophthalmic referral. Local steroidal drops are contraindicated.

24.6.5 Preseptal orbital cellulitis

This is an infection of the eyelids and periorbital region anterior to the orbital septum. It is associated with eyelid trauma, periorbital skin infection, and upper respiratory tract and sinus infection and is usually caused by *S. aureus*, *S. pyogenes* or *H. influenzae* and occasionally anerobic infection. The child presents with warm, swollen, tender, erythematous eyelids and may be toxic. There is no proptosis and vision is unaffected. Initial treatment consists of intravenous antibiotics such as flucloxacillin or tobramycin especially, in severe cases, in children under 5 years and in the immunocompromised. Incision and drainage of a suppurative area may be needed.

24.6.6 Orbital cellulitis

Orbital cellulitis is a purulent infection of the cellular tissue behind the orbital septum. It can be caused by extension of infection from neighboring parts of the orbit, especially ethmoidal and frontal sinusitis, dacryocystitis, mid-facial or dental infection, facial erysipelas or 24–72 hours after a penetrating injury. The predominant organisms are *S. pneumoniae* and other streptococcal infections, *S. aureus* and *H. influenzae*. Occasionally the infection is polymicrobial and Gram-negative organisms are a cause in infants.

The cellulitis is usually unilateral with rapid onset of fever, pain and eyelid swelling, pain on downward and lateral eye movement and proptosis. The fundus is difficult to examine. A CT scan of the orbits and the brain may show an intraorbital or subperiosteal abscess. Complications include cavernous sinus thrombosis, meningitis and exposure keratopathy.

Treatment consists of admission for intravenous antibiotics, which should be started empirically, for example with clindamycin and ceftazidime to cover Gram-positive and Gram-negative organisms. The antibiotic can be changed on the basis of bacteriological results and metronidazole can be added for anerobic cover. Tetanus prophylaxis must be brought up to date and a specialist ENT opinion sought for problems such as drainage of sinuses or abscesses.

24.7 **Other emergencies**

24.7.1 Strabismus

Strabismus presenting to the ED is often the transient strabismus common in the first 2–3 months of life, resolving by 4 months. Constant strabismus can be a presentation of serious pathology such as retinoblastoma or cerebral tumor and requires referral for investigation and management.

24.7.2 Papilledema

This is a sign of raised intracranial pressure, usually from a head injury, but occasionally from other causes such as an intracranial tumor. It is often not present in the early stages of raised intracranial pressure when the anterior fontanelle is open.

24.7.3 Birth trauma

Delivery can be associated with periorbital and ocular trauma, in both a normal and a traumatic delivery. Signs include eyelid edema and bruising, corneal edema and abrasion, hyphema and vitreous and retinal hemorrhage. It usually resolves with no active management, but some patients need observation to check for long-term sequele.

References

1. Gilliland, M.G.F., Luckenback, M.W. (1993) Are retinal hemorrhages found after resuscitation attempts? A study of the eyes of 169 children. *Am. J. Forens. Med. Pathol.* **14:** 187–192.
2. Green, M.A., Lieberman, G., Milroy, C.M., Parsons, M.A. (1996) Ocular and cerebral trauma in non-accidental injury in infancy: Underlying mechanisms and implications for pediatric practice. *Br. J. Ophthalmol.* **80:** 282–287.
3. Meadow, R. (1997) *ABC of Child Abuse*, 3rd edn. London: BMJ Publishing Group.

Further reading

MacCumber, M.W. (1997) *Management of ocular injuries and emergencies.* Philadelphia, PA: Lippincott-Raven.
Nelson, L.B. (1998) *Pediatric Ophthalmology.* London: WB Saunders Company.

Chapter 25

Emergencies of the ear, nose and throat

Patricia O. Brennan

Contents

25.1 Introduction

The pediatrician must be familiar with emergency presentations of ear, nose and throat problems and their management. These fall into two main categories, infections and trauma. Most can be treated within the Emergency Department (ED) on an ambulatory basis, but some are more serious and even life threatening and require the urgent attention of an otolaryngologist and an anesthetist. This chapter covers clinical presentation and management of the commonest ear, nose and throat problems presenting to the ED.

25.2 The ear

25.2.1 Common symptoms

Earache

Young children often present with earache. It can originate from the ear or be referred from local structures and the history and examination must therefore cover the whole head and neck. The commonest causes are acute bacterial or viral otitis media or from otitis externa but it can also be caused by dental inflammation, sinusitis, cervical lymphadenopathy and pharyngitis.

Sudden hearing loss

This is an uncommon but distressing complaint. Sudden conductive hearing loss results from head injury or ear infection. The cause of sudden sensorineural loss is often less clear. It can occur after damage to the vestibular or cochlear nerve in head injury or in severe barotrauma such as an aeroplane flight or in scuba diving where a rupture in the round window or the stapes footplate causes leakage of inner ear fluid into the middle ear. The patient experiences fluctuating hearing loss and vertigo. Urgent repair of the leak is needed. Sudden hearing loss can also occur from viral infections like measles and mumps with complete or partial recovery after several weeks.

Vertigo

Vertigo occurs in children with damage to the vestibular system. Acute suppurative labyrinthitis leads to a profound sensorineural deafness but there is no cochlear deafness from labyrinthitis associated with otitis media. Other causes of vertigo include vestibular neuronitis, measles and mumps infections, migraine, head injury and barotrauma.

25.2.2 Infective ear emergencies

Otitis externa

Otitis externa takes two main forms, a localized staphylococcal abscess of a hair follicle in the outer two-thirds of the external auditory canal or a diffuse infection by *Pseudomonas aeruginosa*, staphylococci, fungi or a polymicrobial infection. The canal can also be affected by eczema, psoriasis and chemicals, and children who swim a lot are particularly prone.

On examination, pressure on the tragus in otitis media, pulling the ear backwards and chewing all give pain. The skin of the canal appears red and edematous with a foul smelling discharge. A mucoid discharge always signifies a perforation of the drum. If pus obscures the tympanic membrane and there is difficulty in distinguishing between otitis externa and otitis media with a ruptured tympanic membrane, pulsation of the pus on coughing indicates a rupture of the membrane. Pseudomonas and skin flora are usually isolated from the discharge.

Treatment with gentle toilet of the canal and the instillation of antibiotic and steroid ear drops, such as polymyxin B, neomycin, hydrocortisone drops, is usually effective. If the drum is perforated, the child will also need oral antibiotics such as amoxycillin or a cephalosporin.

Otitis media

Otitis media is defined by the presence of inflammation and fluid in the middle ear accompanied by at least one sign of acute illness.[1] It is a common infection of the middle ear and mastoid air system occurring mainly in children under the age of 8 years (peak incidence 3–36 months) when Eustachian tube function is relatively poor. Surveys have shown that at least 50% of children have had at least one episode of acute otitis media before the age of 3 years.[2] It can develop rapidly and the tympanic membrane can rupture within 1 hour of onset, giving relief of the ear pain. Persistent effusion is seen after acute otitis media in 50% of children after 1 month and 10% after 3 months. Suboptimal treatment can lead to deafness resulting in delayed speech in infants and poor performance in school.

The most common causative organisms in otitis media are *S. pneumoniae, H. influenzae* and less commonly Group A hemolytic streptococci, *Moraxella catarrhalis* and respiratory viruses. Gram-negative infections can occur in the very young and in the immunosuppressed.

Otitis media *presents* with malaise, ear pain and occasionally discharge in the older child. The frequency of associated symptoms varies greatly and acute otitis media cannot be differentiated from upper respiratory tract infection on the basis of symptoms alone. Young children may present with less specific signs and symptoms such as irritability or lethargy, pyrexia, poor feeding, vomiting and ear pulling. Clinical signs may be misleading, but usually the ear drum will be red and dull and bulging or perforated with a grey/white discharge exuding from the middle ear. Otitis media with an effusion (glue ear) may be asymptomatic but the serous effusion will give a dull grey tympanic membrane on examination. The child may develop hearing problems and delayed language development.

Examination with an auriscope can be difficult in a fractious young child. The child should be held in a hug sideways on the parent's knee, with one arm round the parent's back and the other included in the parent's hugging arm. The child's knees are held between the parent's legs to prevent kicking. The parent uses the free hand to gently and firmly hold the child's head sideways onto their chest, giving the examiner access to one ear. The author finds that the child will accept examination with the auriscope if his or her ear is tickled with the finger first. The best auriscopic view of the drum is obtained if the pinna is pulled downwards in an infant and upwards and backwards in an older child. The child must be completely rotated through 180° to examine the other ear.

Treatment of symptoms includes antipyretics and analgesics such as paracetamol. Recent work has shown that oral antibiotics prescribed at first presentation reduce the probability of an extended time of pain in one out of 17 children treated and a similar chance of side effects directly attributable to the antibiotics[3]. The need for oral antibiotics has been debated recently. No major benefit has been consistently demonstrated in controlled trials and some experts recommend watchful waiting for 48–72 hours before starting antibiotic therapy if symptoms can be controlled with analgesics alone. However, most physicians would prescribe broad spectrum antibiotics such as amoxycillin as first-line treatment, for children who:
• are under 24 months of age
• are unwell
• look toxic
• have a history of more than 24 hours.

Amoxycillin-clavulanate should be reserved as a second-line treatment for those who do not respond to amoxycillin. All children who have had otitis media should be reviewed 7–10 days later by their primary care practitioner. Up to 10% of children will have an effusion 3 months postacute otitis media. These should have their hearing tested.

Complications from otitis media include:
- perforated tympanic membrane
- conductive hearing loss
- serous or bacterial labyrinthitis
- acute mastoiditis
- facial nerve palsy
- meningitis.

Acute mastoiditis
Acute mastoiditis is an infection of the mastoid air spaces behind the ear. It occurs with otitis media particularly in infants and is usually caused by streptococcal and staphylococcal species, *Klebsiella pneumoniae* and *Pseudomonas aeruginosa*. All children with acute mastoiditis must be admitted for intravenous antibiotics. Indications for mastoid drainage include severe toxicity, intracranial spread of infection and failure of rapid resolution on conservative treatment.

Facial palsy
Bell's palsy is the commonest cause of facial weakness in childhood. Its etiology is unclear, but reactivation of HSV or inflammatory edema with compression of the nerve at the stylomastoid foramen have been suggested. It presents with sudden onset of unilateral facial weakness over 1–2 days, often associated with a recent viral infection. There is sometimes retroauricular pain and hyperacusis, but 85% of children regain good function within 6 months. Steroids given early have an immunosuppressant and anti-inflammatory effect.

Facial palsy occasionally occurs in association with other conditions:
- Local causes
  - otitis media
  - facial or temporal lobe trauma
  - neoplasms
- Systemic causes
  - Lyme disease
  - Kawasaki disease

25.2.3 Trauma to the ear

Injuries to the pinna
Accidental injuries to the pinna are fairly rare as the ear is protected by the triangle of the shoulder, skull and base of the neck.

Bruising of the ear can occur from a direct blow. It is commonly seen in non-accidental injury when it may be associated with bruising of the scalp behind the ear and with cheek bruising. Occasionally ear injury causes a large bleed separating the cartilage of the ear from the perichondrium. Untreated, pressure of the hematoma on the cartilage can cause necrosis resulting in an unsightly deformity. Attempts at aspirating the blood invariably fail. All cases need urgent referral to an otolaryngologist who will cut a window in the cartilage and put in a small suction drain to evacuate the hematoma.

Lacerations of the pinna must be assessed carefully. Most are superficial and can be sutured in the ED. Those involving or exposing the cartilage require meticulous wound toilet and antibiotic cover as infection leads to perichondritis and cartilage destruction. Lacerations of the helical rim crossing skin and cartilage require accurate three-layer closing with positioning of the rim to avoid unsightly notching.

Embedded earrings can be removed in the ED after topical anesthesia of the ear lobe. Ear piercing, particularly in the upper part of the pinna, can become infected. This requires prompt treatment with antibiotics to avoid perichondritis.

Burns to the pinna occur in 90% of severe facial burns. Those resulting in exposure of the cartilage should be treated with topical antibiotics, such as sulphur sulfadiazine, to avoid chondritis. Later they might need debridement and sometimes reconstructive surgery.

Injuries to the drum and middle ear

The tympanic membrane is injured by direct trauma, when an object such as a cotton wool bud or a hair grip is inserted into the external auditory meatus to clean or scratch the ear. Rarely, trauma penetrating directly into the middle ear can result in fracture of the ossicles. Simple perforation usually heals spontaneously within 1–3 months. Treatment with analgesics or antibiotics is only needed if the injury is painful or involves contamination for example by water. Barotrauma can also result in a ruptured drum most commonly after a slap to the ear and also after flying in an aeroplane, diving or exposure to an explosion.

Bleeding from the ear or behind the tympanic membrane (hemotympanum) may indicate a fracture in the bony roof of the middle ear cavity. Any trauma to the ear which results in vertigo, sensorineural deafness or facial nerve palsy should be referred urgently to an otolaryngologist. Fractured skulls should also be referred to the appropriate specialist according to local protocols.

Aural foreign body

Removal of an aural foreign body, commonly stones, beads or small bits of paper, may be delayed as the child has few, if any, symptoms. Insects creeping into the auditory canal are particularly distressing and should be drowned with alcohol or olive oil before removal. If the child is co-operative and the foreign body is visible through an auriscope, then removal with forceps or syringing can be attempted in the ED. Syringing should not be used if the foreign body is of vegetable matter as it may swell and forceps should not be used for smooth objects which may be pushed in further. If removal is unsuccessful, the child should be referred to the next ear, nose and throat clinic.

Before discharging the patient, the ear should be checked for further foreign bodies and for damage to the tympanic membrane and otitis externa.

25.3 Mouth and oropharynx

25.3.1 Infections

Stomatitis

Children of all ages can suffer from stomatitis. Monilial or candidal stomatitis (thrush) is common in infants and in immunosuppressed children, herpes simplex and Coxsackie virus infection at any age, and aphthous ulcers in school-aged children.

Thrush is a fungal condition mainly affecting the tongue, buccal mucosa, gums and palate. It forms white plaques surrounded by inflammation, which bleed when scraped. Extensive infection leads to feeding difficulties and occasionally a perianal rash. Thrush rapidly responds to oral nystatin suspension, 100 000 units four times per day.

Herpes simplex virus causes a primary infection of the buccal mucosa, tongue and lips, usually in children of 2–6 years of age. A gingivitis precedes the vesicles, which ulcerate and form white plaques. Occasionally, the child will inoculate the virus on to the skin of their fingers or great toes and develop a herpetic whitlow. The patient is usually toxic and in pain and is reluctant to eat and drink. The condition is self-limiting and resolves spontaneously in 10–12 days. Treatment is mainly symptomatic with an antipyretic and analgesic such as paracetamol or ibuprofen and encouragement of fluids. Acyclovir may shorten the length of the illness in immunocompromised children.

Coxsackie virus causes ulcerating lesions of the mouth and pharynx and may be associated with similar lesions on the palms of the hands and the soles of the feet (hand foot and mouth disease). It is self-limiting.

Aphthous ulcers are the commonest oral infection. They are painful and although usually single, may be multiple and even confluent. The cause is unknown, but is believed to be infectious. They resolve spontaneously in 1–2 weeks but may recur.

Tonsillitis

Tonsillitis is common, particularly in the 4–6 year age group and may be associated with an upper respiratory tract infection. The majority of infections are caused by viruses including the adenovirus, influenza and parainfluenza viruses, Coxsackie virus and echovirus. Group A β hemolytic streptococcus is particularly common in children over the age of 3 years and may be associated with a petechial rash on the palate and occasionally with post-streptococcal nephritis. Rheumatic fever is now rare in developed countries.

Tonsillitis presents with a sore throat and occasionally food refusal in young children. There may also be headache, fever, cervical lymphadenopathy, pain radiating to the ear, a rash, signs of a coryza and occasionally abdominal pain. On examination, there is a pyrexia, tachycardia and red swollen tonsils. Both viral and bacterial infections can produce a tonsillar exudate. Koplik's spots, white nodules with surrounding erythema on the mucosa of the cheek and palate, are associated with measles. Occasionally one tonsil appears much larger than the other. This can be due to asymmetrical anatomical position, atypical infections such as actinomycosis, fungal or atypical mycobacterial infections and rarely a lymphoma.

Investigations are usually unnecessary for uncomplicated tonsillitis. However, a full blood count showing atypical lymphocytes and a positive Monospot test will help to distinguish infectious mononucleosis, and viral antibodies can be helpful if the tonsillitis becomes chronic.

Children who are systemically unwell or who have marked tonsillar involvement should be treated with an antipyretic and analgesic such as paracetamol and a 10-day course of penicillin or erythromycin.

The differential diagnoses of tonsillitis are listed in *Box 25.1*.

Upper airway obstruction

Upper airway obstruction is more common in children than in adults because the small calibre airways block more easily. It is very frightening for both the patient and the parents and is a frequent cause of presentation to the ED. Stertor is caused by supralaryngeal obstruction and stridor by laryngeal or upper tracheal obstruction. The child with upper airways obstruction needs a brief assessment:

> **Box 25.1** Differential diagnoses of tonsillitis
>
> - **Scarlet fever** (erythrogenic β hemolytic streptococcus) uniform red rash, sore 'strawberry' tongue, striae on flexor surface of elbows, peeling hands
> - **Infectious mononucleosis** (Epstein–Barr virus) especially in adolescence, malaise, often lasting for months, measles type rash, lymphadenopathy, enlarged spleen. Monospot positive
> - **Herpangina** (Coxsackie virus) vesicles or ulcers on the fauces
> - **Pharynoconjunctival fever** (adenovirus) headache, conjunctivitis and pharyngitis
> - **Quinsy** (Group A streptococcus, or anaerobes) peritonsillar abscess, giving muffled voice, drooling, trismus and a bulge in the soft palate and deviation of the uvula. Treat with penicillin and clindamycin. May need surgical drainage

1. NEVER EXAMINE THE THROAT OF A CHILD WITH STRIDOR
2. Assess the work of breathing – respiratory rate, recession, accessory muscles

   N.B. No airflow = no stridor
   N.B. Slowing of respiratory rate, reduced recession may herald arrest

3. Assess the circulation – a raised pulse may signal increasing hypoxia
4. Assess oxygenation (pulse oximetry) – increasing drowsiness or agitation and cyanosis are signs of hypoxia

Quinsy and severe tonsillitis are among the causes of upper airway obstruction, more of which are listed below:

Epiglottitis

This septicemic illness is always an emergency but is fortunately becoming rare in countries with an immunization programme against *H. influenzae* type B. The child is pale, anxious, ill and feverish with quiet snoring stridor caused by rapid swelling of the epiglottis, obstructing the larynx. The painful throat prevents talking or swallowing and the child has drooling of saliva. He or she sits up, leaning forward with the chin elevated to optimise airway opening. On examination there is tachypnea, tachycardia and sternal recession. Once the diagnosis is suspected, the child should be disturbed as little as possible as sudden respiratory obstruction may ensue. Oxygen may be given by facemask. The throat should not be examined and no upsetting investigations should be undertaken at this stage.

Senior anesthetic and otolaryngology help must be summoned as the child will need expert intubation and a tracheostomy if intubation is unsuccessful. Once the airway and ventilation are secured, then blood cultures and an epiglottic swab are taken and intravenous ceftaxime started. Most children recover and can be extubated within 2–3 days.

Retropharyngeal abscess

A retropharyngeal abscess is a potentially life-threatening but rare emergency caused by an infection by Group A streptococcus, anerobes or staphylococci in the potential space between the anterior border of the cervical vertebrae and the posterior wall of the esophagus. The clinical picture of a toxic child with stridor and drooling is very similar to epiglottitis and the initial management of the patient is the same. The child's throat should not be examined, but the fluctuant mass obstructing the larynx and esophagus would be difficult to see clinically anyway. Lateral neck X-rays, taken once the airway has been secured, reveal an increased width of soft tissues anterior to the cervical vertebrae. Antibiotic treatment with intravenous penicillin and cefazolin is effective. Surgical drainage may be necessary.

Other causes of upper airway obstruction are listed in *Box 25.2*.

General measures for management of airways obstruction include:
1. Prevent agitation – settle child on parent's lap and do not disturb.
2. Improve oxygenation by giving high concentration oxygen by facemask.
3. Get senior help appropriately.
4. Nebulized epinephrine (adrenaline) 2 ml 1/1000 with oxygen gives transient improvement (see Chapter 5).
5. If intubation is necessary, it should be carried out by an experienced anesthetist. Intravenous cannulation, blood tests, fluids and drugs should be given after intubation.

Box 25.2 Other causes of upper airway obstruction

- **Croup:** common and often presents in the evenings
- **Bacterial tracheitis:** life-threatening *H. influenzae* or *S. aureus* infection; presents as croupy cough in a toxic child
- **Diphtheria:** rare in unimmunized children
- **Angioedema:** acute laryngeal swelling with an anaphylactic reaction, treated with epinephrine (adrenaline), antihistamines and steroids
- **Laryngeal foreign body:** see Chapter 2 for management

Infected lesions in the neck

Cervical lymphadenitis is a bacterial infection of the lymph nodes in the neck. It presents with fever and a painful erythematous swelling. *S. aureus* and Group A streptococcus are the commonest organisms, treated with flucloxacillin or cephalexin. Collections of pus might need incision and drainage. A chronic unilateral cervical lymphadenitis can be caused by *Mycobacterium tuberculosis* or an atypical mycobacterial infection.

A *thyroglossal cyst* develops along the line of descent of the thyroid gland and can occur anywhere from the base of the tongue to the sternal notch. The cyst can become infected, and present with a red tender swelling, which moves up when the child swallows or puts out the tongue. Treatment is by oral antibiotics and occasionally by incision and drainage of the cyst.

25.3.2 Trauma to the mouth and oropharynx

Lacerations to the lips

Lacerations to the lips are common, particularly from dog bites or falls on to the face, when the teeth may penetrate the lips. If the laceration is through the whole thickness of the lip, all three layers must be closed. It is important that the position of the cut edges and landmarks of the lips are aligned exactly on suturing as even a slight misalignment of 1 mm of the vermilion border will give a disfiguring deformity. Difficult cases should be referred to a plastic or faciomaxillary surgeon.

Injuries to the tongue

The tongue is a large muscle mass with a copious blood supply. It may be injured in falls and when the child bites his or her own tongue. X-rays should be taken in any case where a laceration of the tongue is associated with chipped teeth to look for a foreign body. Even small tongue lacerations bleed briskly although the bleeding has often ceased by the time the child attends the ED. Minor lacerations usually heal spontaneously. Ice lollipops and ice cream may relieve the pain and reduce swelling. Indications for referral for suturing, under general anesthetic, include lacerations which are:
• deep
• > 1 cm long
• continuing to bleed
• gaping and through the tongue edge

The movement of the tongue muscle mass will tend to make the sutures cut out and so they should take a deeper bite into surrounding tissues.

327

Accidental mouth injuries in young non-mobile babies are very rare and injuries to the tongue and frenulum of the upper lip may indicate non-accidental injury.

Palatal injury

Children sometimes fall while sucking a pencil, sustaining a puncture wound of the palate. Trauma to the central palate is unlikely to involve vascular structures in the neck and superficial small wounds need no treatment. However, lateral palatal wounds or postpharyngeal wounds may involve major vessels such as the carotid artery or the jugular vein. In addition, an expanding hematoma of the neck from a puncture wound may present with reduced neck pulses and intraoral bleeding. All but the small superficial lacerations of the central palate should be referred for possible exploration.

25.4 The nose

25.4.1 Nasal discharge

Nasal discharge is a symptom of many conditions in children, the commonest of which are discussed below.

Upper respiratory tract infection

On average, children suffer from four upper respiratory tract infections per year. The youngest child in a family may get many more for a period when their older siblings start nursery or school. The child has sneezing, a runny nose and is mildly unwell. Symptomatic treatment only is needed with plenty of fluids and an antipyretic and analgesic if necessary. Complications include tonsillitis, otitis media and sinusitis.

Sinus infection

The ethmoid and maxillary sinuses are present at birth, but the frontal and sphenoidal sinuses are undeveloped until 4–6 years of age. Sinus infections usually involve the frontal and maxillary sinuses in older children. They can be caused by a range of organisms including *H. influenzae*, Group A streptococcus, *S. pneumoniae* and *Moraxella catarrhalis*. Presentation is with headaches, yellow green thick nasal discharge, and pain and tenderness over the maxillary and frontal sinuses. Ethmoidal sinusitis may cause pain referred behind the eyes.

Treatment includes an antipyretic and analgesic such as paracetamol and oral decongestants. Local decongestants such as ephedrine can cause rebound congestion and are not advised. A 10-day course of an antibiotic is prescribed if there is systemic upset and amoxycillin-clavulanate, cefaclor or erythromycin are all effective. Rarely, with severe or recurrent problems the sinuses might need surgical drainage.

Allergic rhinitis

The symptoms of allergic rhinitis are often associated with atopy and may be seasonal, or due to specific allergens in the environment. It presents with persistent nasal obstruction and profuse watery nasal discharge, sneezing and itching of the nose and eyes. Investigations are rarely done, but occasionally serum IgE and RAST (radioallergosorbent tests) are helpful in guiding treatment.

Management includes separation of the child from the allergens if possible and local steroid insufflations with beclomethasone or fluticasone. Oral antihistamines and topical sodium cromoglycate prophylaxis can also be useful.

25.4.2 Nasal trauma

Blunt trauma

The nose is often injured in children who fall on to the face or who sustain a direct blow to the nose. It may be an isolated injury, or associated with other fractures of the middle third of the face.

The child presents with swelling, tenderness, bruising and deformity of the bridge of the nose, sometimes with periorbital edema and subconjunctival hemorrhage. Careful assessment is needed to guide the management (*Box 25.3*).

Box 25.3 Assessment in blunt trauma to the nose

- **Septal hematoma:** a cherry red swelling inside the nose. It can cause pressure necrosis of the nasal septum and collapse of the nose and may progress to a septal abscess. It needs immediate referral for incision and drainage under general anesthetic
- **Septal deformity:** occasionally the septum is deviated to one side, needing referral
- **Nasal deformity:** fracture without displacement needs no treatment. Deformity should be assessed 7–10 days after the injury when the swelling has settled. Reduction may then be necessary within the next few days
- **Thickening of the bridge:** this is often slow to settle but needs no active treatment

---

X-rays are not routinely taken in nasal injury as they often do not alter management and they inevitably irradiate the lens. They are indicated if there are:
• breaks in the skin (potential compound fracture)
• other associated facial injuries
• medicolegal reasons

A clear watery discharge after nose injury may indicate a CSF leak from a fracture of the base of the skull, passing through the cribriform plate.

Epistaxis

Nose bleeds can be troublesome in childhood but are rarely serious. The bleeding usually occurs from the anterior part of the nasal septum, Little's area at the site of a plexus of vessels. By far the most common causes are traumatic, particularly a blow to the nose and nose picking, which often causes bleeding on the side of the dominant hand. Less frequent causes are listed in *Box 25.4.*

Assessment involves a full history of the bleeding and assessment of the cardiovascular state of the child, and sites of local and systemic cause for the bleeding. Rarely, profuse bleeding may occur with pallor, sweating, a raised pulse, low blood pressure and anemia. Blood should be grouped and cross-matched and a coagulation screen undertaken when necessary.

To stop the bleeding, the child should sit leaning forward with the mouth open. The soft parts of the nose should be pressed between the fingers for 15 minutes. A cotton wool roll under the upper lip puts pressure on the labial artery and helps stop the hemorrhage. If the bleeding is

---

Box 25.4 Causes of epistaxis

• Local causes
  ◦ allergic rhinitis
  ◦ local infection
  ◦ foreign body
  ◦ rarely tumors
• Systemic causes
  ◦ increased venous pressure e.g. with severe cough of cystic fibrosis or pertussis
  ◦ sickle cell anemia
  ◦ leukemia
  ◦ clotting disorders

persistent, referral will be needed for admission and a nasal pack. Continued bleeding may necessitate cautery and even ligation of vessels.

Rebleeding can be prevented if infection, ulceration and crusting in the anterior nose is reduced by topical antibiotic and barrier cream such as chlorhexidine/neomycin cream.

Nasal laceration

Lacerations of the thick skin of the nasal alae can result in an unsightly notched scar. It is important that the cartilage is not left exposed as infective chondritis can result. The junction of the skin and mucosa must be apposed and sutured accurately. All but the most minor lacerations should be repaired by a plastic surgeon or otolaryngologist.

Nasal foreign body

Nasal foreign bodies, usually paper, sponge or food, are potentially dangerous owing to the possibility of inhalation and must be removed. Some present quickly if the child tells an adult what they have done or if they are observed. Others may present late with a foul smelling unilateral nasal discharge.

Nose blowing or stroking the nose will occasionally expel the foreign body. If these are unsuccessful, it is worth having one attempt to remove the object in the ED. The child should be immobilized, preferably by being hugged by a parent in a similar way to that used to examine the ears. The foreign body can usually be hooked out by inserting a blunt hook above the foreign body and extracting it against the nasal floor. Vegetable matter is more difficult to remove as it may swell on absorbing the nasal secretions. Topical antibiotic may be needed if the mucosa is injured during the procedure or is infected. If removal is unsuccessful, the child should be referred to an otolaryngologist.

References

1. Klein, J.O. (1994). Otitis media. *CID* **19**: 823–833.
2. Pukander, K., Karma, P., Sipila, M. (1982) Occurrence and recurrence of acute otitis media among children. *Acta Otolaryngol.* **94**: 479–486.
3. Moyer, V.A., Elliott, E.J., Davis, R.L. *et al.* (2000) *Evidence-based Pediatrics and Child Health*. London: BMJ Books.

Suggested reading

Bull, P.D. (2002) *Lecture Notes on Diseases of the Ear, Nose and Throat*. Oxford: Blackwell Science.

Cotton, R.T., Myer III, C.M. (1998) *Practical Pediatric Otolaryngology.*
    Philadelphia, PA: Lippincott-Raven Publishers.
Fleischer, G.R., Ludwig, S. (2000) *Textbook of Emergency Pediatrics.*
    Philadelphia, PA: Lippincott Williams and Williams.

Chapter 26

Dental emergencies

Patricia O. Brennan

Contents

Dental emergencies in childhood fall into three main categories, trauma, infection and bleeding.

26.1 Trauma

In the 1993 UK Children's Dental Health Survey of over 19 000 children, 26% showed signs of dental trauma by the time they were 15 years of age. In addition, some children will have had tooth and soft tissue oral injuries that will have healed leaving no signs, giving an estimated 30% of children sustaining oral or dental injuries. The peak incidence of this trauma occurs in children between the ages of 1 and 3 years when they are learning to walk, and 8 and 11 years when their activities become more boisterous and less cautious. The upper central incisors are most vulnerable to injury. Risk factors include:
• protruding front teeth
• hyperactivity
• physical handicap
• contact sports

26.1.1 History

In addition to a general medical history, the history of when, where and how any injury happened is important. Details of first aid given and any previous dental trauma will help to guide management. If a tooth is broken, all fragments should be accounted for. They could be inhaled, ingested or remain embedded in a laceration.

Dental and oral injuries inconsistent with the history given should arouse suspicion of non-accidental injury (see Chapter 27).

26.1.2 Examination

The examination in dental trauma must be wider than just the teeth. The injury may be associated with facial trauma, particularly in serious accidents such as road traffic accidents when assessment and management of the dental trauma will have to wait until any life-threatening injuries have been treated. The examinations are listed in *Box 26.1*.

Suspicion of ingestion or inhalation of lost tooth fragments should be checked by X-ray of chest and upper abdomen. Lacerations of the mouth and lips associated with chipped and lost teeth should also be X-rayed to exclude a foreign body in the wound.

Box 26.1 Examination for dental trauma

- **Extra-oral**
  - General examination
  - Head and neck
    - soft tissue injuries
    - bony tenderness
    - bony margins, especially mandible and maxilla
    - movement, especially of temporomandibular joint
- **Intra-oral**
  - Soft tissue injuries
    - cheek
    - tongue
    - palate
- **Dental**
  - Bony tenderness
    - gingival margins
  - Teeth
    - tenderness
    - chipping
    - looseness
    - displacement
    - avulsion

26.1.3 Investigation

Children should be referred to a dentist who will check for vitality of teeth and also take appropriate X-rays.

26.1.4 Trauma to primary teeth

Trauma to the teeth is particularly common as young children learn to walk and fall forwards, causing a range of injuries. The immediate damage to teeth is considered in the ED and the dentist will later consider the sequele of this damage and the indirect effects on permanent teeth.

Concussed teeth are tender but need no active treatment.

Subluxed and loosened teeth rapidly re-attach without splinting. Teeth which are displaced labially or palatally should be gently replaced. *Displacement* of primary teeth with a fracture of the alveolar plate is more likely than crown or root fractures in this age group, as the alveolar bone is relatively thin and elastic.

Teeth pushed apically into the gums, *intrusion*, will re-erupt within a few weeks. The injury may appear to be minor, but hypoplasia, hypermineralisation or aberrant eruption of permanent dentition can occur from contact with or apical infection from the root of the intruded tooth. *Completely avulsed* primary teeth should not be replaced because of the possibility of damage to the underlying developing permanent tooth.

Crown fractures can vary in severity from minor chips or crazing of the enamel to fracture of enamel, dentine, pulp and cementum. Treatment varies from smoothing of rough areas to pulp treatment and reconstruction of the tooth. This is difficult in most young children and the dentist's preferred option is often regular review of the progress for minor injuries or extraction for more serious injuries. *Root fractures* with a stable coronal fragment should be left to heal, but those with a very mobile coronal segment will be treated by extraction.

General treatment of oral and dental injuries in young children will include oral antibiotics and a soft diet and analgesics for painful injuries. Tetanus prophylaxis must be adequate for any open wound or bleeding. All dental injuries should be regularly monitored for long-term sequele.

26.1.5 Trauma to secondary dentition

Trauma to secondary dentition is particularly distressing for both child and parent. With the present low caries rate, a traumatic injury can be particularly devastating to an otherwise perfect smile, with consequent psychological sequele. A summary of the management of dental trauma is shown in *Table 26.1*.

First aid treatment of an avulsed tooth consists of:
1. Clean tooth gently by licking or putting in milk or tap water. Do not scrub or damage the membrane around the root or use antiseptic or soap.
2. Replace the tooth gently in the socket in the correct orientation.
3. Stabilise the tooth by getting the child to bite on a handkerchief.
4. Seek immediate dental help.

If there is reluctance to replace the tooth, the child and the tooth should be brought directly to a dentist or ED. The tooth should be transported in the buccal sulcus of the child or parent if possible. Otherwise it should be put into milk or contact lens solution at room temperature. The tooth should be replaced, preferably within 30 minutes, but certainly within 2 hours to have a chance of re-implantation. It will need splinting for 7–10 days and may need root canal treatment later.

Table 26.1 Summary of management of trauma to secondary teeth.

Injury	Signs	Treatment
Concussion	Tender with bleeding around gingival margin	Reassure
Intrusion	Pushed apically into gum – needs a large force. Tooth may re-erupt if minor displacement, but otherwise needs orthodontic repositioning. May result in pulp necrosis and infection	Refer to Orthodontics
Subluxation	Tender loose teeth with bleeding of gingival margin. Most rapidly become firm. 12% lose vitality	Soft diet and analgesics
Lateral luxation	Displaced loose tooth	Realign and splint for 7–10 days
Avulsion	Lost tooth	Re-implant. May need root treatment. See later
Fractured teeth	Cracked and fractured enamel	Smooth sharp edges
All more serious fractures should be urgently referred to a dentist		
	Dentine fracture	Threatens vitality. Dentist will dress with calcium hydroxide and seal with a restoration
	Exposed pulp	As for dentine fracture, but may need root treatment
	Root fracture – mobile or displaced tooth	Reduce and splint but prognosis depends on the position of the fracture

General care of all dental trauma is to give analgesics and soft diet for painful teeth and to make sure that the child is fully immunized against tetanus. All injuries to the secondary dentition will need regular monitoring by a dentist to detect and treat long-term sequele.

26.2 Dental infection

A dental infection can be localized with redness and swelling of the gum and sometimes pointing to the labial sulcus. However, infection in a child is likely to be more extensive with facial swelling and cellulitis. Deep infection can lead to spread to the submaxillary spaces, a submandibular abscess and even cavernous sinus thrombosis. The abscess should be drained. The infected tooth will need root canal therapy, apicectomy or even extraction. A broad spectrum antibiotic should be prescribed.

Infections in tissues of the head and neck can present as pain and discomfort in the mouth. These include: mumps and suppurative parotitis, herpes simplex stomatitis and candida.

26.3 Bleeding tooth socket

Occasionally children present with a bleeding tooth socket after a primary tooth has come out or after extraction of a tooth by a dentist. The clot should be removed from the socket and the child encouraged to bite for 10 minutes on a small roll of sterile gauze. If bleeding continues, a dental opinion should be sought as the socket may need suturing. If the bleeding is extensive or prolonged, a bleeding or clotting screen must be carried out to look for disorders of hemostasis.

26.4 Tongue piercing

Piercing of the tongue and lips is becoming more popular. Patients should be counselled that tongue piercing can lead to problems, in particular:
• airway obstruction secondary to swelling
• aspiration of jewellery
• infection resulting in Ludwig's angina
• prolonged bleeding
• chipped or fractured teeth
• difficulties with speech, mastication and swallowing

Suggested reading

Andreasen, J.O., Andreasen, F.M. (1994) *Textbook and Colour Atlas of Traumatic Injuries to the Teeth*. Copenhagen: Munksgaard.

Dental Practice Board for England and Wales. (1999) National Clinical Guidelines and Policy Documents. In: *Pediatric Dentistry*. Eastbourne: Dental Practice Board for England and Wales.

Roberts, G., Longhurst, P. (1996) *Oral and Dental Trauma in Children and Adolescents*. Oxford: Oxford University Press.

Chapter 27

Child abuse

Patricia O. Brennan

Contents

27.1 Introduction

Child abuse was described in 1946 by Caffey and in *The Battered Child* by Henry Kempe in 1962. Since that time, it has been increasingly recognised in various forms as a cause of acute injury, permanent damage, disability and even death. Any of these may present to an Emergency Department.

This chapter seeks to help the emergency pediatrician to learn about the range of abuse, to differentiate non-accidental injury from accidental injury, to undertake initial management and protection of the child and refer on to the appropriate professionals. The assessment and management will be guided by local child protection procedures and be in a multiprofessional forum. The emphasis must be that the welfare of the child is paramount.

27.2 Definition and incidence of abuse

Child abuse is the avoidable impairment of health, development and welfare of a child resulting from 'parental' (or care-giver at the time) action or inaction. It involves treatment of a child in a way that is unacceptable in a given culture at a given time. [1] Thus, the definition varies from culture to culture and through the ages in any given culture. It is proper therefore that the final diagnosis of 'child abuse' is not left to one individual, but rests with a local multidisciplinary group including doctors, social workers, police and health visitors amongst others.

There will be a spectrum across every type of abuse. This is exemplified in physical abuse by the spectrum:

acceptable corrective trauma ↔ deliberate cruelty

The incidence of abuse is very difficult to define. Few surveys are comparable in study group or methodology. It is said to occur in 15 per 1000 American children. [2] In the UK, at least 1:1000 under 4-year-olds suffer serious physical abuse, at least 1:10 000 children are thought to die of abuse and in 1995, over 35 000 children were on Child Protection Registers.

Referrals for investigation have risen over recent years. It is not clear whether this reflects an increase in the actual incidence of abuse. What is clear, is that in many countries, society is increasingly willing to recognise the existence of child abuse and try to do something about it.

There are recognised risk factors for abuse in both individual children and for families (*Boxes 27.1* and *27.2*).

Box 27.1 Risk factors for abuse in children

- Under 4 years or preschool children
- Unwanted pregnancy
- Doubtful paternity
- Separation in the newborn period, with inadequate bonding
- Physically or mentally handicapped children – remember to include those with serious medical conditions

---

Box 27.2 Risk factors for child abuse in parents

- Substance and alcohol abuse
- Young, immature parents
- Few skills
- Emotional stress and unstable relationships
- Financial stress and unemployment
- Poor mothering experience or abuse of parents as children
- Violent reaction to stress
- Mother pregnant or premenstrual
- Learning difficulties
- Parental mental health problems
- Domestic violence

27.3 Types of abuse

Individual cases of abuse fall along a spectrum, but for ease of categorization, these are separated into broad groups:
- physical abuse
- sexual abuse
- neglect
- emotional abuse
- other sorts of abuse such as Munchausen syndrome by proxy

If a child has been a victim of one sort of abuse, then he or she is more likely rather than less likely to also be the victim of the others. The assessment of any case must therefore include an assessment of the whole child.

27.3.1 Physical abuse

Trigger factors for an incident of physical abuse may be a family crisis or period of difficult behavior in the child such as prolonged crying, difficult feeding or wetting or soiling. It is important to remember that the degree of danger to the child is not related to the severity of the presenting injury, but to the situation within the family. A young baby with minor cheek bruising may well be at grave risk of severe life-threatening injury in the near future.

Physical injury is probably the commonest presentation of child abuse to the ED. Experience in accidental injuries gives a good foundation for judging the non-accidental injury. Both accidental and non-accidental injuries usually present with one or more of the following:
• bruising
• burns
• other soft tissue injuries
• fractures

In order to differentiate the accidental from the non-accidental, consider: **Does the injury fit the history given?**

Take the history of any injury, from both parent and child if possible. Record every explanation for each injury, carefully and verbatim, without medical interpretation. Worrying features include those listed in *Box 27.3*.

Box 27.3 Significant features in the history

• A history which is not consistent with the physical findings
• A changing, vague or absent history
• Delay in presentation, particularly with a painful injury
• A history of assault from the child
• Strange affect or behavior of parents or child when giving the history
• Frequent previous attendances

The child is then examined. No child should be examined against his or her will or repeatedly. Consent must be obtained from someone with parental rights, even if a child is brought in by social workers. This rule should only be overturned in an acute medical emergency, where urgent lifesaving treatment of the child is needed. Young children should be examined in the presence of a parent, but older children and young people should be given the choice of who is present.

Bruising
Children sustain bruising throughout their childhood and the number of bruises varies from child to child. Accidental bruises vary with the

stage of development and mobility, the activities undertaken and even the personality of the child. Energetic children have many bruises and grazes, especially on shins, knees, elbows, forearms, occasionally over spinous processes and over the forehead in toddlers. Unusual but accidental bruises have a specific explanation.

Bruising is one of the commonest presentations of both accidental and non-accidental injuries and various aspects must be considered:
• the site
• the shape and size
• the pattern of the bruises
• the age
• the number

Some of the patterns suggestive of abuse include:
• *unusual sites* of bruising such as the soft part of the cheek, the ears, inside of the arms and inner thighs, the neck and small of the back and chest, the upper arms and shoulders and the genitalia and buttocks
• *bruising from hands*, such as the fingertip clusters of round bruises, the arc-shaped bruise around finger ends, and the parallel bruises or petechie of the fingers in slap marks, pairs of bruising from pinching
• *specific patterns of bruising* from implements or artifacts such as crescentic bite shaped bruises
• *various ages* of bruises
• *an unusual number* of bruises

Each bruise should be carefully drawn on a body chart, and described with details of color and size of each injury. Take particular care when marking right and left. Research has found ageing of bruises by color to be less specific than previously thought. The only dogmatic statement now made is that any bruise with yellow discoloration is at least 18 hours old and probably more than 3 days old. All other colors have been recorded at any stage from when the injury was sustained until the time of resolution. [3]

Burns and scalds

The depth of a burn depends on the temperature and duration of exposure. At 65.5° C (150° F) adult skin sustains a full thickness burn in 2 seconds. A child's skin can burn in a quarter of the time. It is estimated that 1–16% of burns presenting to EDs are inflicted injuries. In addition, neglected children may be scalded or burnt or even suffocated in house fires due to poor supervision. A small number die from deliberate abuse. Diagnosis is difficult.

Accidental scalds often have splash marks, follow the lines of clothing and are of variable depth. Accidental contact burns usually involve the palms and forearms. Peak incidence of accidental burns and scalds is the second year of life. The peak age for inflicted burns and scalds is in the third year of life. The characteristics of inflicted scalds and burns described are:

- *contact burns in unusual sites*, e.g. dorsum of the hand, back, buttocks
- *dipping scalds*, sharply demarcated glove and stocking scalds of uniform depth with no splash marks – the soles are spared if the foot is pressed on the bottom of the bath
- *some buttock/perineal burns*, especially with central sparing
- *cigarette burns*, especially of the stubbing, circular punched out full-thickness type rather than the oval or triangular brushing burns, or
- *that child's development* is such that alleged mechanism is impossible, e.g. 6-month-old climbing into a bath of hot water.

Other unusual burns such as friction burns or chemical burns can sometimes be inflicted. Deep burns and scalds leave scars – a permanent sign of abuse.

Fractures
Fractures are common accidental injuries in childhood, especially in school-aged children, but fractures of most bones have at some time been a presentation of non-accidental injury. Certain types require further investigation, especially in the under 2-year-olds and even more especially in the non-ambulant infants and those associated with intracranial injuries (*Box 27.4*).

Fractures in child abuse often present late. Knowledge of the normal healing process is important. Callus is visible 10–14 days after the fracture (earlier in infants) and matures over the following weeks. The bone then remodels and gradually returns to normal within the next 1–2 years.

If one suspicious bony injury is detected, the child needs a skeletal survey in order to look for others. Plain X-rays are superior for detecting skull fractures, but these are difficult to date. A bone scan is better for detecting rib fractures and for the early detection of minor injuries of long bones. Fractures at various stages of healing denote repeated assaults.

Head injuries
Accidental head injuries, especially from road traffic accidents are the commonest cause of death in children over 5 years of age. They are

---

Box 27.4 Bony injury requiring further investigation

- **Skull fractures:** especially large, wide, multiple or complicated fractures which cross suture lines, occipital and depressed fractures and those associated with intracranial injury
- **Rib fractures** (less so in preterm babies in the neonatal period where porotic bones fracture more easily). These are more easily seen after 7–10 days when callus develops. Posterior and anterior fractures may be caused by squeezing and lateral fractures by direct blows. It is doubtful whether cardiopulmonary resuscitation causes rib fractures
- **Spiral or long bone fractures** (excluding the spiral tibial fracture in a toddler), and bilateral or multiple fractures, especially those at various stages of healing indicating fractures of different ages
- Any fracture in a child **under 1 year of age**
- **Metaphyseal fractures** (corner or bucket-handle fractures) at the ends of long bones from rotatory or traction forces causing disruption close to the physis, often multiple and at the elbows, wrists, knees and ankles. They appear to cause little pain and may be associated with subperiosteal new bone in the more severe injuries
- **Old fractures** with delayed presentation or those found incidentally
- **Unusual fractures**, e.g. of the sternum and scapula
- **Spinal injury** from hyperflexion/extension with defects in the anterior superior edges of the vertebral bodies and narrowed disc spaces often in the lower thoracic and upper lumbar areas

---

also common in physically abused children and may include bruising to the face or head, skull and facial fractures, subgaleal and intracranial hemorrhage, cerebral edema and contusion, and diffuse axonal injury. In infants, 95% of serious head injuries are associated with abuse when external head injury can be associated with intracranial injuries. Permanent, serious mental and physical disabilities can result.

A direct impact to the head from blows or from throwing the child against a hard object, can cause a fracture and very occasionally, an extradural hematoma, from bleeding of the middle meningeal artery. The fractured skull may, some hours later, be associated with gross soft boggy swelling of the scalp on the associated side. A similar swelling can occasionally result from hair pulling.

Young infants may be the victims of the *shaken baby syndrome*. The child is held around the chest, facing the assaulter, who has the fingers at the back near the costovertebral junction and the thumbs anteriorly. The hands squeeze and rotate slightly, putting a rotatory force. This fractures the ribs both posteriorly on the costospinal junction and anteriorly at the costochondral junction, and raises the intrathoracic pressure and therefore the venous pressure. The child is then shaken vigorously, causing an anterior/posterior movement of the head with a rotatory movement. The brain moves inside the skull. The acceleration/deceleration forces shear the bridging veins between the brain surface and the dura, causing a subdural hematoma, often bilaterally. During the shaking, the arms and legs flail around, causing metaphyseal fractures at the ends of the long bones of the limbs.

In addition, the infant may be thrown on to a bed or against a firm surface, increasing the shearing forces and occasionally causing a fracture. Infants with an extradural or subdural hemorrhage present with signs of raised intracranial pressure with irritability, vomiting, fits, drowsiness, apneic attacks and occasionally unconsciousness and a bulging fontanelle. Bilateral fundal hemorrhages are particularly associated with a subdural hematoma, but may occur in its absence. Children with serious head injuries with fractures and intracranial hemorrhage may well have no external signs of injury.

In all small babies with bruising and a fracture, even without cerebral signs, a CT scan of the brain should be performed in the acute stages to exclude extradural, subdural, subarachnoid and intracerebral hemorrhages, and cerebral edema. MRI is more effective in detecting posterior fossa and non-hemorrhagic intraparenchymal trauma and shearing injuries.

Other soft tissue injuries
Other soft tissue injuries suggestive of non-accidental injury include:
- *torn frenulum* from forceful feeding with a bottle or from a blow; in older infants, this can be associated with chipped teeth
- *tongue and palatal injuries*
- *hair loss* from pulling, with scalp swelling and tenderness
- *abdominal injuries* from a kick or a punch presenting as a shocked child with splenic or hepatic damage or even rupture of the gut.

27.3.2 Child sexual abuse

Child sexual abuse is any abuse of children for the sexual gratification of adults. It is common and increasing numbers of cases are referred to pediatricians for assessment. Defining incidence and prevalence is difficult, as sampling techniques and methodology vary. What is clear is that child sexual abuse is common, both of girls and boys. In reported studies, prevalence varies from 12–17% in girls and 5–8% in boys in the UK. Perpetrators are usually, but not exclusively, male, often mother's cohabitee, a male relative or a neighbor. Child sexual abuse entails all types of sexual activity, often with escalating intrusiveness as the child gets older from oral/oral or orogenital contact or fondling in the young, to anal or vaginal penetrative sex in older children. Cases present to the ED in four main ways:

- physical signs, injury
- chronic physical problems such as vaginal discharge or soreness, anal or vaginal bleeding or perineal warts
- disclosure of abuse by the child or by someone else – treat allegations about parents who are in dispute about access arrangements to their child with caution
- behavioral problems as a long-term sequel to sexual abuse, e.g. self-harm, encopresis, enuresis or sexualized behavior.

Before assessing any case, the emergency pediatrician should know about local procedures.

Genital injuries

Children can injure the genital area accidentally. There is usually a specific history such as falling astride a bath or a bicycle cross-bar. In such instances, the girls usually (but not always) injure the anterior vulval region sustaining pubic and clitoral bruising and small mucosal abrasions. Occasionally the injury is more posterior. Boys can also sustain genital bruising from fights, falling toilet seats or from getting the penis caught in a zip fastener.

In any child with a history of perineal trauma with significant anogenital bleeding, a brief examination should be undertaken to exclude severe blood loss requiring emergency surgical management. In every case where the history is not entirely consistent with the injury, the child should then be referred for a more senior pediatric opinion. Very occasionally the child needs an examination under general anesthetic. The pediatrician will arrange a joint examination with a forensic pediatrician (for collection of forensic evidence) and referrals to police and social services as appropriate according to local protocols.

The medical part of the investigation will include a history, including a family history and a history of bladder and bowel problems. After consent has been obtained, a full examination and appropriate investigations are carried out.

In sexual abuse, there may be suggestive signs of physical trauma such as bruising to the thighs, neck and upper arms. The anogenital examination, usually carried out using a colposcope, may show signs of recent trauma (*Box 27.5*).

There may be signs of more chronic abuse (*Box 27.6*).

Box 27.5 Genital signs of injury in recent sexual abuse in girls

- Hymenal and vaginal lacerations, edema, bruising
- Lacerations to the labia minora and posterior fourchette
- Anal fissures, particularly deep fissures crossing the anal margin, swelling of the skin around the anus and bruising

---

Box 27.6 Genital signs of chronic sexual abuse in girls

- A rolled edge to a widened hymen, possibly with asymmetrical notches of old healed tears
- Scarring especially of the posterior fourchette
- The thickened, brawny skin of the labia majora from intracrural intercourse
- The asymmetrical rugae of healed anal fissures and lax sphincter, scarring and occasionally reflex anal dilatation
- Infective conditions related to sexual abuse such as anal warts, and infections with herpes and gonorrhea

---

If any signs suspicious of sexual abuse are found fortuitously during an examination, the doctor should quietly complete the examination, carefully document the findings and ask for more senior help promptly.

It must be remembered, however, that many cases of child sexual abuse have no abnormal physical signs and that, even in 3.5% of cases of penile penetrations confirmed by the victim and the perpetrator and in 57% of cases of confirmed digital penetration, no abnormal physical signs are detected. [4] A case of suspected sexual abuse, even without physical signs requires a full multi-agency investigation. The examination often reassures a child who feels that she or he has been harmed.

At the end of the joint physical examination, the pediatrician can then take over the care of the child and family and consider other factors such as an infection check, postcoital contraception, medical follow up and counselling and communications with general practitioners and health visitors.

Disclosure

Children may disclose sexual abuse shortly after the incident. However, many disclose some time later when they feel it is safe to tell someone. As soon as parents know, they often become extremely distressed and seek urgent help. They may present to the ED, where a short history should determine the likely type and timing of abuse and a judgement can be made on the urgency of referral to the social services, police and specialist pediatrician. Often in these cases, the medical examination is best deferred until after the interviews with child and family, in a calm daytime clinic when all the resources are to hand.

Behavioral problems

Child sexual abuse can leave lasting emotional and psychological damage. The child may present to the ED, even years later, with depression, substance abuse (including alcohol abuse), other self-harm and behavior problems.

As stated, the investigation of child sexual abuse is the domain of the trained specialist. If a child presents to the ED, with signs or symptoms of sexual abuse, the pediatrician should:

1. Take a history
2. Undertake any urgent medical management needed
3. Calm the family and assure them the case will be carefully considered, and let them know of any local procedures
4. Refer on to an experienced pediatrician
5. Refer on to local social services and police

27.3.3 Neglect and emotional abuse

Cases of neglect and emotional abuse occasionally present to the ED or they may be identified in children presenting with other problems. It is important that they are identified for what they are, so that help can be accessed for the child and family. Neglected children tend to fail to thrive and may fail to achieve full potential in other parameters of development. Classically they have dry sparse straight hair and a protuberant abdomen and cold extremities and frozen watchfulness, but signs are often more subtle. Children with exceptionally short stature with no detectable organic disorder may be failing to grow due to longstanding abuse and neglect. Chronic undernutrition can cause poor growth and despite a proper diet thereafter, these children may remain significantly smaller than their peers. A separate group of children suffering from chronic emotional abuse may have hyperphagic short stature. [1] Neglected children might also suffer mild to moderate learning difficulties.

Occasionally the relationship between a child and parent or between child and the professionals leads to a suspicion of emotional abuse. Children are noted to be quiet, sad, withdrawn or overfriendly and attention seeking, overactive with a very short attention span. Older children can present, for example as self-harmers. The role of the ED pediatrician in each case is to undertake urgent medical treatment and then refer the child for psychiatric assessment and long-term management. The child psychiatrist will need to understand the nature of the underlying problem to offer treatment for the child and family.

27.3.4 Other forms of abuse

Munchausen syndrome by proxy (MSBP)
Children with MSBP may present to the ED with coma, drowsiness, apnea or fits. A few of these have been intentionally poisoned or suffocated. Munchausen syndrome by proxy also presents as factitious or induced illness, such as bleeding per rectum, hematuria, poisoning, or other illnesses, such as fits, which are never witnessed by anyone other than the care-giver. It occurs mainly in preschool children and is thought to have an incidence of at least 3 per 100 000 in children under 1 year of age in the UK; 95% are abused by their mothers. The abuse is twofold, by the actions of the mother and by the investigations arranged by the medical staff. The diagnosis is difficult to make and the cases are difficult to manage. It is important that records of all attendances of each child to the ED are kept together and are available at each new attendance to give the total picture over time. This will help in the overall evaluation of each child.

Poisoning
Accidental poisoning is common, but occasionally children present to an ED with non-accidental poisoning, two-thirds of which occur in the context of MSBP. The possibility of non-accidental poisoning with drugs or other substances, such as salt, should be considered in the differential diagnosis of a child presenting with unexplained illness, or inexplicable signs and symptoms, and in children who are brought in moribund or suffer sudden unexplained death. Blood for electrolytes, blood gases and toxicology, and urine specimens for toxicology, should be taken and a history should be sought of any source of drugs or medicines, both prescribed or bought over the counter.

Smothering
Sudden infant death syndrome (SIDS) is a label given where a previously healthy child dies suddenly and unexpectedly. A proportion (10–20%) of these babies is now thought to have been smothered with no charac-

teristic clinical signs or autopsy findings. Warning features of this sort of abuse are:

- previous apneas or near miss cot deaths occasionally leading to anoxic brain damage
- previous unexplained disorders affecting the child or siblings
- previous sudden infant deaths in the family
- a parent who predicted the child's death
- a parent who has an unusual response/reaction to the episode

Miscellaneous

In children with chronic medical conditions, failure to administer prescribed treatment can be a form of abuse. Other parental behavior causes concern, such as over-anxious parents and those who shop their child around several doctors for more and more medical opinions.

27.4 History and examination of children with suspected abuse

The 'whole child' should be assessed and full history and examination must be carried out on all children who are thought to have been abused (*Box 27.7*).

27.4.1 Examination

The examination must assess the whole child. It includes:
- height, weight, head circumference and nutrition
- demeanor and behavior and interaction of child
- developmental assessment, including language and social skills
- general appearance – cleanliness, infestation, appropriate clothing

---

Box 27.7 History in suspected child abuse

- History of current injury/complaint including when, where and how it happened and any first aid given
- Past medical history, including all ED attendances and hospital admissions
- Family history and social history, including details of people living in the household, parental mental illness, substance and alcohol abuse, domestic violence, previous cohabitees etc., previous episode of abuse or sexual offences within the family
- Developmental history, including progress at school if appropriate
- Behavioral history, including friendships, temper tantrums etc.
- Systemic review, including appetite, urinary and bowel problems

---

- general examination, including ears, nose, throat, eyes, respiratory system, cardiovascular system, abdomen, central nervous system
- all injuries, both reported and unreported, which should be measured, charted and described and if possible photographed
- observation of behavior of carers and their interaction with the child

Height and weight

Children who are thought to have been abused may also be suffering from non-organic failure to thrive. All assessments should include accurate height, weight and head circumference. These should be recorded on centile charts and ideally related to the parental heights to judge whether the child's growth is within normal limits. Sequential measurements are useful to follow the child's growth before and after any intervention.

Ear examination

The ears should be carefully and extensively examined. Bruising behind the ears can either be due to a direct blow to the ears, or due to bleeding associated with a basal fracture of the skull. Accidental bruising of and behind the pinna is quite uncommon and usually has a specific history. It is rarely if ever bilateral. Unilateral or bilateral bruising of the pinna occurs frequently with other injuries in non-accidental injury. It can be caused by a blow, when it often extends from the cheek, in or across the pinna and on to the mastoid, and even on to the scalp behind the ear. Bruising on both sides of the rim of the pinna can be caused by pinching. In addition, the ear drum can be ruptured in a child who has had a severe, blunt blow to the ear.

Eye examination

The eyes can show signs of both recent and previous non-accidental injury. A thorough examination should always be undertaken. Further examination outside the expertise of the emergency pediatrician should be carried out by an ophthalmologist, who can perform indirect ophthalmoscopy and get a better view of the anterior section of the fundus, the site of many non-accidental fundal hemorrhages. The eyes can demonstrate signs that could be due to abuse (*Box 27.8*).

Permanent damage to vision can be a result of child abuse. Occasionally sexually transmitted diseases manifest with ocular signs such as purulent gonococcal conjunctivitis or the intraocular inflammation of syphilis.

Box 27.8 Eye signs associated with child abuse

- Periorbital hematoma: black eye
- Conjunctival or subconjunctival hemorrhage
- Anterior segment injury – hyphema
- Intraocular hemorrhages – retinal, preretinal, subretinal and hyaloid hemorrhage, often associated with shaken baby syndrome
- Retinal detachment – acutely from a hemorrhage or chronically from scarring
- Papilloedema and occasionally late optic atrophy
- Squint, acutely from a raised intracranial pressure and chronically from poor vision

---

27.5 Investigation

27.5.1 Screens for 'easy bruising'

Any child who is assessed for bruising should have a full blood count (hemoglobin, white cell and platelet counts) and examination of a film by a hematologist, and clotting screen (prothrombin time, activated partial thromboplastin time, thrombin time and fibrinogen), performed to exclude most medical causes for 'easy bruising'. Just occasionally, children with bruises from idiopathic thrombocytopenic purpura or leukemia are initially thought to have been abused. If a suspicion of a bruising problem remains, then further investigations such as platelet aggregation studies, factor assays, the bleeding time and Von Willebrand screen should be done after advice from a hematologist.

27.5.2 Skeletal survey

A proper skeletal survey (not a babygram) should be carried out on all children who are being assessed who:
- are physically abused children under 3 years, and especially infants
- are presented with a fracture thought to be due to abuse
- are older children with severe soft tissue injury
- have unexplained signs or symptoms, particularly neurological problems
- suffer sudden unexplained death

A follow up skeletal survey 10–14 days later can be very useful and show healing fractures not obvious in the initial survey. The differential diagnosis of unexplained bony injury includes normal variant, osteogenesis imperfecta, copper deficiency, osteomyelitis, or osteoporosis, for example associated with cerebral palsy and rickets. Osteogenesis imperfecta is rare but must be considered. It can occur with a spectrum of severity, but the mild type IVA, accounting for approximately 5% of all cases, is a particularly difficult diagnosis as it is associated with normal teeth and sclera.

27.5.3 Photography

Injuries should be photographed wherever possible, to document the findings, which will change over time, for case discussion between colleagues and for teaching. This is in addition to, not instead of the injury chart. A ruler included in the photograph, adjacent to an injury, helps to give an idea of its true size. Any photograph taken for medicolegal purposes must have a chain of evidence, with verification of the identity of the child and documentation of who took the photograph and when. Ideally the photograph should be taken by a police photographer or the official hospital medical photographer. Consent should be obtained for photographs from someone with parental responsibility and from the child themselves if appropriate.

27.6 Child Protection Register check

During the investigation of an incident, the local Child Protection Surveillance system should be checked for previous episodes of child abuse in the family. In the UK, Child Protection Registers are kept of all children who have been abused and who are still thought to be at risk.

27.7 Differential diagnoses

There are many medical conditions that can masquerade as child abuse in all its forms (*Box 27.9*). This list is by no means exhaustive.

27.8 The ED pediatrician's role

The suspicion of child abuse is usually raised by a combination of factors from both the history and the examination. ED nursing and medical staff must be alert to the possibility of non-accidental injury and know how to manage any case that presents. They should progress logically through history, examination, provisional diagnosis and the decision-making as in any other case.

All clinical records must be contemporaneous, dated and signed. They may be needed as evidence in a Court of Law. They should include records of conversations with parents or caretakers and it is wise to have another member of staff present at all times when dealing with the case.

Box 27.9 Differential diagnoses of child abuse

- **Bruising**
  - idiopathic thrombocytopenic purpura
  - Henoch–Schönlein purpura
  - erythema nodosum
  - leukemia
  - folk medicines – coining, cupping
  - hemangioma
  - Mongolian blue spot
  - clotting disorders such as hemophilia
- **Fractures/bony changes**
  - osteogenesis imperfecta
  - fractures in porotic bones, e.g. of myelomeningocoele
  - congenital syphilis
  - scurvy
  - copper deficiency
  - rickets
- **Burns and scalds**
  - impetigo
  - other staphylococcal skin infections
- **Failure to thrive**
  - cystic fibrosis
  - coeliac disease
- **Anogenital signs**
  - lichen sclerosus et atrophicus
  - perianal and vulval moniliasis
  - scratching from threadworms

Each unit has its own guidelines to help the emergency pediatrician decide when to refer the case to a pediatrician with special interest and expertise in child protection. The doctor is often faced with the difficult task of what and how to tell the parents at this stage. To impart suspicions that might not be supported by a more experienced pediatrician may lose the confidence and cooperation of the parents. It is important not to lie. If challenged, it is right to be honest and admit that the signs are not consistent in your opinion and that you are seeking the advice of a more senior doctor. It can be difficult to know when to alert the social services and police. A knowledge of emergency legislation such as the Emergency Protection Order in the UK is necessary, to ensure the child's safety when the parents withdraw their cooperation. The emergency pediatrician can have an important role in writing reports and statements and attending the Case Conference and the Court to give evidence of details of the initial presentation of the child.

It is important to detect abuse if it is present, to protect the child and support the family and prevent further abuse. However, it is also important not to overinvestigate as a multi-agency investigation of an accidental injury is traumatic for the family. It is right to be cautious but not afraid to seek senior advice if in doubt.

In summary, it is the role of the emergency pediatrician to:
1. be alert to the possibility of child abuse
2. take a good history
3. do a full medical examination
4. chart and photograph any lesions
5. document the findings and date and sign all records, including the body charts
6. do bleeding and clotting screens
7. order a skeletal survey when appropriate
8. undertake any other investigations indicated by the examination
9. check any local Child Protection Register
10. consider whether there are any other children at risk in the family
11. report the case to the local authority and work with social workers and police to protect the child and investigate the case
12. write reports or statements and appear in Court if necessary.

References

1. Meadow, S.R. (1997) *ABC of Child Abuse*. London: BMJ Publishing Group.
2. Ludwig, S. (2000) *Child Abuse. Pediatric Emergency Medicine*. Philadelphia, PA: Lippincott Williams and Wilkins, pp. 1669–1704.
3. Knight, B. (1996) *Forensic Pathology*. London: Arnold Publishing, pp. 143–144.
4. Muram, D. (1989) Child sexual abuse: relationship between sexual acts and genital findings. *Child Abuse Neglect* **13**: 211–216.

Further reading

Caffey, J. (1946) Multiple fractures of the long bones of infants suffering from chronic subdural hematoma. *Am. J. Roentol.* **56**: 163–173.
Hobbs, C.J., Hanks, H.G.I., Wynne, J.M. (1999) *Child Abuse and Neglect. A Clinicians Handbook*. London: Churchill Livingstone.
Kempe, C.H., Silverman, F.N., Steel, B.F., Droegmuller, W., Silver, H.K. (1962) The battered child syndrome. *J. Am. Med. Ass.* **181**: 17–24.
Kleinman, P.K. (1998) *Diagnostic Imaging of Child Abuse*. Missouri: Mosby.

Chapter 28

Animal bites and stings

Lisa M. Evered

Contents

28.1 Introduction

Animal bites, which range from minor to potentially life or limb threatening, are a common cause of visits to the Emergency Department. Caring for the bitten child requires an understanding of the types and locations of injuries, and of the potential outcomes. This chapter addresses the Emergency Department management of animal bites, including some controversial aspects of care.

28.2 Statistics

It is estimated that one half of all North Americans will be bitten by an animal or another human being in their lifetimes. Only one sixth to a quarter of bites are reported and these include mainly those which have become infected or which have not healed and those occurring during crimes or unprovoked attacks. Dog bites occur with an estimated frequency of 1–3 million per year in the USA, and account for approximately 1% of visits to the ED. Most victims are children falling in the age range of 5–14 years old.

Animal bites have a significant impact on health. The annual mortality from dog bites in the years between 1979–1988 was found to be 6.7 per 100 million people, with pit bull terriers accounting for 47% and German shepherds for 11%. Death is usually from exsanguination.

The forces generated by the jaws of a dog can vary from 150 pounds per square inch (psi) in untrained German shepherds, to 2000 psi in K-9 rottweilers. This is enough to tear through sheet metal.

28.3 Types and locations of bites

For children under 5 years old, 88% of bites are to the head, a pattern that reflects both the height and the defensive behaviors of the victim (*Table 28.1*).

It is crucial to rule out abuse whenever a human bite is encountered in a child. It has been demonstrated that the distance between the canine teeth of primary teeth is less than 3 cm, which allows discrimination from those inflicted by another child vs an adult if a mark has been left.

There are three categories of human bites, outlined in *Box 28.1*.

Rats are the perpetrators in about 2% of animal bites, with an infection rate of approximately 2%. Skunks, raccoons, bats, foxes, woodchucks, livestock, ferrets, other rodents (including hamsters), lagomorphs, alligators, camels, cougars, wolves, primates and squirrels are all animals that account for a minor percentage of animal bites.

Table 28.1 Sites of bites

Cause of bite	Total bites (%)	Common sites
Dog bites	80–90	54–85% extremities, esp. upper 15–27% head and neck 10% trunk
Cat bites	5–15	60–67% upper extremities 15–20% head and neck 10–13% lower extremities <5% trunk
Human bites	3.6–23	Male: especially hand, arm, shoulder Female: breast, genitalia, leg, arm
Rat bites	2	

Box 28.1 Bite human categories

Occlusional/simple
- Teeth sunk into skin, anywhere other than hand
- No more dangerous than any other laceration

Occlusional bites to the hand
- Higher risk for infection and complication

Clenched fist injuries – 'fight bite'
- Most serious due to joint involvement and pathogens involved
- 3–8 mm puncture or laceration of skin overlying the third metacarpophalangeal joint or back of hand
- Should be evaluated by a hand surgeon

28.4 Injuries and outcomes

Injuries that must be considered when evaluating a child that has been bitten include injuries that compromise airway and breathing, vascular and/or nerve damage, soft tissue injuries, fractures, and injuries to tendons or joints. Particularly concerning are injuries to eyes, dural tears with or without intracranial hemorrhage and, of course, amputations.

Potential sequele that may not be initially considered include those listed in *Box 28.2*.

28.5 Infection

As one of the more common potential complications of a bite, infections warrant further discussion.

> **Box 28.2** Sequelae to animal bites
>
> - Infection
> - Blood transfusion
> - Compartment syndrome
> - Post-traumatic stress disorder
> - Death

28.5.1 Risk factors

Box 28.3 outlines the types of risk factors for bite infections. Of note is that puncture wounds account for up to 40% of animal bite infections, and have a two-fold increased risk compared with lacerations. This is partly due to the fact that they are difficult to clean.

28.5.2 Infection rates

The rates of infection of animal bites vary significantly, dog bites being the lowest at 2–20%, and cat bites being high, with rates ranging from 30–80%. Human bites fall in the middle, infecting 10–50% of the time. Of interest, in the pre-antibiotic era, 33% of victims seen more than 1 hour after injury required amputation of the affected part because of severe infection.

> **Box 28.3** Risk factors for bite infection
>
> **Species of animal:** Cat, human, pig, possibly primate
> **Location:** Hand, foot, over major joint, scalp or face of infant
> **Wound type:** Puncture wounds, crush injuries, contaminated wound, treatment delay > 12 h
> **Patient characteristics:** Immunosuppression, corticosteroids, asplenia, diabetes mellitus, vascular disease

28.5.3 Infecting pathogens

An animal bite is a polymicrobial process, commonly a mix of aerobic and anerobic pathogens. In one study, a median of five bacterial isolates were isolated per culture (range, 0–16). One of the most common bacteria is *Pasteurella multocida*, which has been found in 77% of cat bites and 13% of dog bites. *Capnocytophaga canimorsus* can cause severe infection in immunocompromised bite victims. *Bartonella henselae* is the usual cause of cat-scratch disease. *Acinetobacter* has a reported association with hamster bites. *Eikenella corrodens* is the most significant pathogen that arises in human bites.

With the rising popularity of reptiles as pets, the ED must be aware of the association with unusual subtypes of *Salmonella*, with carriage rates in iguanas ranging from 36–77%.

Certain infections develop in bites by non-domesticated animals. *Streptobacillus moniliformis* is the infecting agent in rat-bite fever, and bites by rabbits and squirrels can result in tularemia, in which the causative agent is *Francisella tularensis*.

Some rare but deadly infections, such as rabies, can occur in victims of bites: 2–8 weeks after sustaining a bite from a rabid animal, there is a 20% chance of contracting rabies, with 100% mortality if the patient is infected. The virus occurs in every continent except Australia and Antarctica. Some areas such as the UK and Scandinavia have negligible or very low risk, but others, such as parts of Asia and Africa and Latin America, have a high risk. The most common animal reservoirs in the USA are skunks, raccoons, foxes and especially bats. The disease presents in humans with a headache and fever followed by spasms, hydrophobia and hallucinations, paralysis and death usually from respiratory paralysis. The management will be addressed later in the chapter.

Wound bacterial counts decrease over time (up to 96 hours) in wounds that are left open, which is why bites that are at high risk for infection are not to be sutured.

28.6 **The bitten child**

28.6.1 ABCs

The first aspect to approaching any pediatric patient is resuscitation of life and limb. Particularly important considerations in bite victims are injuries to the airway, any compromise of breathing (as may occur in anaphylaxis if the patient has a severe allergy to the animal), and circulatory compromise by anaphylaxis or hemorrhagic shock. It is also critical to address bite wounds that may have potentially endangered perfusion to a limb.

28.6.2 History

Taking a complete history of the bite involves a complete description of the bite (what was bitten, where is the bite, when did it happen, how did the bite occur, why was the child bitten, in which country the bite took place if the child was on holiday?). Information on the animal must also be collected, if possible, including who the owner is, the immunization status of the animal, how the animal was behaving, and the circumstances surrounding the attack. Risk factors for infection should be elucidated, bearing in mind rabies and tetanus in particular.

Any symptoms that occur must be noted, particularly pain, paraesthesia, weakness, and loss of function of any limb. The history should also include any treatment that was given prior to arrival in the ED, including irrigation. As with all patients, a complete medical history should be obtained, focusing on bleeding disorders, immunosuppression by medication or disease, asplenia, diabetes, and arterial or venous disease. Any prior injuries, pre-existing disability or deficits, or tendency to form keloids should be noted. Allergies, particularly to anesthetics, analgesics or antibiotics, the tetanus immune status and a history of medication, particularly anticoagulant use, are all important. A psychosocial history can be relevant, with emphasis on handedness, and vocation.

It is important to stress that all open wounds over the knuckles should be considered human bite wounds unless otherwise confirmed. Patients are often not forthcoming with information about 'fight bites', for various reasons. The danger of misdiagnosing this limb-threatening injury must be stressed.

28.6.3 Physical examination

Ensure the vital signs are stable, as outlined above. The wound is evaluated for entrance and exit sites, laceration length and depth, and any potential crush injury. Nerve and tendon function must be assessed, and vascular integrity be established. Underlying joints and bones need to be examined for penetration, and the wound should be searched for any foreign bodies or contamination. Exploration is key, when anatomically feasible. To avoid missing significant joint involvement, 'fight bites' must be examined in the position the injury occurred, usually a clenched fist. The wounds should be photographed or diagrammed.

28.6.4 Investigation

If the wound is clinically infected, it should be cultured for aerobic and anerobic microbes. X-ray should be made of all crush injuries, suspected fractures, and in order to locate any potential foreign bodies. Joint injection, and vascular imaging can be considered if indicated.

28.6.5 Management

Cleaning
Irrigation is the most valuable aspect of caring for bite wounds. Saline or copious water irrigation are adequate. Povidone–iodine solution may decrease the rate of rabies but can damage tissue. Chlorhexidine, hydrogen peroxide, benzalkonium chloride and detergent-containing products cause tissue damage and are possibly less effective antimicrobials than saline.

Irrigation with 50–100 ml cm^{-1} of wound should be carried out with a 20 ml syringe and 18 G needle or a port device spiked into an i.v. bag of saline, along the direction of the wound; 5–8 psi pressure is ideal to give adequate irrigation without tissue damage. Splash-back of infected material on to the health worker should be prevented.

Devitalized or crushed tissue and any foreign material should be removed, but no aggressive probing and coring is recommended, nor is debridement of puncture wounds. Excessive debridement can lead to a defect that cannot be closed, which results in poor cosmesis.

Closing the wound

Most lacerations can be closed safely within 8–12 hours of wounding. Some wounds may be safely closed up to 24 hours after injury with appropriate cleansing, debridement and prophylactic antibiotics (as indicated).

Primary closure may be indicated in bites to the face and head, and low-risk bite wounds. It should be avoided in deep puncture wounds, clinically infected wounds, contaminated injuries and bites to the hand. Wounds examined more than 24 hours after the bite occurred should not be sutured.

If the wound is not closed immediately, delayed primary closure is indicated for all clinically uninfected high risk wounds 72 hours after initial treatment.

Certain wounds should be allowed to close by secondary intention, including: deep puncture wounds, wounds examined more than 24 hours after injury, clinically infected wounds, and some hand bites.

All significant wounds should be immobilized in a position of function, and kept elevated.

28.6.6 Prophylaxis: antibiotics, vaccines, and immunoglobulins

Antibiotics

There is some controversy around which patients should receive antibiotic prophylaxis. Although each bite must be evaluated on a case-by-case basis, there are certain 'rules of thumb'. General indications for antibiotic use are noted in *Box 28.4*.

When deciding which antibiotic to use in a patient with indications for prophylaxis, remember the polymicrobial nature of bite wounds (*Table 28.2*).

> **Box 28.4** Indications for antibiotics
>
> **Antibiotics indicated**
> - Involvement of joints, tendons or bones
> - Hand or lower extremity bites
> - Devitalized tissue or significant contamination
> - Deep puncture wounds
> - Moderate or severe wounds
> - Impaired host immune response
> - Impaired host circulation (e.g. diabetes)
>
> **Antibiotics not indicated**
> - Face bites (that do not require closure)
> - Superficial injuries (e.g. abrasions)
> - Types of bites with a low infection rate (see *Box 28.3*)
> - Shallow puncture wounds

The recommendation for dog, cat and human bites is 3–5 days' treatment with amoxycillin/clavulanic acid. Clindamycin with trimethoprim/sulphamethoxazole may be used if the patient is allergic to penicillin. These recommendations are empirical, as there are no definitive studies comparing amoxycillin-clavulanic acid with penicillin or first-generation cephalosporins in mammalian or human bites.

The most important thing to remember about antibiotic use in animal bites is that it is not a substitute for proper local wound care!

Vaccines and immunoglobulins

Rabies: In wounds from a potentially rabid animal, prompt, thorough wound irrigation with soap or iodine solution reduces the development of rabies by up to 90%, and the rabies vaccine/immunoglobulin combination is virtually 100% effective. There are clear guidelines on when to use these, as outlined in *Box 28.5*. $20 \, IU \, kg^{-1}$ of human rabies immune globulin (HRIG) is given on day 0. As much HRIG as practically feasible should be infiltrated locally, and the rest given intramuscularly. HRIG is contraindicated if the patient has been previously vaccinated. There are three vaccines available, all equally effective: human diploid cell vaccine (HDCV), rabies vaccine adsorbed (RVA) or purified chick embryo cell culture (PCEC). The vaccine should be given intramuscularly on days 0, 3, 7, 14 and 28, unless the patient had been previously vaccinated (in which case, the dose would be given only on days 0 and 3). HDCV also may be given intradermally.

Reactions to the vaccine include the local reactions of pain and redness and systemic reactions of headache, fever, muscle aches, vomiting and

Table 28.2 Antibiotic use in animal bites

Antibiotic	Organisms covered	Organisms not covered
Amoxycillin/ clavulanic acid	*Staphylococcus aureus, Escherichia corrodens,* anaerobes, *Pasteurella multocida,* and *Captocytophaga canimorsus*	*Pseudomonas aeruginosa*
Cefuroxime	*S. aureus,* most *E. corrodens,* anaerobes, and *P. multocida*	*P. aeruginosa*
Ceftriaxone	*S. aureus, E. corrodens,* most anaerobes, *P. multocida, C. canimorsus* and *P. aeruginosa*	
Penicillin	*P. multocida,* and also covers *E. corrodens* (produces β-lactamase), *C. canimorsus*	poor coverage against *S. aureus*
Cephalexin	*S. aureus*	*P. multocida, E. corrodens, P. aeruginosa*
Dicloxacillin	*S. aureus*	*P. multocida, P. aeruginosa*
Trimethoprim/ sulphamethoxazole	*E. corrodens, P. multocida*	*C. canimorsus*
Clindamycin	*C. canimorsus*	*E. corrodens*

urticarial rashes. Anaphylaxis has also been reported. The three-dose course of human diploid cell vaccine should be offered routinely to those working with imported animals.

Tetanus: As with all unclean wounds, tetanus must be considered and prophylaxis given when indicated (see Chapter 29).

28.6.7 Follow up

The patient should be seen again by a healthcare professional if there is any concern or risk of infection, the timing dependent on each individ-

---

Box 28.5 Rabies vaccination guidelines

Dog/cat bite
- If healthy, observe animal for 10 days and give HRIG and vaccine to the patient only if signs of rabies develop in the animal
- If suspected rabid animal, give HRIG and vaccinate

Skunk, raccoon, bat, fox, woodchucks
- Give HRIG and vaccine unless animal proven to be negative or geographic area is free of rabies
- Consider strongly even if only exposed to a bat

Livestock, ferrets, rodents, lagomorphs
- Consider individually
- Rarely requires prophylaxis

Abbreviation: HRIG, human rabies immune globulin

---

ual case. In any case, discharged patients should be sent home with good instructions for wound care and signs of infection. Healthcare professionals should also take this opportunity to counsel on prevention, to help reduce the chances of future bites.

28.7 When to admit to hospital

Rarely, animal bites lead to complications that necessitate hospitalization. Some indications are listed in *Box 28.6*.

28.8 Conclusions

To summarize: dog bites present to the ED most frequently, while cat bites have a higher rate of infection. The chief management issues include assessing for underlying injury, irrigation with copious normal saline, suturing low-risk bites and providing prophylaxis for high-risk bites. Last but not least, do not forget the preventables (rabies and tetanus).

28.9 Other bites and stings

Various other bites and stings occur in various parts of the world. The common types of problems in each ED depend on the local fauna, and each department will have appropriate local guidelines. An example of a local guideline is that for managing bites from the major venomous brown, tiger, copperhead and red-bellied snakes of Victoria, Australia (*Figure 28.1*). Other examples from around the world are listed below in *Table 28.3*.

Box 28.6 Indications for admission to hospital

- Systemic manifestations of infection (fever, chills)
- Severe cellulitis
- Injuries requiring reconstructive surgery
- Significant bites to the hand
- Penetration of a joint, nerve, bone, tendon, or central nervous system
- Infection refractory to oral or outpatient therapy
- Likelihood for non-compliance
- Presence of peripheral vascular disease
- Immunocompromised or diabetes mellitus

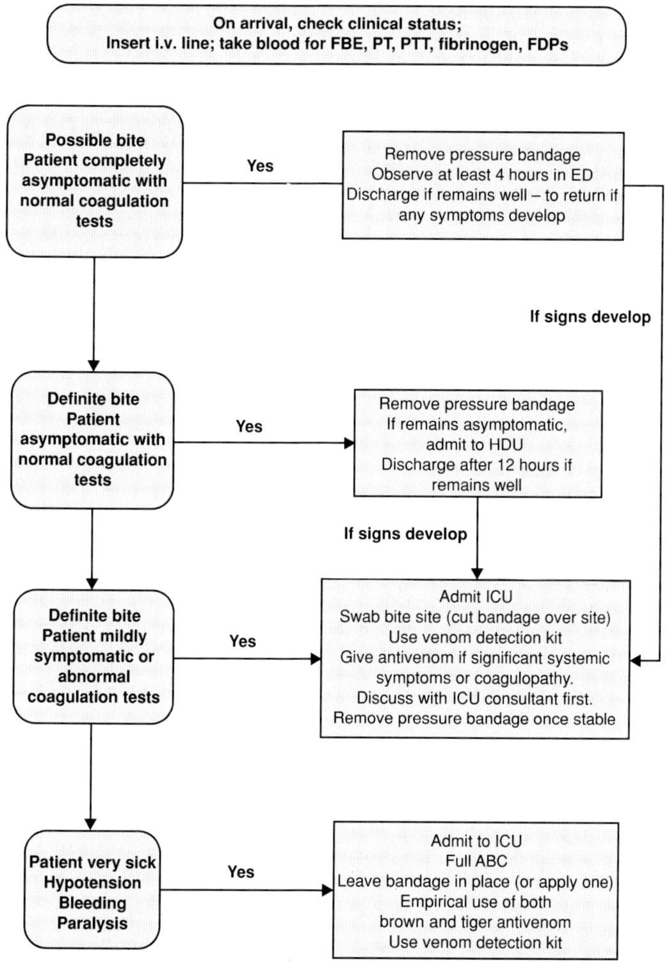

Figure 28.1 Guidelines for management of snake bites in Victoria, Australia. Abbreviations: FBE, full blood evaluation; FDP, fibrin degradation products; HDU, high dependency unit; ICU, intensive care unit; PT, prothrombin time; PTT, partial thromboplastin time

Table 28.3 Various bites and stings

Animal	Clinical characteristics	Usual treatment
Snakes – rattlesnakes (Crotalidae)	*Local:* stinging, progressive edema, subcutaneous hemorrhage *Systemic:* paraesthesias, fasciculations, progressive paralysis	Remove constrictive clothing, immobilize extremity, no tourniquet, Antivenom as indicated i.v. fluids. ID snake. Tetanus prophylaxis as indicated. Antibiotic prophylaxis as indicated
Scorpions (Centruroides)	Pain, local hyperaesthesia ± CNS stimulation, respiratory distress, dysrhythmias	Cold compresses + local anesthetic for mild. Monitor for systemic symptoms
Spiders		
Brown recluse (*Loxosceles reclusa*)	Dermonecrotic: local infarction/necrosis ± autoimmune reaction; edema, target lesion or vesicles, pain	Local potent corticosteroid ointment t.i.d. for mild; dapsone for severe Consider debridement, antibiotics, hyperbaric O_2
Black widow (*Latrodectus mactans*)	Neurotoxic: pain radiating up extremity, cramps, paralysis, hypertension	Diazepam + analgesics for mild. Antivenin (skin test first) for painful muscle contraction or hypertension
Red back spider (*Latrodectus hasseltii*) (Australia)	*Local:* pain, erythema, edema *Systemic:* gradual onset nausea, vomiting, hypertension, muscle weakness	Analgesic with generalized symptoms, give antivenom after premedication with norepinephrine (noradrenaline)
Bees (UK)	*Local:* pain, swelling, erythema *Systemic:* occasionally cause anaphylaxis. The swarm may settle on the child causing widespread stings. African bees are more	Symptomatic treatment only unless anaphylaxis Remove the sting

Wasps (UK)	aggressive than UK ones and are spreading across Europe and South America *Local*: pain, swelling, erythema *Systemic*: occasionally cause anaphylaxis. Causes airway problems if sting is in the mouth or throat	Symptomatic treatment only unless anaphylaxis
Echinodermata (sea urchins, starfish, sea cucumbers)	*Local*: burning pain, swelling, erythema *Systemic*: weakness, syncope, paraesthesias/paralysis	Immerse in hot (45°C) water; Remove pincers and easily removable spines Consider antibiotics as needed
Blue-ringed octopus (*Hapalochlaena maculosa*) (Australia)	Rapid onset of paralysis	Pressure and immobilization for affected limb. There is no antivenom. Admit to ICU and ventilate if necessary
Elasmobranch (stingrays)	*Local*: ragged laceration with pain/edema *Systemic*: cramps, vomiting, diarrhoea, weakness, diaphoresis, dysrhythmias, hypotension, rarely death	Irrigate wound, immerse in hot water, remove foreign material Consider antibiotics Supportive care
Scorpaenidae (lionfish, stonefish, scorpion fish)	*Local*: ischemia/cyanosis/necrosis, pain, edema, paraesthesias *Systemic*: gastrointestinal, seizures, weakness, delirium, dysrhythmias, heart failure, hyper/hypotension, rarely death	Immerse in hot water; remove foreign material Consider antibiotics Supportive care

Key references

Fleischer, *et al.* (2000) *Textbook of Pediatric Emergency Medicine*, 4th edn. : Lippincott Williams & Wilkins, Chapter 91.

Talan, D.A. (1999) Bacteriologic analysis of infected dog and cat bites. Emergency Medicine Animal Bite Study Group. *N. Engl. J. Med.* **340**: 85–92.

Further reading

Griego, R. *et al.* (1995) Dog, cat and human bites: a review. *J. Am. Acad. Dermatol.* **33**: 1019–1029.

Knapp, J.F. (1999) Updates in wound management for the pediatrician. *Pediatr. Clinics N. Am.* **46**: 1201–1213.

Chapter 29

Immunization

Patricia O. Brennan

Contents

Immunization is one of the most cost-effective and safest interventions in medicine. Since Edward Jenner demonstrated that cowpox gave protection from smallpox 200 years ago, immunization has made an enormous impact on the incidence of many infections around the world. From the 19th century until 1946 in the UK, vaccination of children was enforceable. Immunizations are now voluntary and parental permission is needed to immunize a child according to current schedules. The 1996 Government Guide to immunization states that:

> It is every child's right to be protected against infectious diseases. No child should be denied immunization without serious thought as to the consequences, both for the child and the community.

29.1 Types of immunity

Immunity can either be passive or active. *Passive immunity* results from injection of human normal immunoglobulin from donors who are negative to hepatitis B surface antigen (HbsAg) and to antibodies to human immunodeficiency viruses types 1 and 2 (HIV) and hepatitis C. It is heat treated to kill viruses and has antibodies against infectious agents that are currently prevalent in the general population. Specific immunoglobulins are available for tetanus, hepatitis B, rabies and varicella-zoster. These are prepared from the pooled plasma of donors who have a high titre of antibody following infection or immunization.

Active immunity results from inactivated or attenuated organisms or their products. They work by inducing cell-mediated immunity and serum antibodies (IgM and IgG).

29.2 Types of vaccine

There are four main types of vaccine available. These are shown in *Box 29.1*.

Following a course of immunization (from one or more doses depending on the infection), the antibody or antitoxin remains high for some time, usually from months to years. It then declines, but a challenge from further immunization or infection usually causes a rapid rise.

Each country has its own routine immunization schedule for children. This is updated in line with the latest research and the prevalent infections. The current UK schedule is shown in *Table 29.1*.

A recent schedule for USA children, also includes the following:

Box 29.1 Types of vaccine

Inactivated organisms against
- pertussis
- typhoid
- poliomyelitis (OPV)

Live attenuated organisms against
- mumps
- measles
- rubella
- poliomyelitis (IPV)
- BCG

Toxoids
- tetanus
- diphtheria

Other immunizing components
- influenza
- pneumococcus

Table 29.1 The current UK childhood immunization schedule

Vaccine	Timing	Age
Diphtheria/tetanus/pertussis	1st dose	2 months
Hemophilus influenzae type b (Hib)	2nd dose	3 months
Poliomyelitis	3rd dose	4 months
Meningococcus C		
Measles/mumps/rubella		12–15 months
Diphtheria/tetanus		3–5 years
Poliomyelitis		
Measles/mumps/rubella		
BCG		10–14 years
Tetanus/low-dose diphtheria		13–18 years
Poliomyelitis		

- 3 doses of hepatitis B vaccine at birth or 1 month, 2 months and 6 months
- varicella vaccine at 15–18 months and again at 14–16 years if still susceptible
- a second dose of measles, mumps and rubella vaccine at 11–12 years

There are few absolute contraindications to immunization. These include:
- an acute illness – postpone immunization
- *severe* local or general reaction
- live vaccines in pregnancy or in patients who are immunosuppressed from chemotherapy, radiotherapy, following bone marrow transplant, steroids or for any other reason

Children who are positive for HIV will need individual advice. The most relevant immunizations in the ED are tetanus, hepatitis B and rabies.

29.3 Tetanus immunization

Clostridium tetani is present in soil and will never be eradicated. It can contaminate and grow anerobically even in very small wounds. It produces toxins and in 4–21 days after contamination can cause muscle rigidity and severe, very painful spasms (tetanus). It remains common in some areas of Africa and Asia from contamination of the neonate's umbilical stump. Tetanus is becoming rare in countries with an effective infant immunization programme.

A primary course of tetanus immunization consists of three doses of adsorbed tetanus toxoid given by deep subcutaneous or intramuscular injection at monthly intervals, starting at 2 months of age. Reinforcing doses are given at age 3–5 years and a further dose 10 years later. Older unimmunized children should have the same primary course of three doses at monthly intervals together with two reinforcing doses at 10-yearly intervals. For adults who have had all five doses, further doses are not recommended except at the time of tetanus prone wounds, as there is an increased risk of severe local reactions.

If a child presents with an open wound, tetanus prophylaxis should consist of the following steps.
1. Thoroughly cleanse and irrigate the wound
2. Assess the risk of tetanus contamination:
   - low risk – wound < 6 hours old
   - high risk – wound > 6 hours old, infected or sustained in high-risk environment such as a stable
3. Assess current tetanus status of patient and treat accordingly (*Table 29.2*)

Adverse reactions to tetanus immunization are listed in *Box 29.2*.

29.4 Hepatitis B immunization

Hepatitis is a viral infection acquired parenterally or sexually. Staff working in an ED are particularly at risk as a result of contact with bodily

Table 29.2 Tetanus prophylaxis in wounds

Immunization status	Type of wound	Treatment
No immunization	Low risk	Start active immunization programme
	High risk	Tetanus specific immunoglobulin plus start active immunization programme
3 or more doses within 5 years	Low risk	No treatment needed
	High risk	No treatment needed
3 or more doses within last 5–10 years	Low risk	No treatment needed
	High risk	Reinforcing dose of tetanus toxoid

Box 29.2 Adverse reactions to tetanus immunization

Local
- redness, pain, swelling around injection site

General
- pyrexia, headache, myalgia
- urticaria and anaphylaxis
- rarely peripheral neuropathy

fluids and from needlestick injuries and bites. Patients present following accidental needlestick injuries, particularly when children play with syringes and needles discarded by drug misusers (see also later section in this chapter).

Hepatitis B itself can range from a subclinical illness through a generalised illness with anorexia, nausea, vomiting and arthralgia to a fulminating hepatic necrosis; 2–10% of infected adults become carriers, but carrier rate is higher in infected children and reaches 90% of those infected perinatally.

The vaccine available for active immunization contains HbsAg adsorbed on to aluminium hydroxide adjuvant. Specific hepatitis B immunoglobulin (HBIG) is available for passive immunization.

Staff should be actively immunized with three doses of hepatitis B vaccine on day 0 and 1 month and 6 months later, before starting work in the department.

Patients or unimmunized staff who sustain a high-risk wound such as a needlestick injury, after the wound has been cleansed well with soap and water, should be immunized as in *Box 29.3*.

Box 29.3 Immunization schedule against hepatitis B after high risk wound

Day 0: single dose of hepatitis B immunoglobulin and 1st dose of hepatitis B vaccine
1 month later: 2nd dose of hepatitis B vaccine
2 months later: 3rd dose of hepatitis B vaccine
1 year later: 4th dose of hepatitis B vaccine

The vaccine does have some side effects such as local pain and redness or a generalised flu-like illness with fever, arthritis and myalgia.

29.5 Rabies immunization

The rabies virus occurs in every continent except Australia and Antarctica. Some areas such as the UK and Scandinavia have negligible or very low risk but others such as parts of Asia and Africa and Latin America have a high risk. Guidelines on the recognition and management of rabies are given in Chapter 28.

29.6 Needlestick injuries

Staff in the ED are at risk of needlestick injuries and should be immunized against hepatitis B before taking up a post. A number of patients will carry blood-borne pathogens and be a real threat to staff. There is a legal duty to have safe working practices and these should be taught on an induction programme. In practice you must assume that all patients are potentially infected and take the necessary precautions:
• All staff must be immunized against hepatitis B
• Wear gloves when examining wounds (and consider goggles in a high risk patient)
• Dispose of sharps safely immediately after use
• Always dispose of needles according to local good practice guidelines

Human immune deficiency (HIV) is less easily transmitted than hepatitis, but has a high mortality. It is transmitted through inoculation of infected blood into the tissues.

Further reading

Fleisher, G.R., Ludwig, S. (2000) *Textbook of Pediatric Emergency Medicine.* Lippincott Williams and Wilkins.

Jenner, E. (1996). *Immunisation against Infectious Disease.* London: HMSO.

Chapter 30

Pain management

Patricia O. Brennan

Contents

30.1 Introduction

Many children who attend the Emergency Department (ED) whether with trauma or illness, are suffering from pain. An important role of the ED is to detect and assess the pain and manage it appropriately to minimise the distress and discomfort of treatment. Each child is different, having his or her own pain threshold and reaction to pain. This is influenced by the child's developmental stage, culture, gender, personality, family and previous experience of pain. The myth that infants and young children do not suffer pain, or forget it, has been dispelled.

Any investigation or procedure must be essential to patient management. Staff must question whether any uncomfortable investigation or procedure is really necessary in order to treat the child. Often minor conditions require neither investigation nor treatment. Aspects of any attendance can cause distress by invoking fear and anxiety. Preparation of the child by both parents and staff can minimise this. Pain increases anxiety and anxiety increases pain. It is important always to be honest with children. Thus, it is better to assure the child that he or she will be kept as comfortable as possible while getting better rather than promising complete pain relief.

Safe pain management will depend on careful selection of patient and method, good emergency pain management protocols, full documentation of drugs given and regular staff training and audit.

30.2 Assessment of pain

Young children have difficulty in communicating that they have pain, let alone in describing the site, nature or severity of the pain. Pain assessment therefore presents a unique challenge in childhood and is an essential ingredient of triage. Assessment must be repeated throughout the attendance and the patient managed accordingly. Parents are not always the best ones to define the level of the child's pain. Knowledge and experience need to be combined to provide a holistic approach to assessment, which consists of at least the key elements below:
- **inference:** experienced professionals can predict how painful certain conditions such as displaced fractures are likely to be
- **discussion:** the child or parent can often tell you how bad the pain is and how it responds to any treatment you give
- **observation:** a complaint of pain, visible distress and crying, raised pulse and respiratory rate can all be due to pain

- **self report scales:** the use and type of scale varies with the age and cognitive ability of the child, the time for education in its use and the nursing knowledge about the scale, e.g. faces scale, visual analogue scale
- **physiological scale:** observing changes such as raised pulse and respiratory rate, changes to blood pressure, crying and bronchospasm may all indicate pain

30.3 Methods of pain management

Each ED should have protocols to guide the physician to superimpose the pain score onto a pain ladder to prescribe the appropriate pain relief as soon as possible. Many methods of pain management are available to the emergency physician (*Figure 30.1*).

Children with recurrent severe pain such as those with sickle cell anemia should have a written schedule of analgesia available in the Emergency Department records. All children given analgesics should be monitored to ensure effective pain relief and to detect problems and manage them effectively.

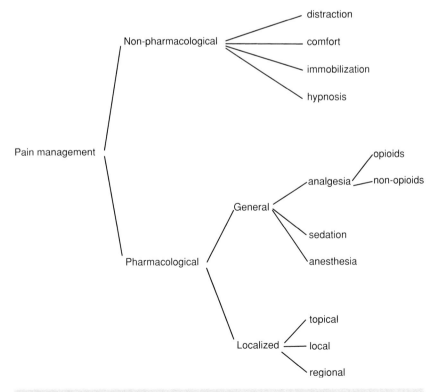

Figure 30.1 Methods of pain management.

30.4 Non-pharmacological techniques of pain management

Non-drug techniques of pain control do not actually reduce pain, but dull the child's perception of it and help the child to cope. They are commonly used in conjunction with pharmacological methods. Children are often frightened by the unknown. Attendance at an ED can be traumatic, but some of the anxiety can be dispelled if the department has the décor and facilities to put children at their ease and the staff have a caring approach to the patient. Parents need help to control their own anxiety so they can assist staff and support their child. Older children may like techniques which increase their sense of having some control, such as relaxation and breathing control.

Most non-drug techniques fall into two main groups: counter-irritation (such as stroking, heat, cold and vibration) and psychological methods. The latter, such as distraction, support, relaxation and music, are most used in the emergency situation and can be combined with even greater effect.

30.4.1 Distraction

This puts pain at the periphery of awareness and helps both the pre-school and school-aged child cope with relatively short pain and distress such as procedural pain. It works best if it involves something of interest to the child that stimulates hearing, vision, touch and movement together, preferably where the parents can become involved. Common strategies include:
• blowing bubbles
• reading pop-up books
• holding a familiar object such as a blanket or pillow for comfort
• getting the child to talk through a favourite experience/outing

30.4.2 Relaxation

This can help with procedural pain. Young children can be cuddled or rocked, while massage, aromatherapy and music and breathing control help older children. Very young infants have been shown to get some analgesia from sucking sweet-tasting solutions.

30.4.3 Restraint

Occasionally some crying or shouting has to be accepted. Some children actually find this is a distraction. If after all your efforts, a child does have to be restrained, this should be done by a person, preferably a parent.

There is no place for tying children down, or using straight jackets, although arm splints are occasionally needed to prevent a child from removing equipment such as an i.v. cannula.

30.4.4 Other techniques

Hypnosis has been effective in helping children cope with acute pain but it needs a clinician who can use the techniques and these are rarely available.

Heat and cold may reduce pain. Cold reduces bruising and swelling and slows chemical reactions and may reduce pain. Warmth relieves stiffness and muscle spasms and may particularly help mobilization after an injury.

Play can be used for distraction or relaxation but is most use as an educational tool to prepare young children for procedures.

30.5 Pharmacological techniques of pain management

Drugs can be used to reduce or control pain in several ways.

30.5.1 Analgesics

Several analgesics with various modes of action are available. In any ED it is good practice to develop guidelines for pain management with a limited number of drugs, together with their dosages, on a pain ladder. An example of an acute pain ladder is given in *Figure 30.2*.

In the ED, oral and intravenous analgesics are usually the preferred options. Intramuscular analgesia should only be used if venous access is impossible and oral analgesics are inappropriate. Children particularly dislike intramuscular injections and older children dislike rectal drugs. Adequate and regular pain relief is essential. There is no place any longer for analgesics 'p.r.n.'. Opioids are excellent in severe pain and are not addictive when used in children.

Table 30.1 shows the range of analgesic drugs, all of which have a place in the management of acute pain in children.

30.5.2 Local anesthetics

These act locally on nerves, providing complete local anesthesia. Their use may allow lower doses of analgesics but adequate analgesia must be prescribed to act as the local anesthetic wears off. There are two main

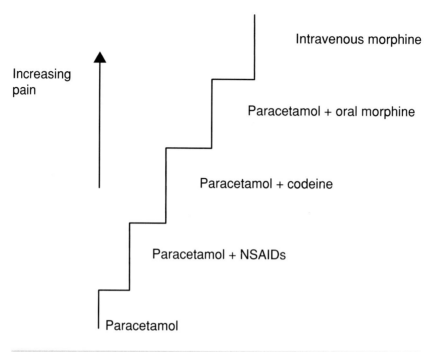

Increasing pain

Intravenous morphine

Paracetamol + oral morphine

Paracetamol + codeine

Paracetamol + NSAIDs

Paracetamol

Figure 30.2 An acute pain ladder.

groups: the amides (lignocaine/lidocaine, prilocaine and bupivacaine) and the esters (amethocaine and cocaine). Toxicity results from excessive doses with increased absorption or from inadvertent i.v. injection. It presents with circumoral numbness, dizziness and slurred speech and can progress to fits or seizures, coma, respiratory arrest and cardiac arrhythmias. Use of a vasoconstrictor such as epinephrine (adrenaline) reduces toxicity and extends duration of action but should not be used in digital or penile blocks, or in the tips of the nose or ear lobes. Various local anesthetic agents are detailed in *Table 30.2*.

Topical anesthesia
Several topical anesthetics have been used over the last 20 years. Initial ones containing cocaine were used on open wounds and acted rapidly, but led to reports of death. Newer preparations such as EMLA (Eutectic mixture of 5% lignocaine and prilocaine) and Ametop gel (amethocaine) are safe, but are only for use on unbroken skin and take up to 1 hour to be effective. Open wound preparations include LET (lidocaine/epinephrine (adrenaline)/ tetracaine) and TAC (tetracaine/epinephrine (adrenaline)/cocaine).

Local anesthetic wound infiltration
1% lignocaine is usually used at 3 mg kg^{-1}. A solution warmed to body temperature and buffered with 1 part 8.4% sodium bicarbonate to 9

Table 30.1 Analgesics for use in children

Drug	Use	Preparation	Contraindication/side effects	Comments
Paracetamol	Mild analgesic Antipyrexial	Oral, acts in 60 min Rectal acts in 90–120 min	After major surgery, liver disease	Very safe Central antipyretic effect blocking prostaglandin synthetase action in the hypothalamus Peripheral analgesic effect owing to blocking of impulse generation at bradykinin sensitive chemoreceptor Complements the effects of NSAIDs and opioids
NSAIDs (non-steroidal anti-inflammatory drugs) ibuprofen, diclofenac or naprosyn	Mild analgesic Antipyrexial Anti-inflammatory	Oral – ibuprofen, diclofenac Rectal – diclofenac	Causes GI bleeding or irritation, decrease in platelet activity and renal blood flow Hepatic dysfunction. Only under supervision to asthmatics	Acts by inhibition of prostaglandin synthesis peripherally. Complements the effect of paracetamol
Opioids Codeine phosphate	Moderate pain	Oral	Causes constipation, respiratory depression in preterm infants, nausea/ vomiting	Best used with paracetamol or NSAIDs Acts centrally and peripherally Has a ceiling for analgesic effect but not for respiratory depression

Table 30.1 Analgesics for use in children – *continued*

Drug	Use	Preparation	Contraindication/side effects	Comments
Opioids – *continued*				
Morphine	Severe pain	Oral, subcutaneous, intravenous	As for codeine plus sedation Not in raised intracranial pressure Respiratory depression Use with caution in hypovolemia and hypotension	Regular monitoring of conscious state, respiratory rate, heart rate and blood pressure is needed Naloxone and equipment for artificial ventilation must always be available when morphine is used
Entonox (nitrous oxide 50% and oxygen 50%)	Emergency situations such as application of splints or positioning for X-rays Rapidly effective analgesic with weak sedative effects	On-demand inhalation	Occasionally causes vomiting and euphoria Do not use with head or chest injuries containing air or in bowel obstruction	Must be given 50% with 50% oxygen. Good analgesia, some sedation

parts 1% lignocaine injected slowly through a small bore needle into the wound will lessen the pain of injection. Buffering cannot be used with epinephrine (adrenaline)/local anesthetic mixtures. *Table 30.2* shows a range of local anesthetics for use in children.

30.5.3 Nerve blocks

These can be useful ways of providing good pain relief in the ED. Digital nerve blocks for repair of finger or toe fractures and lacerations and femoral blocks for fractured femurs and facial blocks are particularly useful. Other blocks used in some hospitals include those listed in *Box 30.1*.

Vasoconstrictors such as epinephrine (adrenaline) must not be used with lignocaine in fingers, toes or penile blocks as arterial spasm would cause damage.

Intravenous regional blocks
Intravenous regional blocks with prilocaine or lignocaine using a double pneumatic tourniquet by a suitably trained doctor, are used by many to provide short-acting anesthesia of a limb. Equipment must be available to deal with side effects. A Bier's block to reduce a displaced fractured forearm is particularly useful in older children. The tourniquet should not be let down until at least 20 minutes after the local anesthetic has been given to minimise the risk of potentially toxic blood levels of local anesthetic.

Box 30.1 Nerve blocks

Sciatic block: analgesia to lower leg and foot for fractured tibia or fibula
Posterior tibial block: sole of the foot
Saphenous block: medial aspect of the foot
Superior peroneal block: most of the dorsum of the foot
Sural nerve block: lateral aspect of foot
Medial cutaneous branches of the posterior tibial nerve: posterior heel
Ulnar nerve block: medial third of palm, little finger and metacarpal; medial side of ring finger
Median block: whole tip and anterior half of thumb, index and middle fingers, lateral half of ring finger and lateral aspect palm
Infraorbital nerve block: upper lip and cheek from midline and tip of nose
Mental nerve: lower lip and jaw to midline
Supraorbital nerve: forehead and scalp

Table 30.2 Local anaesthetics for use in children

Drug	Use	Benefits	Disadvantages
Lignocaine	Finger blocks Wound infiltration (Topical in EMLA) Maximum dose 3 mg kg^{-1}	Fast onset and safe Less cardiotoxic in overdose Addition of epinephrine (adrenaline) prolongs action and reduces bleeding	Short action (2 h) Can be painful – see text
Prilocaine	Bier's block in older children. Topical in EMLA	Fast onset Least toxic	Occasionally toxic to young children
Bupivacaine	Epidural blocks	Long duration	Cardiotoxic
Amethocaine	Topical – Ametop Eye drops	Absorbed through skin	Irritant if left on too long
Cocaine	Nose drops	Well absorbed	Toxic
EMLA (eutectic mixture of local anesthetic)	For i.v. cannulation Put under occlusive dressing for 1 hour	Vasoconstrictor	Not for open wounds or on anus
Ametop (amethocaine gel)	In i.v. cannulation, under occlusive dressing for 45 min	Vasodilatation (can help i.v. cannulation)	Irritant if left too long
Lidocaine-epinephrine (adrenaline)-tetracaine (LET) gel	For repair of open wounds up to 4 cm in length. Takes 30–60 min to take effect	Most effective for facial lacerations (80% effective) Less so for extremity lacerations (<50%)	Though some have used it on mucosal membranes, most practitioners avoid this out of concern for tetracaine overdose
Tetracaine-adrenaline (epinephrine)-cocaine	As for LET gel, can take 30–60 min to take effect. Wounds up to 4 cm	As above	The cocaine in this preparation makes storing it logistically complicated

30.5.4 Sedatives

Conscious sedation is sometimes used in conjunction with analgesics to relieve pain and anxiety in fractious and frightened young children. It should not be used in airway obstruction and may be less effective in children taking anticonvulsants. The child should be monitored while under sedation as the drug may cause respiratory depression. Hypoxemia can be a cause or an effect of the agitation sometimes caused by the drug. Skills and equipment for airway management must be available whenever sedation is used. See *Box 30.2* for types.

Box 30.2 Types of sedatives

Chloral hydrate: a traditional, safe sedative, acting in approximately 40 minutes. It may cause an agitated response. It has no analgesic properties. It is very effective in children under age 2 years
Midazolam: An amnesic sedative with no analgesic properties and can be used intravenously, intramuscularly, orally and intranasally. It occasionally causes agitation and respiratory depression and can be reversed by flumazenil. Frequent sedation failure
Temazepam: can be used for children weighing over 30 kg
Ketamine: an analgesic and sedative that can, rarely, cause laryngospasm. It should not be used after a head injury and might cause hallucinations and nightmares. It is a rule in some countries that it should only be used by a consultant anesthetist. However, this is not a general rule and it is relatively frequently used by emergency pediatricians in North America

---

Box 30.3 illustrates a protocol for conscious sedation used in North America.

30.5.5 General anesthetics

General anesthetic remains the best option for relief of pain and anxiety in the management of some children in the ED. It must be given in a properly equipped area, with facilities for monitoring and resuscitation by a properly trained anesthetist.

30.6 Examples of pain management

30.6.1 Laceration closure

There are many ways of minimizing pain and anxiety on closure of lacerations.
• Does the wound really need closing (e.g. many tongue lacerations can be left open)?

> **Box 30.3** Regime for conscious sedation
>
> **INDICATION 1 Sedation but no need for pain control**
> *< 2 years old*: chloral hydrate 50 mg kg^{-1} up to 1000 mg orally or p.r.
> *> 2 years old*: midazolam parental solution 0.5 mg kg^{-1} up to 12 mg
> p.o. Warn parent that this only lightly sedates the child and the
> patient will still be aware and responsive
>
> **INDICATION 2 Sedation plus analgesia**
> *< 10 years old*: ketamine sedation 2 mg kg^{-1} i.v. Draw up in one
> syringe with atropine (0.1 mg kg^{-1} to control ketamine's
> secretagogue effects). Administer over a 2–3 minute period stopping
> administration when the child's eyes become glazed
> *> 10 years old*: midazolam and fentanyl sedation:
> • midazolam: draw up 3 syringes of 0.05 mg kg^{-1} of i.v. midazolam
> • fentanyl: draw up 3 syringes of 1 µg kg^{-1} of i.v. fentanyl
> • naloxone and flumazenil must be kept at the bedside
> • give midazolam over 2 minutes then fentanyl over 2 minutes.
>   Continue alternating midazolam and fentanyl until adequate
>   sedation. If all 6 syringes are given without adequate sedation, then
>   QUIT sedation and consult the anesthetist
> Both of these techniques require:
> • full, regular BP monitoring
> • continuous pulse, respiratory rate and oxygen saturation
>   monitoring
> • that the sedator and the nurse must have airway skills
> • that airways equipment must be available
> • that the child must be nil by mouth for 2–4 hours prior to
>   sedation
> • that full informed consent is gained
> • recovery in a quiet darkened room
> • discharge when the child can walk or is interactive

• Can you use alternative skin closure techniques (e.g. Steristrips, histoacryl skin glue)?
• Explain the nature of any procedures to child and family.
• Get the help of a play specialist to use non-pharmacological techniques.
• Can you use topical anesthesia with LET gel?
• If local anesthetic is necessary, use warmed, buffered solution and inject slowly through the wound with a small bore needle.
• Consider sedation or general anesthetic if the child is very distressed.
• Splint any sutured wound under tension.
• Give adequate postprocedure analgesia.

30.6.2 Fracture management

The pain from fractures can be divided into three phases:

Initial pain management
- immobilization of the limb with a splint or sling
- adequate analgesia – from paracetamol in minor fractures ascending up the pain ladder to intravenous opioids for displaced fractures

Definitive treatment. This covers the spectrum from:
- immobilization in a backslab or plaster for minor fractures after adequate paracetamol with or without NSAIDs
- reduction under an intravenous regional block such as a Bier's block or with conscious sedation with either ketamine or a combination of midazolam and fentanyl for forearm fractures in a cooperative child
- reduction under general anesthetic

Post-treatment pain management
- elevation of the injured limb will help to reduce pain and swelling
- adequate analgesia following the pain ladder given in adequate amounts and for an adequate length of time

30.6.3 Intravenous cannulation

The discomfort from i.v. cannulation can be minimized by the application of EMLA cream (1 hour) or Ametop gel (approximately 45 minutes) under an occlusive dressing. EMLA causes vasoconstriction. Ametop causes vasodilatation, aiding cannulation, but has a higher incidence of skin irritation.

30.6.4 Lumbar puncture

Topical anesthesia followed by local infiltration with local anesthetic is used in all children including neonates. Correct positioning of the child minimises the risk of a needle hitting bone, causing extra pain.

30.6.5 Burns

All burns are painful. In the ED, superficial burns need:
- rapid oral analgesia, e.g. with oral paracetamol
- rapid wound dressing to exclude the air – this reduces pain even more rapidly than anesthetics
- rarely, sedation with ketamine in addition to analgesia for dressing changes

More severe burns require intravenous opioids (not intramuscular) before the patient is transferred to a Burns Unit.

30.6.6 Major trauma

Children who have multiple trauma require a primary survey and then management of the airway, breathing and circulation. They are usually in pain and its assessment and management are part of the secondary survey. Opioids must be used with care in small boluses with continuous monitoring, as in major burns. Relative sparing of the brain blood flow occurs in hypovolemic patients, so opioids have a relatively greater effect. Low muscular blood flow reduces drug uptake, reducing the apparent effect of the drug. Once circulation improves, a large bolus of opioid is released with the risk of respiratory depression.

30.6.7 Eye injuries

Corneal and conjunctival abrasions and foreign bodies in the eye are painful. Amethocaine eye drops are instilled to ease the assessment and management of eye injuries and removal of foreign bodies in the eye. They should not be used after assessment, as repeated doses are toxic to the corneal epithelium and may delay healing. In addition, an anesthetised eye is at risk of further undiagnosed injury. Blinking over an abraded cornea is painful. Blinking can be prevented by a soft eye patch.

30.6.8 Sickle cell anemia

Children with recurrent severe pain such as those with sickle cell anemia should have a written schedule of analgesia available in the ED records.

30.7 Pain management in the ED

- Ask the child how much pain they have
- Use a pain assessment tool
- Involve the parents
- Observe any physiological/behavioral signs of abuse
- Take the cause of the pain into account
- Use distraction/psychological approaches, plus a range of analgesics
- Use written information leaflets for the parents
- Re-evaluate the pain at the appropriate interval and treat
- Be aware of the side effects of drugs

Further reading

McKenzie, I., Gaukroger, P.B., Ragg, P., Brown, T.C.K. (1997) *Manual of Acute Pain Management in Children*. London: Churchill Livingstone.

Royal College of Pediatrics and Child Health. (1997) *Prevention and control of pain in children: a Manual for Health Care Professionals*. London: BMJ Publishing Group.

Twycross, A., Moriarty, A., Betts, T. (1998) *Pediatric Pain Management*. Oxford: Radcliffe Medical Press.

Chapter 31

Transport of the seriously ill child

Gale Pearson

Contents

31.1 Introduction

Critically ill children present to the Emergency Department (ED) requiring resuscitation. During or after this process they frequently need to be moved whilst closely monitored and/or dependent on cardiovascular and respiratory support. This move may be to another department in the hospital, such as the operating theatre or X-ray department, or to another hospital for specialist care, such as neurosurgery or pediatric intensive care if not available on site. In many ways the principles that apply to all of these scenarios are the same. They follow both from each other and from the recognition that transfer exposes the patient to risks (*Box 31.1*).

The principal risk is of spontaneous or induced deterioration in the clinical condition occurring in an environment that is not as well equipped as the resuscitation area or intensive care unit. Since the need to move the patient is entirely predictable, local protocols can be worked out well in advance and the appropriate preparations made in terms of equipment and training in order to minimize the risk. There are effectively two scenarios:

Primary transport: in this situation the resuscitation is incomplete or a definitive life-saving procedure has not been performed and the patient needs to be relocated as an emergency in order to achieve this. Clearly time is of the essence and an appropriate level of speed and urgency should be applied. A typical example would be getting a critically ill patient to hospital in the first place from home or the scene of an accident. However, the same approach and priorities apply to relocating patients within the hospital system with extremely urgent conditions such as expanding intracranial hematomas or severe thoracic vascular trauma.

Secondary transport: in which a patient is being routinely relocated within the health system for the next stage in their care. Most referrals to

---

Box 31.1 Principles for the transport of critically ill children

- The safety of the patient is the prime concern
- The number of transports required by an individual patient should be kept to a minimum.
- The transport of critically ill children should be performed by specifically trained and equipped staff
- They should be prepared for deterioration in the patient's condition or other emergencies during the transfer

---

intensive care, both within and between hospitals, are secondary transports in that they occur after resuscitation and stabilization have been completed.

31.2 Who should perform the transport?

The most experienced staff available should inevitably perform primary transports and appropriate arrangements made to cover their other duties while they are absent. However, in the context of primary transport, 'age-appropriate' training takes second place to the airway and resuscitation skills of the accompanying clinical staff.

Secondary transports should be performed by specifically trained and appropriately equipped teams, usually attached to the referral center. As might be expected from the assumptions made in the basic principles of transport listed above, the evidence suggests that such an approach dramatically reduces the risk and consequences of critical incidents during transport. Lead centres for pediatric intensive care and for superspecialist services should provide a retrieval service (24 hours a day 7 days a week) for children who require intensive care within their agreed catchment area. In other circumstances, e.g. a stand-alone retrieval service, the quality of the service should be endorsed by these centers. The provision of a retrieval service must not compromise the care of the patients in the receiving center. It should therefore be appropriately staffed, and the staff need to be appropriately indemnified for the additional hazards to which their jobs will expose them.

31.3 Arranging transport

No transfer should ever occur without clear referral of the patient made by consultant to consultant prior to departure. Furthermore the choice of destination for the transfer should be made for the right reasons. Primary transport for emergencies such as neurosurgical intervention for an expanding intracranial hematoma, should not be deferred or rerouted as a result of actual, declared or suspected availability of a pediatric intensive care bed. The patient should be transferred to the nearest centre capable of performing the life-saving procedure and a pediatric intensive care bed should then be sought when the patient's condition has been stabilized, e.g. postoperatively.

31.4 Protocols

Patients should be resuscitated in an appropriately equipped and age-appropriate high dependency area. Parents have a right to be present if they so wish but should not be obligated to be present. The patient remains the clinical responsibility of the existing medical team until the transfer team (if relevant) arrive and take over. During this time advice can be sought and received by telephone enquiry to a relevant referral centre but the obligations, decisions and standards of care are the responsibility of the doctors attending the patient. Nevertheless, it makes sense for compatible protocols to be developed between the receiving and referring hospitals.

If the transfer team are in any way different from the resuscitating team, then an appropriate formal handover between the senior medical and nursing staff must occur at or near the bedside. Once this handover has occurred and not before, the transport team assumes clinical responsibility for the patient and takes charge of the proceedings. All other clinical staff should then step back or at least defer to them from that moment on.

The transfer team should then formally review the patient and examine them fully in order to anticipate possible causes of deterioration during transport. This assessment, like resuscitation, should adopt an ABCDE approach (airway, breathing, circulation, disability, exposure). All critical access points for support and monitoring should be secured to their satisfaction recognising the importance of protocol in terms of style of fixation and access.

A secure airway is essential. Patients in borderline respiratory failure should usually be pre-emptively intubated and ventilated prior to transfer. This will require knowledge and skill in the appropriate technique of anesthetic induction. Nasal intubation is more stable than oral and it is not appropriate to move a patient if you are unfamiliar with the fixation that has been applied to the endotracheal tube. Additional vascular access may be required prophylactically. Central venous access is easier to secure than peripheral, and arterial pressure monitoring is more reliable than oscillometric cuff, but the delay in establishing and securing such access needs to be weighed against the clinical situation both in terms of their justification and necessity. The philosophy of secondary transfers is often described as 'stay and play' rather than 'swoop and scoop' (as in primary transfer), but this does not mean that non-essential procedures should be performed in an environment that is alien to the transport team. Infusions should be kept to a minimum. Monitoring lines can be flushed intermittently and anesthetic agents chosen to allow bolus administration without large fluctuations in depth of anesthesia. In general terms ventilated patients should be paralysed for transport. All vascular access lines should be clearly labelled on the patient and syringe and the label should characterise the access (central i.v., peripheral i.v., arterial) as well as the contents of the infusion. Monitoring equipment should be solid state and selected for adequate battery life and robust enough for transport conditions.

All appropriate documentation, test results and X-rays should accompany the patient to save time and reduce the risk of duplication at the other end of the transfer. Furthermore, the choice of investigations to be performed prior to transfer should be made shrewdly and balanced against the time delay involved. Is a cranial CT really necessary prior to transfer on this occasion when the hospital has no neurosurgical service or pediatric intensive care?

The transport team should carry sufficient equipment and supplies (e.g. oxygen, drug infusions and blood) to last beyond the expected duration of the transport and to deal with emergencies as and when they occur, although a degree of minimalism is essential to control the quantity/volume (and weight) of the 'transport' equipment and baggage. The team needs to be familiar with the idiosyncrasies of their equipment and the transport vehicle(s) being used. Such knowledge needs to be sufficient to lift them to a level of technical proficiency and problem solving that would be delegated to others in a normal hospital environment.

A clear hierarchy is essential amongst the transport team and between the clinical team and the staff associated with the vehicle at each stage. Appropriate clinical requests (not commands) should be made where necessary to adjust speed, route and altitude where necessary, but the ultimate decision on such parameters may not be medical. The safety of the team as well as the patient has to be borne in mind.

31.5 **Hazards**

There is frequently restricted access to the patient during transport either because of the precautions taken to prevent hypothermia or because of the vehicle being used. Poor ambient light may compound the difficulty and reduce the team's sensitivity in detecting changes in the patient's condition. Coarse movement may dislodge patient and equipment, which both need to be adequately secured. Vibration and noise confound monitoring equipment and acceleration and deceleration forces may have pronounced physiological effects on hemodynamics and intracranial pressure. Altitude has pronounced physiological effects and will expand the volume of fixed quantities of gas. This is of particular importance in pneumothorax, bowel obstruction and ventilation, e.g. cuff size in endotracheal tubes and the tidal volume delivered by pressure-controlled ventilation.

When you are faced with a clinical problem during a transport, it is best to optimise the environment while trying to determine the cause and effect a resolution. If possible stop moving the patient, switch off engines, switch on lights and expose the patient sufficiently to perform the relevant clinical examination. Conditions should then be optimal (beggar's choice) for any necessary procedure(s).

31.6 Training

There is no substitute for practical training in the transport of critically ill patients. This best takes the form of supervised transports performed by the trainee in the presence of the trainer. Training opportunities are limited, however, since it is rarely possible to take more than one trainee at a time and there are, by coincidence and design, a limited number of occasions when patients need to be transported.

Furthermore 'good judgement comes from experience but experience comes from bad judgement.' It is often the history of previous critical incidents that contributes most to future safe practice. It is important to avoid having to learn these lessons more than once. Appropriate audit and critical incident reporting and analysis are essential components of a service that is used with any regularity.

Further reading

Holbrook, P.R. (1993) *Textbook of Pediatric Critical Care*. London: W.B. Saunders.
Pearson, G.A. (2001) *Handbook of Pediatric Intensive Care*. London: W.B. Saunders.

Chapter 32

The dead and dying child

Patricia O. Brennan

Contents

32.1 Introduction

In developed countries, the death of a child is a rare event. In 1991, for example, in England and Wales, there was a total of 3060 deaths in children aged 1–14 years. The common causes of death vary significantly depending on the age of the child.

32.1.1 Sudden infant death syndrome

In infants, sudden infant death syndrome (SIDS) remains one of the commonest postneonatal causes of death. In the UK, the incidence has fallen dramatically since the 1991 'Back to Sleep' campaign, where parents were encouraged to put babies to sleep on their backs rather than their fronts or sides. Recent research has revealed causes of death in some infants who were thought to have been SIDS victims. These include metabolic defects and child abuse. However, SIDS deaths still occur and studies from many countries have shown a similar epidemiological profile (*Box 32.1*).

32.1.2 Accidental deaths

Accidents remain the commonest cause of death in all ages after infancy and are more common and more often fatal at all ages in boys than in

---

Box 32.1 Epidemiology of SIDS

Baby
- Prematurity
- Low birth weight
- Multiple births
- Boys more vulnerable than girls
- Admission to neonatal intensive care unit

Death
- Uncommon in first month
- Rising to peak at 10 weeks
- Rare after 1 year
- Especially at night, in winter

Mothers
- Young
- Poorly educated
- Smoke
- Little interval between pregnancies
- Low socio-economic status

Fathers
- Absent
- Unemployed

---

girls despite continuing primary, secondary and tertiary prevention work.

For the parents, the sudden death of a child invokes extreme grief reactions with a double loss, for what is lost (the child they know) and for what might have been (the child growing up with a life of promise). However good our management, nothing will restore the family to the pregrief state. The recent theory of adjusted bereavement tells us what we should be aiming to help the family achieve: 'that the resolution of grief involves continuing bonds that survivors maintain with the deceased and that these continuing bonds can be a healthy part of a survivors life.' [1]

A dead or dying child brought into an ED is fortunately a relatively rare event and so the staff can be inexperienced in the management of the child and the family. There is no place for rapid certification of the child and immediate transfer to the mortuary. This child and the family need proper care, time and attention. This chapter focuses on the scenario of a dead or dying child brought into an ED and seeks to help staff develop good practice. Throughout the chapter, the child will be referred to as male (he, his) and the doctors and nurses as female (she, her). *Figure 32.1* shows one UK ED's management flow chart of the dead and dying child.

32.2 **Reception/resuscitation**

Once the ED staff are informed of the impending arrival of a dead or dying child, the resuscitation team should prepare both themselves and the resuscitation area. Pediatricians, anesthetists and others should be called as appropriate for the unit.

The ambulance should be met on arrival and child and paramedics conducted to the resuscitation area. Resuscitation is continued while the initial assessment is carried out by a senior doctor. Information on the child and his condition is collected as rapidly as possible from any available source, such as relatives, paramedics and existing hospital records. Rapid management decisions have to be made, often before all the information is available. Staff must be supported in these decisions, even if they are later criticised by others who have all the relevant information available to them.

The presence of parents in the resuscitation room is still debatable and should be decided by parents and staff on an individual basis. Increasingly, parents do not want to be separated from their child, leaving him with strangers. With proper support and explanations from a

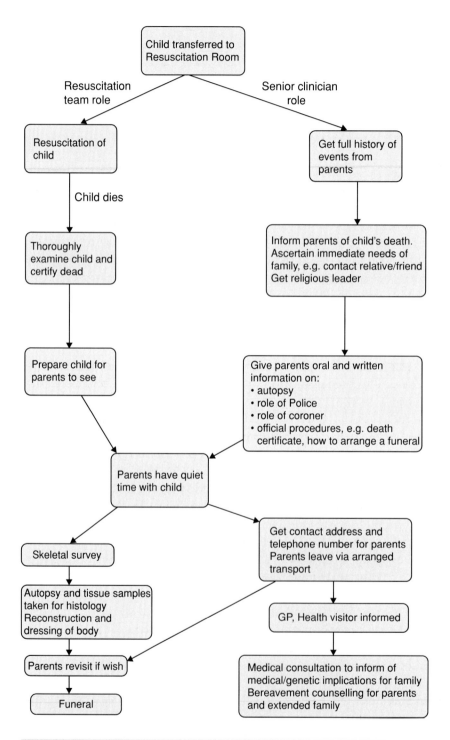

Figure 32.1 Management of the dying child and his family in the ED (in one UK department).

dedicated mature member of staff, parents usually feel able to remain with their child, at least for short periods, with some breaks. Staff may be anxious with the parents present, but usually cope well after training.

Resuscitation is stopped once a senior doctor has decided that it is no longer reasonable to continue. Acceptance should be gained from all present. An ECG trace is recorded and death certified.

A thorough examination is fully and meticulously documented, with both positive and negative findings. It includes the temperature, any skin marks, the state of cleanliness and clothing, any discharge from mouth or nose and fundal changes in the child. The clothes and any nappies or other belongings brought with the child are collected and stored in a plastic bag to help the investigation into the cause of death. Swabs and any other specimens needed to investigate the death are taken. In our own department, with the agreement of the local coroner, the child can then be cleaned and redressed in clean clothes so that when the family come, they see their child presented as well as possible.

It is important that all medical procedures undertaken during resuscitation are documented and any physical signs resulting from the resuscitation noted so that, at post mortem, there is no confusion as to their origin. In our city, the coroner will not allow removal of the endotracheal tube, as tracheal abrasions may be present and need to be interpreted. However, he will allow nurses to cut the endotracheal tube just inside the lips so that its presence is not distressing to the relatives. Nasogastric tubes can similarly be dealt with. Intraosseous needles and cannule can be removed so long as their site is marked.

Once the child is redressed, he is usually laid on the resuscitation room trolley, wrapped in a blanket or shawl to await a visit from the relatives. The child is not left alone, but a nurse is left by his side. Research has shown that parents usually wish to be with the child where he died so that they can feel closer to the child's death. If the parents wish, however, the child is brought to them into the relatives' room.

32.3 Care of the parents

Throughout the resuscitation, the parents are building a relationship with their dedicated nurse. No parent should be without support of family or friends at this time and one early role of the nurse is that of asking a relative or friend of a lone parent to come to the hospital as soon as possible. When this supporter arrives, the nurse may be the appropriate person to inform them of the circumstances of the incident, to spare the parent. In addition, some families will need help from interpreting services or signers for the deaf.

32.3.1 Breaking the bad news

Parents often prefer to be in a room near, but not with, their child during resuscitation. When resuscitation has ceased and the death is certified, it is the role of the senior doctor to inform the parents that the child has died. Even if the child was brought into the department obviously dead, this will need to be confirmed to the parents. The doctor should sit at the same level as the relatives, probably lean forwards and not be afraid to make eye contact. She should always use the child's name and should break the news kindly but simply. She can express regret for the circumstances which have led to the family's attendance, but should never utter platitudes such as 'It'll be all right.' The parents and relatives may appear to be unaware of their surroundings or of what is said to them at this time of grief. [2] However, research has shown that they can often later describe the room and staff in great detail and appear to have heightened or more acute perception of what was said to them. A thoughtless remark can cause pain whereas caring ones are remembered.

Euphemisms for death such as 'We've lost him' can be misconstrued by relatives. The parents may still hope – their child came in an ambulance with a blue light flashing and was taken into a room full of 'high tech' equipment – any of us would hope for a miracle. They must therefore be told directly that their child has 'died' or is 'dead'. The parents' reaction to the news varies widely, from stunned silence to anger and loud outpouring of grief. The staff breaking the bad news can also have a range of powerful emotions (*Box 32.2*).

If no history has yet been taken, then a full one needs to be taken now (*Box 32.3*). This may seem harsh, but the staff, the pathologist, and above all the parents, need to know why the child died, and the history is an important part of the investigation. Once this is explained, the parents normally agree. The history may take time and has to be taken at the parents' pace. By using the child's name and asking in detail sensitively about his life, you are building up a rapport with the parents and developing with them a picture of their child as an individual.

During the history, the parents sometimes start to express their guilt. One mother said to me: 'Do you know what I've done? I put the kettle on before I checked the baby.' Her guilt was overwhelming and, while I was unable to put her mind at ease, I was able to let the bereavement counsellors, who were to see her later, know about her feelings of guilt.

Box 32.2 Reactions to bad news

Initial reactions of receiver
- Withdrawal
- Denial
- Anger
- Isolation
- Bargaining
- Inappropriate responses
- Guilt
- Crying, sobbing, weeping
- Acceptance

Reactions of news breaker
- Anxiety
- Fear
- Panic
- Anger
- Helplessness
- Failure
- Sadness
- Despair

Box 32.3 History to be taken

- Events leading up to death
- When the child was last seen alive and by whom
- How and when the child was found
- Any resuscitation carried out and by whom
- Antenatal history
- Birth and neonatal history
- Previous medical history, previous illnesses, e.g. fits, including hospital and ED attendances
- Feeding pattern
- Sleep, including position
- Development
- Allergies
- Medication
- Immunizations
- Family history

32.3.2 Religious/cultural needs

The staff need to ask about any special needs at this point. Some families would like a religious leader to come to them at the hospital and to have a blessing service. Others wish religious customs around death to be observed (*Box 32.4*) and staff should support families in carrying these out within the limits of any legal investigation into the cause of the death.

Box 32.4 Examples of religious customs around death

Muslim
- Distress may be caused if the body is touched after death by a non-believer (disposable gloves can be used to touch the body)
- Post mortems are forbidden unless ordered by the Coroner
- Removal of a lock of hair would be offensive
- Funeral within 24 hours of the death

Hindu
- Distress may be caused if the body is touched after death by a non-believer
- Post mortems are problematic

Judaism
- The first acts of shutting the eyes, binding up the jaw and laying the arms straight are traditionally done by a family member
- Funeral within 24 hours of the death

32.3.3 Information needs

We need to tell the parents so much, most of which they won't be able to absorb at the time. We tell them everything, and also give the information in writing. Leaflets from national support organisations such as the Foundation for the Study of Infant Deaths in the UK can be helpful.

The parents are told of the normal Police and coroner's involvement and told about the need for a coroner's post mortem.

32.4 **Police involvement**

In our city, if you dial for an emergency ambulance, the Police are automatically informed and will attend – either at the home or the hospital. This is routine, and not because we think there has been foul play. The parents need to know this. The Police in England and Wales gain information for the coroner, the crown officer who is responsible for investigating the cause of death. They need to see the body and have the child identified. This can be done sensitively and quietly by a policeman glimpsing the parents with their child. In addition, the Police fill in a questionnaire to help the coroner with his enquiries into the cause of death. This includes details of family and living conditions and part of their routine role in these circumstances is to take the bedding and clothing used by the child at the time of death for tests.

32.5 **The role of the coroner**

In the UK, all cases of sudden unexpected death are reported to the coroner. He routinely asks for a skeletal survey and post mortem examination in a child brought in unexpectedly dead or dying to determine the cause of death. This is usually carried out within hours of the child's death. The parents therefore have no time to accept the child's death before they are informed of the post mortem. Their consent is not required for the procedure in a coroner's case nor for the retention of small pieces of tissue for further tests to determine the cause of death. However, their consent is required for the retention of any other tissue, for example for research. The parents need to be informed of the facts, again simply but sensitively. A coroner's post mortem will be carried out and it involves an examination of the outside and the inside of the body, like an operation carried out by a highly qualified doctor.

On receiving the result of the post mortem, if there is no evidence of a criminal cause of the death the coroner will decide whether to hold an inquest and when to release the body for the funeral. He will issue the Death Certificate.

32.6 **Further information**

The family will also need further information, such as:
• Where and who issues the death certificate
• How to register a death
• How to organise a funeral
• How to cope financially and what benefits are available

32.7 **Seeing the child**

The long-term grieving and coming to terms with the loss of a child (not 'getting over it') is improved if the parents see and even cuddle the child before they leave the hospital. [3] The extended family often join in with this vigil. Parents are often reluctant to do this at first, or the mother would like to but her husband or partner think it would be too distressing for her. Others often think that they know what is best for the mother, to save her distress. It is important that the mother is not disempowered at this time.

Once the family enters the room where the child is lying, they can be helped to touch and hold their child by being gently told that they can do so, and by the nurse or doctor picking up the child and passing him to them. The parents, at first tentatively but then more naturally, hold the child, cuddle him and talk to him, often passing him from one family member to another. Although they need privacy, they should not be left completely alone with the child. This relatively short vigil with goodbyes is a healthy way to leave the child for the first time and start the bereavement journey. Families often find it difficult to leave the hospital and go home without him. They may need help to do this.

Before the parents leave, you should make sure that you know the family's General Practitioner, the address to which the parents are going and who will be there to support them. You should ensure that they have safe transport – they should not drive or use public transport in their distressed state. You should consider ordering hospital transport or a taxi for them. In addition, you must ensure that they have a contact name and number at the hospital. They may have questions unanswered and ring for help and advice, or they may wish to visit their child again at any time while he is in the hospital.

32.8 What happens afterwards

Sadly, non-accidental injury is still a cause of death in young children, and the skeletal survey is an important part of the coroner's investigation. This is carried out as soon as the child leaves the ED.

The post mortem itself is extensive, to exclude medical and traumatic causes of death. Pathologists are careful to use incisions on the chest, abdomen and within the hairline of the scalp which will not show once the child is redressed. Small specimens of tissue are taken for histology. After the post mortem, the child is redressed in clothes chosen by the family and is put in a crib or bed in the chapel when the parents visit. They often wish a favorite toy to be left with the child.

Mortuary staff or nurses take keepsakes such as hand and footprints on small cards, or a lock of hair from the child. Photographs are taken once the child has been redressed after the post mortem. Occasionally, families request a family photograph with the child. All these are available. Parents may not want them at first, but staff keep them on file as families have been known to request them several years after the child's death.

The family is told the preliminary results of the post mortem as soon as the coroner gives permission. The parents meet with a consultant pediatrician some time later when the results of the histology and other tests are available. The cause of death and the implications for future pregnancies and other children in the family are discussed. Occasionally the family is referred on for more specialised genetic counselling.

32.9 The needs of the siblings

The siblings of the dead child should be involved with the family during the time of bereavement. [4] The type and amount of involvement of the children will depend on their age and on the family dynamics. They do need to be told that their sibling has died as soon as possible, in the same way as adults are told, sensitively, honestly and clearly. They will need explanations appropriate to their age and understanding. The parents may try to protect their surviving children from distress and conversely, the children may try to protect their parents. It is important to realise that they can sometimes take on the blame for family happenings, even the death of their sibling. They may wonder if they are going to die too. Children need to see their parents' grief or they will not believe the dead child was loved and they may fear that they would not be mourned if they died. They may wish to see their brother and with careful sensitive preparation and support, they normally cope well. As with adults, reality is often more acceptable than imagination.

In addition, the children may wish to attend the funeral and, again, with careful explanations and preparation and the agreement of parents, this is usually right for them. During all this time, they need help to express their emotions. They may cry openly or feel angry. If suppressed, their emotions can be expressed later inappropriately. It helps children if:
- they are told what has happened
- their questions are answered
- their grief is acknowledged
- they are included in the family mourning process
- they have mementoes of the deceased
- they have understanding and reassurance about their feelings and concerns
- parents accept that some behavioral/emotional reaction is normal
- they meet other children who have lost a brother or sister.

They need time to explore their new family environment without their sibling, and time and support to return to a routine.

For school-aged children, schools, friends and teachers might be able to help, recognising signs of grief and supporting the child. The class should be told before the child returns to school and some of the class's questions answered. The child's loss should be acknowledged when they return. School links with home will enable teaching staff to understand the child's reactions better, particularly if signs such as outbursts of temper, mood swings or poor school work result.

Occasionally, parents idolise the lost child and can view the dead child as somehow closer and more accessible than the living. They unconsciously compare the living children and occasionally even reject them. Sometimes parents become overprotective of the surviving children. However, parents are usually a child's best help and support. One parent remarked that answering the questions of her 3-year-old surviving child helped her parents to bring things out into the open. [1] At times like this, parents' own grief can prevent them being able to offer enough. In some families children benefit from talking to someone of their choice from outside the family, e.g. a bereavement counsellor who is understanding without being intrusive.

Other family members are also deeply involved and affected by the death of a child. Grandparents in particular grieve for their grandchild but also for the parents.

32.10 Afterwards – the ED responsibility

The health staff have continuing roles and responsibilities after the parents have left the hospital. In the UK, the ED staff must:
• check the documentation
• inform the hospital mortuary technician who will take over the care and management of the child
• inform the coroner
• inform the family's General Practitioner and encourage a home visit
• inform the local Health Services to cancel future appointments, etc.

The family's General Practitioner is particularly important as someone who can visit and help immediately, for example in suppressing lactation in the mother when the child is a baby, and who can give ongoing care and support.

32.11 The follow up

The parents may wish to visit the child at the hospital after the post mortem and often visit several times, day or night, before the child leaves prior to the funeral, sometimes bringing the extended family. The parents need a telephone number and a named person to request a visit. They may be asked to wait for a short time. The child should be brought from the refrigerator into the chapel as soon as possible, so that the skin does not feel so cold by the time the parents arrive. Occasionally, parents ask for a religious service in the hospital's chapel or faith room.

Once a funeral director has been chosen and the death registered, the body can remain at the hospital or be taken to the funeral directors until the funeral. Again, mourning rituals will be important in most families and cultures. They help to make the loss real and give social recognition to the dead. Many religions have specific customs attached to death. Wherever possible, these should be respected by the hospital staff and funeral directors.

Occasionally, the family request the child's body to be brought home the night before or on the day of the funeral. This can usually be arranged.

The relationship between the child's parents will be tested by the bereavement. Mothers and fathers grieve in different ways and often have little understanding of each other's reactions. Any existing problems in the relationship will be magnified. After the death, the parents will need support and understanding for a long time. Support is usually best given by staff with a long-term relationship with the family, and the Primary Healthcare Team can be particularly important here. Most hospitals have bereavement counsellors, who will meet the parents shortly after the child's death and continue regular contact and counselling should the parents so wish. The parents need to know some of the thoughts and feelings that they may experience, including aching arms, distressing dreams and hearing the child's voice.

There are many organizations who can give support to the bereaved family. In the UK, the Foundation for the Study of Infant Deaths and the Compassionate Friends produce helpful leaflets and can provide a befriending service.

32.12 The needs of the staff

After dealing with a dead or dying child and his family, all the staff involved, from clerical staff, nurses and doctors to police, porters and paramedics, are affected. They should have a short time-out to talk through the case, from presentation and decisions to start and stop resuscitation to the after-care of the child and family. In addition, at the end of the shift, a senior member of staff should check that everyone is coping. Some staff may need further periods to discuss the case with a senior member of staff in the ED and some may need support or counselling from professional counsellors outside the department. This will depend on the characteristics of the case, the member of staff and their personal situation.

32.13 Staff training

Before 1991, when SIDS rates were in the order of 2.0 per 1000 live births in England and Wales, even experienced staff had only occasional experience of dealing with families of children brought in dead or dying. Since 1991, the SIDS rate has fallen dramatically, and experience is even more limited. Teaching and training on how to cope are increasingly necessary. Structured working including receiving the child and parents, resuscitation, certification of death, information about the role of the coroner and the post mortem and other formalities must be covered. However, other aspects are as important and should include:
• variations of parents/family response
• the carers' own needs
• interpersonal skills
• words used associated with sensitivity
• insights into responses
• responses to difficult behavior
• ability to handle stress

We need to be clear what our personal and institutional responsibilities are and we need to be able to manage these occasions, which feel like chaos to ourselves and to the bereaved.

References

1. Klass, D., Silverman, P., Nickman, S. (eds). (1996) *Continuing Bonds: New Understandings of Grief.* London: Taylor & Francis.
2. Wright, B. (1991) *Sudden Death, Intervention Skills for the Caring Professions.* London: Churchill Livingstone.
3. Fleming, P., Bacon, C., Blair, P., Berry, P.J. (2000) *Sudden Unexpected Deaths in Infancy.* London: The Stationery Office.
4. Smith, S.C. (1999) *The Forgotten Mourners – Guidelines for Working with Bereaved Children*, 2nd edn. London: Jessica Kingsley.

Further reading

The CEDI SUDI Studies 1993–1996. London: The Stationery Office.
Hindmarsh, C. (2000) *On the Death of a Child.* Oxford: Radcliffe Medical Press Ltd.

Chapter 33

Medicolegal issues

Patricia O. Brennan

Contents

33.1 Introduction

Wide-ranging medicolegal issues have an enormous impact in the work of the pediatric Emergency Department (ED). Large numbers of patients with unselected problems attend in an unplanned way and the doctors are often under enormous pressure to see patients quickly. In the medicolegal sense, any ED is the most vulnerable department in the hospital. Pediatric emergency medicine has added pitfalls, particularly of consent to treatment and confidentiality. The problems are similar in outline in every country and state, although they may differ in detail according to practice and the law. This chapter aims to outline some of the issues faced by all.

33.2 Who can give consent to treatment?

Consent to examination, investigation and treatment of a child under the age of majority (16 years of age in the UK) in an ED can be given by a parent or legal guardian (occasionally the Local Authority if the child is in foster care) and is usually 'implied' by the very fact that a child has been presented for medical help. Consent can be accepted from someone *in loco parentis*, such as a teacher or grandparent in an emergency if the parent is uncontactable in the UK, for example. Written consent is only required for complex and more major procedures requiring regional or general anesthetic.

The age of majority is now 18 years of age in the UK, but young people from the age of 16 years can legally give their own consent (Family Law Reform Act 1969). However, the law does not prevent a young person below the age of 16 giving consent to his or her own treatment. If a doctor judges that the patient has sufficient maturity to appreciate the significance of the risks of a treatment, then the consent is valid. The doctor should document the factors that he or she took into account in accepting consent and should seek to involve the parent in the decision (see confidentiality section).

In the case of a child requiring emergency treatment in the absence of a parent, the need for consent gives way to the immediate need to save the life or future well-being of the patient. If the doctor acts in good faith in an emergency, the courts will uphold his or her decision.

If the parent or guardian of a child refuses consent for a life-saving procedure or treatment, such as may occur if a Jehovah's Witness patient requires an urgent blood transfusion, the doctor should proceed according to his or her own conscience, with counsel from the hospital administration where possible. In a less urgent situation, the doctor should use the appropriate mechanism such as an emergency court order to allow treatment to take place.

33.3 **Confidentiality**

An ED is usually a fairly open and busy area. Staff must be careful to ensure patient privacy and confidentiality in the working environment. Notes should not be left unattended and discussion about a patient between doctors and nurses managing the case should take place in privacy and not within earshot of anyone else. If medical information is held on a computer, then the patient and parent should be aware of this and should be able to have access to it on request.

A doctor holds many confidences of his or her patients. These belong to the patient not the doctor, who is only a custodian and should only share them under specific circumstances and with specific people:
- other healthcare professionals to ensure continuity of appropriate patient care
- when asked to do so by the patient
- parents, when the patient is a minor (see below)
- under circumstances laid down by law, such as the notification of births and deaths
- when ordered to do so by a court of law
- in the interests of the community

In general, when children and young people under the age of 16 years attend an ED, the parents are important parties to the whole consultation, including history, examination, investigation and treatment. Young persons over the age of 16 years have a right to confidentiality. The General Medical Council of the UK accepts that, if a patient is under the age of 16 years and is judged to be sufficiently mature to appreciate all the circumstances of medical treatment, then the doctor should maintain confidentiality at the patient's request and need not disclose any information to the parents. These issues particularly arise in relation to contraception, pregnancy and abortion.

In child protection cases, if a child discloses an episode of abuse to a doctor, the child must be told that the confidence cannot be kept, but will be shared with the appropriate professionals so that an investigation can be carried out and proper protection for the child can be achieved.

The police sometimes ask for information on patients, particularly in cases of assault but no police officer should give the impression that there is an enforceable right to release of information. As a general rule it should not be disclosed without signed consent from the parent or guardian, or in an older child, from the child themself. There are certain circumstances where this guideline can be over-ruled after discussion with a senior doctor and the doctor's medical protection organisation. Examples are a child protection case where the parent is thought to be the perpetrator, or in a road traffic accident in the UK when a doctor is obliged to disclose the identity of people treated after being involved in the accident. If access to patient information is denied by a doctor, but is judged essential by the police, then a witness order may be sought whereby the doctor can be ordered to provide the information.

Access to medical records should be given only to a child's solicitor or insurance company with the written consent of a parent or guardian. If litigation is contemplated against a medical professional for negligence, then the hospital legal advisers and the doctor's medical defence union may wish to be informed at the same time that any records are disclosed.

33.4 Note keeping

Doctors in an ED often have to work quickly under pressure. As a result, note keeping is often inadequate. The discipline of appropriate, accurate notes made at the time the patient is examined is essential. Taking an appropriate history, doing the examination, investigation, management and writing the notes in a timely fashion is an art that should be taught at the beginning of any job in an ED and should be practised throughout the post. The main reasons for accurate documentation of details of the case are:
- to remind the doctor of the details of the case
- to communicate details of the case to other members of the treatment team
- to enable a different doctor at a subsequent attendance to be able to assess the case appropriately
- to remind the doctor of details in order to be able to write a report or statement – the emergency records are a legal document that might support a patient's claim
- to be able to answer complaints
- to recall details of the case if called to court to give evidence or in the future for audit and research

The notes are a legal document and should not be changed. If they are, the change must be clearly noted and dated and signed. The original wording should remain visible. A patient has a right of access to his or her own notes and, in the case of a child, a parent can request access if the child has consented or if it is in the child's best interest.

Details of history and examination in specific conditions are given in other chapters. The following comments relate to all records. It is useful to start the notes with details of the date and time of the examination and of who was accompanying the child. It is also important to note who actually gave the history, often both child and parent. With an injury, the history should state who gave it, together with details of how, why and where the accident happened. Past medical history, immunisations, allergies and medication are all essential parts of any history in a child, however minor the injury.

The examination should state clearly what part was examined and note positive and negative findings. Details of size, shape and condition of any injury should be noted. A description of a 'fresh bleeding abrasion 12 × 10 cm over the lateral left thigh' gives a much clearer picture of the wound than 'graze L. thigh'. In cases of claims for medical negligence, as far as the lawyers are concerned, '**if it wasn't written, it wasn't done.**'

A record in the examination of a febrile child that 'the whole body surface was examined with no signs of a rash,' gives a doctor a much better defence if the child subsequently develops meningococcal septicemia with purpura and dies. It is important therefore to put negative as well as positive findings.

33.5 Complaints

Complaints about an attendance at an ED are frequent and can be about a range of problems, from the waiting room facilities and waiting time, the attitude of the staff, to a missed diagnosis or the treatment. The service is at risk of complaints because it is trying to cope with:
- the unplanned attendances of patients with a whole spectrum of conditions
- the pressure to see patients quickly but thoroughly whatever the workload
- the stress and distress of patients and parents at the time of the attendance
- the ever increasing expectations of the service

Complaints can be minimised in several ways. The doctor should take time to communicate fully with child and family throughout the consultation. A careful history should be taken and the patient examined, assessed and treated. The doctor should ask for help at any stage if unsure of procedure. He or she should not be deflected from the case in hand by requests about other problems and should write up the episode before starting on the next case. Many complaints can be defused if the staff become aware of dissatisfaction at the end of the consultation and offer to let the parent discuss the issues with a senior member of staff immediately. Each health organisation has its own Complaints Procedures. These must be taken seriously and complaints answered in a timely manner. Looking positively, complaints should be used to identify weaknesses in the health system that can be rectified to give the patients and their parents a better service.

33.6 Police statements

The doctor may be asked by the police to give information about an incident on several levels: as an *ordinary member of the public*, for instance as a witness to a road traffic accident; as a *professional witness*, giving the clinical facts of the case such as when the patient attended and details of any injuries sustained; as an *expert witness* when opinions on the cause and outcome of the injuries would be required.

From work in an ED, a doctor is usually asked by the police to act as a professional witness and to give a statement about a patient. As stated above, in the majority of cases, this should only be given with the parents' consent. There may be exceptions to this rule in child protection cases. The statement should contain:
• the doctor's name, qualifications and occupation
• details of the patient's name and date of birth
• when and where the patient was examined
• who was present
• a short statement as to why the patient presented, to put the examination in context (this will be hearsay and may not be taken into account in criminal proceedings, although it will in civil proceedings)
• a precise description of clinical findings in clear simple language without the use of technical terms if possible
• an opinion as to whether the clinical findings are consistent with the history given (if the doctor has enough experience to do so)

The statement should usually be put on an official statement form. A junior doctor should have his or her statement checked by the consultant in charge of the case before signing in the appropriate place and getting the signature countersigned.

A doctor can give evidence of fact, but should not be pressurised to give an opinion if too junior or inexperienced to discuss alternative diagnoses and justify his or her own opinion. A copy of any statement should be kept securely by the doctor or hospital as information relating to it may be asked for many months or even years later.

33.7 The doctor as a witness in court

Even junior hospital doctors can be asked to give evidence in court, based on cases treated while in the ED, usually those on which police statements have been requested. With proper preparation, this should not be too much of an ordeal.

A few days before the hearing, doctors should obtain the original medical notes and a copy of any statement given to the police. They should refresh their memory, rereading the notes and becoming familiar with the details of the case once again. It helps to go over some questions that may be asked and frame some answers. Reading up on the matter will increase confidence in knowledge of the subject. It is important that junior doctors discuss the case and court procedures with the consultant before the trial.

The doctor should arrive punctually, smartly dressed and with the clinical notes in hand. A short conference may be requested by the lawyers to clarify some issues in the statement. Once called to give evidence, the doctor will be led to the witness box and asked to take the Oath or an Affirmation. Name, qualifications, occupation and experience will be asked for and then he or she will be led through the evidence, giving a factual account of the findings. As in the written statement, it is important to avoid complicated medical terms. If this is unavoidable, an explanation of the terms should be given in simple language. Questioning by the instructing lawyer may be followed by a cross-examination by the opposing lawyer. The doctor may be asked to give an opinion on the causation of the clinical findings. As for police statements, give one only if you have sufficient experience to consider alternative explanations and justify your own conclusions. Otherwise, opinions on causation should be requested from more experienced doctors acting as expert witnesses.

Once the prosecution lawyer has finished questioning, the defence lawyer may wish to cross-examine. The court should release you once your evidence has been heard.

Further reading

Gee, D.J., Mason, J.K. (1990) *The Courts and the Doctor.* Oxford: Oxford Medical Press.

Knight, B. (1992) *Legal Aspects of Medical Practice*, 5th edn. London: Churchill Livingstone.

Emergency formulary

Emergency formulary

Drug	Age	Route	Dose	Frequency per 24 hours	Notes
Acetyl cysteine	<12 years <20 kg	iv inf	150 mg kg⁻¹ in 3 ml kg⁻¹ then	Single dose over 15 mins	Used for up to 24 hours after paracetamol overdose. Thereafter seek advice from a Poisons Advice Center
			50 mg kg⁻¹ in 7 ml kg⁻¹ then	Single dose iv inf over 4 hours	
			100 mg kg⁻¹ in 14 ml kg⁻¹	Single dose inf over 16 hours	
	>20 kg	iv inf	150 mg kg⁻¹ in 100 ml then	Single dose over 15 mins	
			50 mg kg⁻¹ in 250 ml then	Single dose infusion over 4 hours	
			100 mg kg⁻¹ in 500 ml	Single dose inf over 16 hours	
	12–18 years	iv inf	150 mg kg⁻¹ in 200 ml then	Single dose over 15 mins	
			50 mg kg⁻¹ in 500 ml then	Single dose infusion over 4 hours	
			100 mg kg⁻¹ in 1000 ml	Single dose infusion over 16 hours	

Drug	Age	Route	Dose	Frequency	Notes
Activated charcoal	1 month–2 years	oral	1 g kg⁻¹	Single dose	Some poisons may require multiple dose treatment at the same doses
	2 years–12 years	oral	25–50 g	Single dose	4 hourly but ensure there are good bowel sounds
	12 years–18 years	oral	50 g	Single dose	
Acyclovir (herpes simplex)	1 month–2 years	oral	100 mg	5	
	2 years–18 years	oral	200 mg	5	
	<3 months	iv inf	10 mg kg⁻¹	3	Double dose in severly immuno-compromised and in encephalitis if over 3 months of age
	3 months–12 years	iv inf	250 mg m⁻²	3	
	12 years–18 years	iv inf	5 mg kg⁻¹	3	
Adenosine	<1 month	iv bolus	50 µg kg⁻¹ increasing every 2 mins by 50 µg kg⁻¹ to a total dose of 300 µg kg⁻¹	Single dose	Very rapidly acting with a 1/2 life <10 seconds. Give in a large peripheral vein for maximum effect. Efficient and safe for SVT
	1 month–12 years	iv	50 µg kg⁻¹ increasing by 50 µg kg⁻¹ every 2 mins to a total dose of 500 µg kg⁻¹	Single dose	
	12 years–18 years	iv	3 mg increasing by 3 mg increments every 2 mins if necessary to a total dose of 12 mg		
Amethocaine	1 month–18 years	topical	1 tube (approx 1 g)	Single application	
Aminophylline	1 month–12 years	iv inf	5 mg kg⁻¹ (maximum 250 mg)	Single loading dose	Over 20–30 minutes. Do not use if already on theophyllines.
	12 years–18 years	iv inf	250–500 mg	Single loading dose	
	1 month–12 years	iv inf	1 mg kg⁻¹ hour⁻¹	Continuous	
	12 years–18 years	iv inf	500 µg kg⁻¹ hour⁻¹	Continuous	

Drug	Age	Route	Dose	Frequency per 24 hours	Notes
Amoxycillin	<7days	Oral/im/iv	50 mg kg^{-1}	2	Increase iv dose to 100 mg kg in suspected meningitis
	7–21 days	Oral/im/iv	50 mg kg^{-1}	3	
	21 days–1 month	Oral/im/iv	50 mg kg^{-1}	4	
	1 month–2 years	oral	125 mg	3	
	2 years–12 years	oral	125–250 mg	3	Oral dose may be doubled in severe infections
	12 years–18 years	oral	500 mg	3	
	1 month–18 years	iv/im	30 mg kg^{-1} (max 4 g)	3	
Aspirin (Kawasaki disease)	1 month–12 years	oral	20–25 mg kg^{-1} initially for 14 days then 3–5 mg kg^{-1}	4	For 6–8 weeks. Continue if evidence of coronary lesions, but otherwise stop
Aspirin Headache	12 years–18 years	oral	300–600 mg	4	Do not give to younger children as risk of Reye's syndrome.
Atropine sulphate (bradycardia)	1 month onwards	iv/io	20 μg kg^{-1} (min. 100 μg, max. 600 μg	Single dose	Give over 1 minute. Do not use in neonates.
Azithromycin	1 month–12 years	oral	10 mg kg^{-1}	1	For 3 days
	12 years–14 years	oral	400 mg	1	
	14 years–18 years	oral	500 mg	1	

Beclomethasone dipropionate (asthma)	6 months–2 years	Inhaled aerosol	50–500 µg	2	
	2 years–12 years	Inhaled aerosol/dry powder	100–500 µg	2	
	12 years–18 years	Inhaled aerosol/dry powder	Up to 1 mg		
Beclomethasone diproprionate (allergic rhinitis)	6 years–18 years	Nasal spray	2 sprays to each nostril	2	
Benzylpenicillin (penicillin G)	Birth – 1 week	iv	25 mg kg⁻¹	2	Contraindications – hypersensitivity
	1 week – 1 month	iv	25 mg kg⁻¹	3	
	1 month – 12 years	iv	25 mg kg⁻¹	4	Double doses may be given six times daily in severe infection Maximum **14.4g/day**
	12–18 years	iv	300–600 mg	4	
Budesonide (croup)	3 months–12 years	neb	2 mg	Single dose	
Bupivacaine hydrochloride	1 month–12 years	Local infiltration	Up to 2 mg kg⁻¹	Single dose	
	12 years–18 years	Local infiltration	Up to 150 mg	Single dose	

Drug	Age	Route	Dose	Frequency per 24 hours	Notes
Captopril	Birth–1 month	oral	10–50 µg kg⁻¹	Single dose	Test dose with patient supine
	1 month–12 years	oral	100 µg kg⁻¹	Single dose	Monitor blood pressure every 15 minutes for 1–2 hours
	12 years–18 years	oral	6.25 mg	Single dose	Start at the lowest dose and titrate up to a maximum dose of:
	Then: Birth–1 month	oral	10–50 µg kg⁻¹	3	<1 month – 2 mg kg/day
	1 month–12 years	oral	100 µg–2 µg kg⁻¹	3	1 month–12 years – 6 mg kg/day
	12 years–18 years	oral	12.5–50 mg	2–3	Dose may be doubled in severe infection
Cefaclor	1 month–1 year	oral	62.5 mg	3	
	1 year–5 years	oral	125 mg	3	
	5 years–18 years	oral	250 mg	3	
Cefotaxime	<7 days	iv	50 mg kg⁻¹	2	
	7 days–1 month	iv	50 mg kg⁻¹	3	
	1 month – 12 years	iv	50 mg kg⁻¹	2	May be up to 4 times per day in severe infections
	12 years–18 years	iv	1–3g	2	
Ceftazidime	1 month–2 months	iv/im	12.5–30 mg kg⁻¹	2	Doses of up to 80 mg kg three times per day in severe infection to a maximum of 6 g
	2 months–12 years	iv/im	15–50 mg kg⁻¹	2 or 3	
	12 years–18 years	iv	1–2 g	2 or 3	
Ceftriaxone	1 month–18 years	iv/im	20–50 mg kg⁻¹	1	Maximum dose 4G. Some centers in the UK use 80 mg kg⁻¹ per dose in meningococcal infections
Chloral hydrate	Birth–12 years	oral	25–50 mg kg⁻¹	Single dose	Acts in approximately 45 minutes

Drug	Age	Route	Dose	Frequency	Notes
Chloramphenicol	Birth–4 weeks	iv bolus	12.5 mg	2	Can be doubled in severe infection. NB not used in many countries including North America due to risk of severe bone marrow depression
	4 weeks–18 years	iv bolus	12.5 mg kg⁻¹ (maximum 1g)	4	
Chloramphenicol (eye infections)	1 month–18 years	Eye drops	1–2 drops 0.5%	4–6	NB Not used in some countries
Chlorpheniramine	1 month–2 years	oral	1 mg	2	
	2 years–5 years	oral	1–2 mg	3	
	6 years–12 years	oral	2–4 mg	3	
	12 years–18 years	oral	4 mg	3	
Ciprofloxacin	Birth–18 years	oral	7.5 mg kg⁻¹	2	
	Birth–18 years	iv	5 mg kg⁻¹	2	
Clindomycin	Birth–12 years	oral	3–6 mg kg⁻¹	4	
	12 years–18 years	oral	150–300 mg	4	
	Birth–1 month	iv/im	5 mg kg⁻¹	3	
	1 month–12 years	iv/im	5–7 mg kg⁻¹	3	
	12 years–18 years	iv/im	900 mg	3	Up to 40 mg kg in severe infections or 4.8g/day
Co-amoxiclav (amoxycillin and clavulanic acid)	1 month–1 year	oral	0.266 ml kg⁻¹ of 125/31 suspension	3	May be doubled in severe infections
	1 year–6 years	oral	5 ml 125/31 suspension	3	
	7 years–12 years	oral	5 ml 250/62 suspension	3	
	12 years–18 years	oral	250/125 tablet	3	

431

Drug	Age	Route	Dose	Frequency per 24 hours	Notes
Codeine phosphate	Birth–12 years	Oral/ rectal/im	500 µg mg kg^{-1}	4–6	Maximum daily dose 12–18 year olds – 240 mg
	12 years–18 years	oral/rectal/ im	30–60 mg	4–6	
Dapsone	1 month–18 years	oral	500 µg kg^{-1}	1	Blistering conditions Double in treatment of leprosy
DC shock	Birth – 18 years	DC shock	2 j kg^{-1}	Initial dose	
		DC shock	4 J kg^{-1}	Subsequent doses	
Desferrioxamine (Iron poisoning)	1 month–12 years	oral	5 g	Single dose	Give single dose in 50–100ml water – may need to give through a nasogastric tube as unpleasant taste
	12 years–18 years	oral	5–10 g	Single dose	
	1 month–12 years	im	1 g	Single dose	May be repeated 8 hourly if necessary
	12 years–18 years	im	2 g	Single dose	maximum dose 80 mg kg^{-1} per day
	1 month–18 years	iv inf	15 mg kg^{-1} hour^{-1} reducing after 4–6 hours	continuous	
Dexamethasone (for croup)	1 month–12 years	oral	150 µg kg^{-1} or 150–300 µg kg^{-1}	2 Single dose	
Diazepam (for status epilepticus)	Birth–12 years	iv bolus	300–400 µg kg^{-1}	Single dose	If necessary, repeat after 10 minutes
	12–18 years	iv bolus	10–20 mg	Single dose	
	Birth–1 month	rectal	1.25–2.5 mg	Single dose	
	1 month–2 years	rectal	5 mg	Single dose	
	2 years–12 years	rectal	5–10 mg	Single dose	
	12 years–18 years	rectal	10 mg	Single dose	

	Age	Route	Dose	Frequency	Notes
Diazepam (for short term anxiety relief)	2 years–12 years	oral	2–3 mg	3	Most effective >12 years old
	12 years–18 years	oral	2–10 mg	3	
Dopamine	Birth – 18 years	infusion	5–20 µg kg⁻¹ min⁻¹	Continuous	Inactivated by sodium bicarbonate Several drug interactions Infuse in 5% dextrose or 0.9% sodium chloride via central line
Dobutamine	Birth – 18 years	iv inf.	2–20 µg kg⁻¹ per min	Continuous	Inactivated by sodium bicarbonate Several drug interactions
Cardiopulmonary resuscitation					
Epinephrine (adrenaline)	Birth – 12 years	iv/io	10 µg kg⁻¹ (0.1 ml kg⁻¹ of 1:10,000)	Initial and subsequent doses	If io, flush with 0.9% saline
		ETT	100 µg kg⁻¹ (0.1 mm of 1:1,000)	Single dose	
	12–18 years	iv/io	1 mg (10 ml of 1:10,000)	Initial and subsequent doses	
		ETT	5 mg (5 ml of 1:1000)	Single dose	
Acute anaphylaxis					
	Birth – 12 years	Deep im	10 µg kg⁻¹ (0.01 ml kg of 1:1,000)	Single dose	Double and repeat twice if no response. Give im if not in shock or while iv access is being gained. The give iv as it may not be absorbed from the im route.
	12–18 years	Deep im	0.5 mg of 1:1000	Single dose	
Croup					
	1 month – 12 years	neb	0.5–1 ml of 1,000	Single dose	Monitor with ECG and oxygen saturation

433

Drug	Age	Route	Dose	Frequency per 24 hours	Notes
Erythromycin	Birth – 1 month	0/iv	10–15 mg kg⁻¹	3	Contraindications –hypersensitivity. Raised serum levels with carbemazepam, digoxin, phenytoin, theophylline and midazolam
	1 month – 2 years	o	125 mg	4	
	2 years – 8 years	o	250 mg	4	
	9 years–18 years	o	500 mg	4	
	1 month–18 years	iv	12.5 mg kg⁻¹	4	
Flucloxacillin	Birth–7 days	iv	25–50 mg kg⁻¹	2	Doses may be doubled in severe infections.
	7 days–1 month	iv	25–50 mg kg⁻¹	3	Do not mix with aminoglycosides
	1 month–18 years	iv	12.5–25 mg kg⁻¹ to a maximum of 4G	4	
	1 month–1 year	oral	62.5 mg	4	Dose may be doubled in severe infections
	1 year–5 years	oral	125 mg	4	
	5 years–18 years	oral	250 mg	4	
Flumazenil	1 month–12 years	iv bolus	10 µg kg⁻¹	Single dose	If no response, in 1 minute, repeat with half initial dose every minute for up to 5 minutes until recovery
	12 years–18 years	iv bolus	200 µg	Single dose	
Frusemide	Birth–12 years	iv bolus	0.5–1 mg kg⁻¹	Single dose	Repeat of no response after 2 hours
	12 years–18 years	iv bolus	20–40 mg		

Drug	Age	Route	Dose		Notes
Gentamicin	Birth–7 days	iv	<2 kg in wieght – 3 mg kg⁻¹	1	Do not mix with penicillins, cephalorsporinns, erythromycin. Reduce in renal impairment. Monitor by serum levels 1 hour post dose.
	7 days–1 month	iv	>2 kg in weight – 3 mg kg⁻¹ <2 kg in weight – 3 mg kg⁻¹	2 2	
	1 month–12 years	iv	>2 kg in weight – 3.75 mg 2.5 mg kg⁻¹	3	
	12 years–18 years	iv	1–2 mg kg⁻¹	3	
Glucagon	1 month–2 years	Im/sc iv rapid bolus	500 µg	Single dose	Should be effective in 15 minutes. Can be repeated once or twice if necessary until iv access gained
	2 years–18 years	Im/sc iv rapid bolus	<20 kg in weight – 0.5 mg >20 kg in weight –1 mg	Single dose	
Hydralazine	Birth–12 years	iv bolus over 20 minutes	300–500 µg kg⁻¹	Single loading dose	Repeat 4–6 times per day to a total of 3 mg kg in 24 hours. Reconstituted in 1 ml water and diluted with NaCl 0.9%
	12 years–18 years	iv bolus over 20 minutes	5–10 mg	Single dose	
	Birth–12 years 12 years–18 years	iv inf in inf	12.5–50 µg kg⁻¹ per hour 3–9 mg per hour	continuous continuous	Maximum dose 3 mg kg in 24 hours
Hydrocortisone (severe asthma anaphylaxis)	Birth–1 month	iv/ bolus/ im/io	2.5 mg stat, then 2 mg kg⁻¹ 4 times daily	Single dose Then 4	
	1 month–12 years	iv/ bolus/ im/io	4 mg stat (maximum 100 mg) then 2–4 mg kg⁻¹	Single dose 4	
	12 years–18 years	iv/bolus/ im/io	100–500 mg then 100–500 mg	Single dose 4	

435

Drug	Age	Route	Dose	Frequency per 24 hours	Notes
Hydrocortisone (replacement)	Birth–12 years	oral	4 mg m^{-2}	3	Maintenance
	Birth–12 years	oral	6.6 mg m^{-2}	3	Replacement dose in congenital adrenal hyperplasia
Ibuprofen	1 month–12 years	oral	5 mg kg^{-1}	3–4	
	12 years–18 years	oral	200–600 mg	3–4	Maximum dose 2.4G/day
Immunoglobulin (Kawasaki syndrome)	1 month–12 years	iv	2G kg^{-1}	Single dose	In Kawasaki syndrome give over 10 hours as soon as possible after onset of disease.
Ipratropium bromide	Birth–18 years	inhaled	Up to 120 μg	4	
	1 month–1 year	neb	125 μg	Single dose	can be repeated every 2 hours if necessary
	1 year–5 years	neb	250 μg	Single dose	
	5 years–18 years	neb	500 μg	Single dose	
Isopronterol (Isoprenaline)	Birth – 1 month	iv inf	20–300 nanogram kg^{-1} per min	continuous	Use lowest possible effective dose
	1 month – 12 years	iv inf	20 nanogram– 1 μg kg^{-1} per min	continuous	Compatible with 5% glucose and 0.9% sodium chloride
	12 years – 18 years	iv inf	1–4 μg per min	continuous	
Ketamine (conscious sedation)	<10 years	iv	2 mg kg^{-1}	Single dose	In syringe with atropine 0.01 mg kg to control ketamine's secretagogue effects

Labetalol	1 month–12 years	iv bolus	250–500 µg kg^{-1} loading dose	Continuous	Start at low dose and titrate against blood pressure Total maximum 3 mg kg
		Followed by: iv continuous	1–3 mg kg^{-1} per hour		
Lactulose	1 month–1 year 1 year–5 years 5 years–10 years 10 years–15 years	oral oral oral oral	2.5 ml 5 ml 10 ml 15 ml	2 2 2 2	Starting dose is illustrated, but vary to give a comfortable soft-formed stool
Lignocaine hydrochloride (Lidocaine) (antiarrhythmic)	Birth–12 years	iv bolus	500 µg kg^{-1} then 1 mg kg^{-1} every 5 minutes	Single initial dose Then	With ECG monitoring
	12–18 years	iv bolus	50–100 mg (total maximum 3 mg kg) then 4 mg per min for 30 minutes then 2 mg per min for 2 hours then 1 mg per min reducing further after 24 hours	Single dose	

437

Drug	Age	Route	Dose	Frequency per 24 hours	Notes
Lignocaine (Lidocaine) (local anesthetic)	Birth–12 years	Local infiltration	Up to 3 mg kg^{-1}	Single dose	Repeat no more than 4 hourly
	12 years–18 years	Local infiltration	Up to 200 mg		
Lignocaine and prilocaine (EMLA)	1 month–18 years	Topical under occlusive dressing	Maximum 2 g for a minimum of 1 hour and a maximum 5 hours	Single dose	
Lorazepam (for status epilepticus)	Birth–12 years	iv/rect Sublingual/IO	50–100 μg kg^{-1}	Single dose	
	12–18 years	iv/rect/ Sublingual/IO	4 mg	Single dose	
Methyl prednisolone (asthma)	1 month–18 years	iv	1 mg kg^{-1}	6 hourly	
Metoclopramide	Birth–12 years	Oral/im/ slow iv bolus	100 μg kg^{-1}	2–3	
	12 years–18 years	Oral/im/ slow iv bolus	<60 kg – 5 mg >60 kg – 10 mg	3 3	

	Age	Route	Dose		Notes
Metronidazole	1 month–12 years	iv/oral	7.5 mg kg^{-1} (maximum 400 mg)	3	Oral dose has excellent bioavailability
	12 years–18 years	iv/oral	400 mg	3	
Midazolam for seizures	1 month–18 years	iv	150 µg kg^{-1}	Single dose	Repeat after 5 minutes if seizures continue
Midazolam (for sedation)	1 month–12 years	Im/iv bolus	50–100 µg kg^{-1}	1	Doses up to 300 µg kg may be needed
	12–18 years	Iv bolus	2 mg	1	If after 2 minutes, sedation is not adequate, extra doses of 500 ug–1 mg can be given to a total dose of 5 mg
Morphine sulphate (acute pain)	1 month–12 years	iv bolus over 5–10 minutes	100–200 µg kg^{-1}	Single dose	Dose may be repeated up to 4 times per 24 hours for infants <6 months and up to 6 times in 24 hours in those >6 months
	12 years–18 years	iv bolus over 5–10 minutes	2.5–10 mg	Single dose	
Naloxone	1 month–12 years	iv bolus	10 µg kg^{-1} then 100 µg kg^{-1} (maximum 2 mg)	Single dose Single dose	If no response, give higher dose Repeat as necessary to maintain the reversal of opioid
	12 years–18 years	iv bolus	10 µg kg^{-1} then 2 mg	Single dose Single dose	

Drug	Age	Route	Dose	Frequency per 24 hours	Notes
Noradrenaline		In inf	0.02–1.0 µg kg^{-1} per min	continuous	Better than dopamine, dobutamine or epinephrmne in hypotension due to tricyclic antidepressants
Nystatin	1 month–18 years	oral	1 ml (100,000 units)	4	
Paracetamol	Birth–12 years	oral	10–15 mg kg^{-1}	4–6 hourly prn	Maximum dose 60m <3 months, 80m >3months in 24 hours
	12 years–18 years	oral	500 m –1G	4–6 hourly prn	Maximum dose 4G in 24 hours
	Birth–12 years	rectal	20 mg kg^{-1}	4–6 hourly prn	Maximum dose 90m or 4G in 24 hours
Paraldehyde	Birth–12 years	Rectal	0.4 ml kg^{-1} (max 10 ml)	Single dose	
	12 years–18 years	Rectal	5–10 ml	Single dose	
Penicillin	See benzyl penicillin and phenoxymethylpenicillin				
Phenobarbitone (status epilepticus)	Birth–18 years	iv	15 mg kg^{-1}	Single dose	Loading dose
	Birth–12 years	iv	2.5–5 mg kg^{-1}	2	Maintenance dose
	12 years–18 years	iv	300 mg	2	
Phenoxymethyl penicillin	<1 year	Oral	62.5 mg	4	Contraindications – hypersensitivity
	1–5 years	Oral	125 mg	4	
	6–12 years	Oral	250 mg	4	
	12–18 years	Oral	500 mg	4	
Phenytoin (status epilepticus)	Birth–1 month	iv	20 mg kg^{-1}	Single first dose	
	1 month–18 years	iv	18 mg kg^{-1}	Single first dose	
	Birth–12 years	iv	2.5–5 mg kg^{-1}	2	Maintenance dose given over 30 minutes
	12 years–18 years	iv	100 mg	3–4	

Drug	Age	Route	Dose	Frequency	Notes
Prednisolone acute asthma	1 month–18 years	oral	1–2 mg kg⁻¹ (maximum dose 40 mg)	Daily	For 1–5 days in acute asthma
Prednisolone (nephrotic syndrome)	1 month–18 years	oral	60 mg m⁻²	Starting dose	For 4 weeks, then after at least 3 days free of proteinuria, go on to maintenance
			<u>Then</u> 40 mg m⁻²	Alternate days	For 4 weeks, then stop
Prednisolone (ITP)	1 month–18 years	oral	2–4 mg kg⁻¹	1	For 2 weeks then tapering
Prilocaine 4%	<10 years	Local infiltration	1 ml	Single dose	
	>10 years	Local infiltration	1–2 ml	Single dose	
In anaphylaxis–for relief of urticaria					
Promethazine	1 month – 12 years	O/iv slow bolus	500 µg–1 mg kg⁻¹ maximum 25 mg	4	Caution in < 1 month old because of sudden infant death syndrome
Prostaglandin E1		iv inf	0.01–0.1 µg kg⁻¹ per min		To keep patent ductus arteriosus open – continue until cardiac opinion open
Pyridoxime	Birth–1 month	iv bolus	50–100 mg	Single dose	Test dose. If seizures cease, change to maintenance oral.

Drug	Age	Route	Dose	Frequency per 24 hours	Notes
Rabies human immunoglobulin	Birth–18 years	1/2 infiltrated around wound and 1/2 im	20 iu kg⁻¹	Single dose	For post-exposure passive prophylaxis
Rifampicin	Birth–3 months	neb	10 mg kg⁻¹	1	For treatment of tuberculosis
	3 months–12 years	oral	10 mg kg⁻¹	1	
	12 years–18 years	oral	<50 kg in weight –450 mg >50 kg in weight –600 mg	1	
Salbutamol (for treatment of acute wheezing)	6 months–5 years	neb	2.5 mg	Single dose	
	over 5 years	neb	5 mg	Single dose	
	6 months–2 years	inhaled	Up to 2400 µg	6	
	3 years–4 years	inhaled	up to 3600 µg	6	
	over 5 years	inhaled	up to 7200 µg	6	
	6 months–12 years	iv inf	0.1–1 µg kg⁻¹ per min	continuous	in 5% dextrose or 0.9% saline
Senna	2 years–6 years	granules	2.5 ml	1 at night	Starting dose. Vary to give a comfortable soft-formed stool.
	6 years–12 years	granules	2.5–5 ml	1 at night	
	12 years–18 years	granules	5–10 ml	1 at night	
Sodium picosulphate	2 years–5 years	oral	2.5 ml	1 at night	
	5 years–10 years	oral	2.5–5 ml	1 at night	
	10 years–18 years	oral	5–15 ml	1 at night	

Drug	Age	Route	Dose	Frequency	Notes
Temazepam	1 month–12 years	oral	1 mg kg⁻¹	Single dose	
	12 years–18 years	oral	20 mg	Single dose	
Thiopentone (Status epilepticus)	Birth–18 years	iv bolus	2–4 mg kg⁻¹	Single dose	Ventilation facilities must be available. Should only be used by staff with advanced airway management skills.
Tranexamic acide	1 month–18 years	oral	25 mg kg⁻¹	3	Not for hematuria as can give renal colicc
Trimethoprim	1 month–18 years	Oral/iv	4 mg kg⁻¹	2	Treatment of infections
	1 month–18 years	oral	2 mg kg⁻¹	Once at night	Prophylaxis
Vancomycin	1 month–12 years	iv	15 mg kg⁻¹ first dose then, 10 mg kg⁻¹ per dose	Loading dose then 4 times daily	Total daily dose <2G per day
Vecuronium	Birth–18 years	iv bolus	80–100 µg kg⁻¹	Single dose	Initial dose

Further reading

Advanced Paediatric Life Support – The Practical Approach, Third Edition, 2001, BMJ Books, London

Medicines for Children, 1999, RCPCH Publications Ltd, London

Frank Shann (2001) *Drug doses*. Melbourne Formulary, 11th edn. Collective PTY Ltd.

Index

Note: Page references in *italics* refer to Figures; those in **bold** refer to Tables